Complications in Implant Dentistry

Editor

MOHANAD AL-SABBAGH

DENTAL CLINICS OF NORTH AMERICA

www.dental.theclinics.com

January 2015 • Volume 59 • Number 1

ELSEVIER

1600 John F. Kennedy Boulevard • Suite 1800 • Philadelphia, Pennsylvania, 19103-2899

http://www.dental.theclinics.com

DENTAL CLINICS OF NORTH AMERICA Volume 59, Number 1
January 2015 ISSN 0011-8532, ISBN: 978-0-323-34173-8

Editor: John Vassallo; j.vassallo@elsevier.com
Developmental Editor: Stephanie Carter

Dental Clinics of North America (ISSN 0011-8532) is published quarterly by Elsevier Inc., 360 Park Avenue South, New York, NY 10010-1710. Months of issue are January, April, July, and October. Business and Editorial Offices: 1600 John F. Kennedy Boulevard, Suite 1800, Philadelphia, PA 19103-2899. Periodicals postage paid at New York, NY and additional mailing offices. Subscription prices are $280.00 per year (domestic individuals), $485.00 per year (domestic institutions), $135.00 per year (domestic students/residents), $340.00 per year (Canadian individuals), $628.00 per year (Canadian institutions), $410.00 per year (international individuals), $628.00 per year (international institutions), and $200.00 per year (international and Canadian students/residents). International air speed delivery is included in all *Clinics* subscription prices. All prices are subject to change without notice. **POSTMASTER:** Send address changes to *Dental Clinics of North America*, Elsevier Health Sciences Division, Subscription Customer Service, 3251 Riverport Lane, Maryland Heights, MO 63043. **Customer Service (orders, claims, online, change of address): Elsevier Health Sciences Division, Subscription Customer Service, 3251 Riverport Lane, Maryland Heights, MO 63043. Tel: 1-800-654-2452 (U.S. and Canada). Fax: 314-447-8029. E-mail: journalscustomer service-usa@elsevier.com (for print support); journalsonlinesupport-usa@elsevier.com (for online support).**

Reprints. For copies of 100 or more, of articles in this publication, please contact the Commercial Reprints Department, Elsevier Inc., 360 Park Avenue South, New York, NY 10010-1710. Tel.: 212-633-3874; Fax: 212-633-3820; E-mail: reprints@elsevier.com.

The *Dental Clinics of North America* is covered in *MEDLINE/PubMed (Index Medicus), Current Contents/Clinical Medicine, ISI/BIOMED* and *Clinahl.*

Contributors

EDITOR

MOHANAD AL-SABBAGH, DDS, MS
Chief, Division of Periodontology; Program Director of Graduate Periodontology, Department of Oral Health Practice, College of Dentistry, University of Kentucky, Lexington, Kentucky

AUTHORS

MOHANAD AL-SABBAGH, DDS, MS
Chief, Division of Periodontology; Program Director of Graduate Periodontology, Department of Oral Health Practice, College of Dentistry, University of Kentucky, Lexington, Kentucky

ELIZANGELA BERTOLI, DDS, MS
Assistant Professor, Division of Restorative Dentistry, Department of Oral Health Practice, College of Dentistry, University of Kentucky, Lexington, Kentucky

ISHITA BHAVSAR, BDS
Research Assistant, Division of Periodontology, Department of Oral Health Practice, College of Dentistry, University of Kentucky, Lexington, Kentucky

JOSÉ LUIS CALVO-GUIRADO, DDS, MS, PhD
Faculty of Medicine and Dentistry, Hospital Morales Meseguer, University of Murcia, Murcia, Spain

IGOR BATISTA CAMARGO, DDS, MSc
Research Fellow, Department of Oral and Maxillofacial Surgery, College of Dentistry, University of Kentucky, Lexington, Kentucky; PhD Student in College of Dentistry of Pernambuco, University of Pernambuco, Recife, Pernambuco, Brazil; Captain-Dentistry, Oral and Maxillofacial Surgeon, Brazilian Army, Brazil; Military Hospital Area of Recife, Recife, Pernambuco, Brazil

DOLPHUS R. DAWSON III, DMD, MS, MPH
Assistant Professor, Division of Periodontology, Department of Oral Health Practice, College of Dentistry, University of Kentucky, Lexington, Kentucky

RAFAEL ARCESIO DELGADO-RUIZ, DDS, MSc, PhD
Department of Prosthodontics and Digital Technology, School of Dental Medicine, Stony Brook University, Stony Brook, New York

PINAR EMECEN-HUJA, DDS, PhD
Assistant Professor, Division of Periodontics, Department of Oral Health Practice, College of Dentistry, University of Kentucky, Lexington, Kentucky

RODRIGO FUENTEALBA, DDS
Assistant Professor, Restorative Division, College of Dentistry, University of Kentucky, Lexington, Kentucky

PAUL FUGAZZOTTO, DDS
Private Practice, Milton, Massachusetts

IQUEBAL HASAN, BDS
Assistant Professor, Department of Oral Health Practice, College of Dentistry, University of Kentucky, Lexington, Kentucky

SAMUEL JASPER, DDS, MS
Associate Professor, Division of Periodontology, Department of Oral Health Practice, College of Dentistry, University of Kentucky, Lexington, Kentucky

FAWAD JAVED, BDS, PhD
Engineer Abdullah Bugshan Research Chair for Growth Factors and Bone Regeneration, 3D Imaging and Biomechanical Laboratory, College of Applied Medical Sciences, King Saud University, Riyadh, Saudi Arabia

JORGE JOFRÉ, DDS, PhD
Director, Center for Advanced Prosthodontics and Implant Dentistry, University of Concepcion, Concepcion, Chile

MOHD W. KHALAF, DDS
Private Practice; Orofacial Pain and Oral Medicine Division, Department of Head and Neck Surgery, Kaiser Permanente, Sacramento, California

HYEONGIL KIM, DDS, MS
Associate Professor and Prosthodontics Program Director, Department of Restorative Dentistry, School of Dental Medicine, The State University of New York at Buffalo, Buffalo, New York

AHMAD KUTKUT, DDS, MS
Assistant Professor, Division of Restorative Dentistry, Department of Oral Health Practice, College of Dentistry, University of Kentucky, Lexington, Kentucky

DENIELLE C. MEDYNSKI, DMD
Assistant Clinical Professor, UCSF Center for Orofacial Pain, San Francisco, California

PHILIP R. MELNICK, DMD
Private Practice, Los Alamitos, California

CRAIG S. MILLER, DMD, MS
Professor of Oral Medicine, Department of Oral Health Practice, College of Dentistry, University of Kentucky, Lexington, Kentucky

JEFFREY P. OKESON, DMD
Professor and Chair, Department of Oral Health Science, College of Dentistry, University of Kentucky, Lexington, Kentucky

GITANJALI PINTO-SINAI, DDS
Assistant Professor, Division of Restorative Dentistry, Department of Oral Health Practice, College of Dentistry, University of Kentucky, Lexington, Kentucky

GEORGIOS E. ROMANOS, DDS, PhD, Prof. Dr. med. dent
Department of Periodontology, School of Dental Medicine, Stony Brook University, Stony Brook, New York

RAMTIN SADID-ZADEH, DDS, MS
Assistant Professor, Department of Restorative Dentistry, School of Dental Medicine, The State University of New York at Buffalo, Buffalo, New York

FARHAD VAHIDI, DMD, MSD, FACP
Associate Professor, Department of Prosthodontics, New York University, College of Dentistry, New York, New York

JOSEPH E. VAN SICKELS, DDS
Provost Distinguished Service Professor; Assistant Dean of Hospital Dentistry; Professor of Oral and Maxillofacial Surgery, College of Dentistry, University of Kentucky, Lexington, Kentucky

JUAN F. YEPES, DDS, MD, MPH, MS, DrPH, FDS RCSEd
Associate Professor, Department of Pediatric Dentistry, James Whitcomb Riley Hospital for Children, Indiana University School of Dentistry, Indianapolis, Indiana

Contents

The concept of osseointegration has revolutionized the treatment options for the replacement of missing teeth in both partially and completely edentulous patients. Dental implants are widely used because clinical practice and studies have documented its successful outcomes. However, implants can occasionally fail, and such failures can be classified as early or late. Measures that can aid in the early recognition of failing osseointegrated implants are needed, as are measures that can facilitate appropriate treatment methods aimed at saving failing implants by determining the probable etiologic factors. This article summarizes our current understanding of the local factors that can be linked to implant failure.

Dental implants are an important treatment option for patients interested in replacing lost or missing teeth. Although a robust body of literature has reviewed risk factors for tooth loss, the evidence for risk factors associated with dental implants is less well defined. This article focuses on key systemic risk factors relating to dental implant failure, as well as on perimucositis and peri-implantitis.

Preimplant planning with complex imaging techniques has long been a recommended practice for assessing the quality and quantity of alveolar bone before dental implant placement. When maxillofacial imaging is necessary, static film or digital images lack the depth and dimension offered by computed tomography. Cone-beam computed tomography (CBCT) offers the dentist not only a radiographic volumetric view of alveolar bone but also a 3-dimensional reconstruction. This article reviews the use of CBCT for assessing implant placement and early detection of failure, and compares the performance of CBCT with that of other imaging modalities in the early detection of implant failure.

Placement of dental implants in the maxillofacial region is routine and considered safe. However, as with any surgical procedure, complications occur. Many issues that arise at surgery can be traced to the preoperative evaluation of the patient and assessment of the underlying anatomy. In this article, the authors review some common and uncommon complications that can occur during and shortly after implant placement. The emphasis of each section is on the management and prevention of complications that may occur during implant placement.

Loss of soft and hard tissue is common after tooth extraction. Substantial resorption of alveolar bone compromises esthetics and may result in prosthetic and surgical limitations. Immediate implant placement at the time of tooth extraction is used to maintain alveolar ridge dimensions. Clinical studies support the successful outcome of immediate placement of dental implants in fresh extraction sockets; comparative clinical studies have found that implant survival rates after immediate placement are similar to those after delayed placement. This article addresses surgical techniques for immediate implant placement and the prevention and the management of complications associated with this procedure.

The maxillary posterior edentulous region presents a challenge when planning for restoring missing teeth with a dental implant. The available bone in such cases is often not dense and not adequate for the placement of a properly sized implant because of maxillary sinus pneumatization and alveolar bone loss. Maxillary sinus lift is a predictable procedure to provide adequate bone height for the purpose of implant placement. However, complications are encountered during or after the execution of the sinus lift procedure. In this article, the prevention and management of maxillary sinus complications are discussed.

Many studies have documented the successful outcomes of dental implants, but have also reported the association of sensory disturbances with the surgical implant procedure. Postsurgical pain is a normal response to tissue injury, and usually resolves after the tissue heals. However, some patients who receive dental implants experience persistent pain even after normal healing. This article describes the basic anatomy and pathophysiology associated with nerve injury. The incidence and diagnosis of these problems, in addition to factors that result in the development of chronic persistent neuropathic pain and sensory disturbances associated with surgical implant placement, are discussed.

Nerve trauma caused by dental implant placement is associated with altered sensation and chronic pain. Complete or partial loss of sensation is often reported by patients who have experienced nerve trauma during implant surgery. Some patients report persistent pain and neurosurgery disturbance long after the normal healing time has passed. In addition, neuropathic pain is reported after implant surgery. Practitioners who place dental implants must be familiar with the differential diagnosis, prevention, and management of neuropathic pain. This article provides insights into the prevention and management of neurosensory deficits and chronic persistent neuropathic pain and considerations for patient referral.

The ideal management of peri-implant diseases focuses on infection control, detoxification of implant surfaces, regeneration of lost tissues, and plaque-control regimens via mechanical debridement (with or without raising a surgical flap). However, a variety of other therapeutic modalities also have been proposed for the management of peri-implantitis. These treatment strategies encompass use of antiseptics and/or antibiotics, laser therapy, guided bone regeneration, and photodynamic therapy. The aim of this article was to review indexed literature with reference to the various therapeutic interventions proposed for the management of peri-implant diseases.

Implants are exposed to a diverse oral environment and host responses that contribute to health or disease. For the last few decades, clinicians have relied on standard clinical and radiographic findings to assess the health of implants. However, recent studies involving the pathogenesis of peri-implantitis have identified microbial species and several putative biomarkers that could aid clinicians in this diagnostic process in the near future. This article provides an overview of the microbial species involved in implant health and disease and biomarkers found in oral fluids that relate to the underlying biological phases of a failing implant.

Although osseointegrated dental implants have become a predictable and effective modality for the treatment of single or multiple missing teeth, their use is associated with clinical complications. Such complications can be biologic, technical, mechanical, or esthetic and may compromise implant outcomes to various degrees. This article presents prosthetic complications accompanied with implant-supported single and partial fixed dental prostheses.

Implant-supported removable prostheses improve patients' satisfaction with treatment and quality of life. Improvements in the implant's surface and in attachment elements have made this treatment method very successful. However, some biological and mechanical complications remain. Mechanical complications associated with implant-supported overdentures and implant-supported removable partial dentures are loss of retention of attachment systems, the need to replace retention elements and to reline or repair the resin portion of the denture, and implant fracture. Despite their success, implant-supported removable prostheses require periodic maintenance.

The definition of failure for dental implants has evolved from lack of osseointegration to increased concern for other aspects, such as esthetics. However, esthetic failure in implant dentistry has not been well defined. Although multiple esthetic indices have been validated for objectively evaluating clinical outcomes, including failure of an implant-supported crown, only one author has determined a failure threshold. On the basis of objective indices, esthetic failures in implant dentistry can be categorized as pink-tissue failures and white-tissue failures. This article discusses esthetic failures, the factors involved in these failures, and their prevention and treatment.

DENTAL CLINICS OF NORTH AMERICA

Preface

Complications in Implant Dentistry

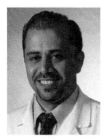

Mohanad Al-Sabbagh, DDS, MS
Editor

The concept of osseointegration, introduced by Brånemark, has revolutionized the clinical practice of dentistry. Because studies have documented their predictability and successful long-term outcomes, dental implants are rapidly becoming an alternative to traditional prostheses and are one of the preferred treatment options for replacing missing teeth in both partially and completely edentulous ridges. Dental implants are a viable alternative for many patients in need of a dental prosthesis and are widely accepted in the field of dentistry because they provide the tripartite objective of function, esthetics, and comfort.

The implant industry has greatly advanced, and new dental implant systems have been introduced into the market. We have seen a huge increase in scientific knowledge about the biological and biomechanical factors associated with implant success. In recent years, the development of bone regeneration and sinus lift procedures and the evolution of implant surface characteristics have made implant therapy one of the most important treatment solutions in contemporary dentistry.

Although dental implants have improved the quality of life of many patients, a wide body of literature has reported their associated morbidity. Studies have also documented the association of complications with surgical implant procedures and prosthetic rehabilitation. Management of complications can be challenging and often requires a combination of surgical and prosthetic approaches.

The current issue of *Dental Clinics of North America* blends knowledge gained from clinical experience with knowledge obtained from the current body of dental literature to establish therapeutic guidelines for preventing and managing implant-associated complications. Through this effort, we aim to assist clinicians in identifying and treating undesirable presurgical, intrasurgical, and postsurgical problems associated with implant placement. In these 13 articles, we have attempted to describe and suggest management options for all of the reported implant complications. This issue is designed to serve as a guide for the thought processes involved in clinical

Dent Clin N Am 59 (2015) xiii–xv
http://dx.doi.org/10.1016/j.cden.2014.09.006
0011-8532/15/$ – see front matter **dental.theclinics.com**

decision-making so that dental practitioners can not only prevent complications but also manage them when they occur.

The article by Drs Al-Sabbagh and Bhavsar summarizes current knowledge about biological, biomechanical, and bacterial factors that have been linked with, or that contribute to, implant failure. Measures for determining the probable etiological factors that can facilitate appropriate treatment methods aimed at saving failing implants are also reviewed.

The next article, by Drs Dawson and Jasper, examines the evidence for systemic, environmental, and genetic risk factors associated with the failure of dental implants and with perimucositis and peri-implantitis.

Drs Yepes and Al-Sabbagh review current knowledge about the accuracy of cone-beam computed tomography (CBCT) for the short-term and long-term evaluation of implant health. The authors also review the use of CBCT in assessing implant placement and detecting implant failure as early as possible. They also discuss the advantages of CBCT over other imaging modalities for evaluating implant placement.

The article by Drs Camargo and Van Sickels elucidates some of the more common and a few of the more severe surgical complications that can occur during or shortly after the surgical placement of dental implants. The article also emphasizes the prevention and management of such complications.

Drs Al-Sabbagh and Kutkut address surgical exploration and the recommendations for osteotomy preparation for immediate implant placement. The authors also propose guidelines for immediate implant placement, provisionalization, and loading, as well as the prevention of complications associated with immediate implant placement.

The article by Dr Fugazzotto and coauthor provides a clinical decision-making protocol aimed at preventing the intraoperative and postoperative complications associated with sinus lift procedures and bone augmentation of the posterior maxillary ridge before dental implants are placed. The article also provides some guidelines for the management of such complications.

Dr Al-Sabbagh and coauthor review the documented association of sensory disturbances with the surgical implant procedure and the development of chronic persistent neuropathic pain and neurosensory disturbance. The article also describes the basic anatomy and pathophysiology associated with nerve injury. Moreover, it discusses the cause and diagnosis of persistent pain after implant placement.

The companion article by Dr Al-Sabbagh and coauthor provides insights into the prevention of nerve injury and the management of patients who report persistent pain long after the normal healing time for dental implant procedures has passed. The authors discuss both pharmacologic treatment and surgical nerve repair of such injuries.

Dr Romanos and coauthor provide information about various proposed therapeutic interventions for the management of peri-implant diseases and suggest guidelines for the management of peri-implantitis. The authors also address the cause of peri-implant diseases and the risk factors associated with these conditions.

The article by Dr Emecen-Huja and coauthor provides an overview of the microbial species found around healthy and diseased implants. It also discusses the biomarkers found in oral fluids that are related to the underlying biological phases associated with disease progression and failing implants.

Dr Sadid-Zadeh and coauthor review indexed publications related to the technical and mechanical prosthetic complications accompanied with implant-supported single and partial fixed dental prostheses.

The article by Drs Vahidi and Pinto-Sinai focuses on mechanical complications and failures associated with implant-supported overdentures and implant-supported removable partial dentures. The authors also provide some insight into the prevention and management of such complications or failures.

Finally, Drs Fuentealba and Jofré review some indices that determine the esthetic success or failure of implant-supported crowns. The article also reviews the more common pink-tissue esthetic failures and the less common white-tissue esthetic failures. It discusses the factors involved in these failures and their prevention and management.

Because our understanding of implantology is increasing and the biomedical literature is voluminous and constantly expanding, our knowledge is in a continual state of flux. The increasing volume of scientific literature makes it extremely difficult for busy clinicians and academicians to keep up with their professional reading. This difficulty is complicated by the fact that all clinicians have a responsibility to keep up with general medical advances, not just those related to their own specialty (if for no other reason than the ever-increasing array of drugs taken by our patients). This issue of *Dental Clinics of North America* can serve as a resource in clinical matters for our readers.

It is the editor's goal to provide readers with a systematic method of assessing the complications associated with implant placement or restoration, to offer guidelines for selecting the most appropriate management method for dealing with specific complications, and to present suggestions for preventing surgical or restorative complications. Because of the clinical emphasis of the 13 articles presented in this issue, they should be of immense value to our readers.

Mohanad Al-Sabbagh, DDS, MS
Division of Periodontology
Department of Oral Health Practice
College of Dentistry
University of Kentucky
800 Rose Street
Lexington, KY 40536-0297, USA

E-mail address:
malsa2@email.uky.edu

Key Local and Surgical Factors Related to Implant Failure

Mohanad Al-Sabbagh, DDS, MS*, Ishita Bhavsar, BDS

KEYWORDS

• Local factors • Implant failure • Dental implants

KEY POINTS

• Clinicians should critically evaluate the patient's oral hygiene, compliance, motivation, and risk factors before suggesting dental implant treatment.

• Achieving primary stability is important for successful implant placement.

• Host-related factors, operative-related factors, and implant-related factors may influence the outcome of implant treatment and should be thoroughly evaluated during treatment planning.

• Practitioners treating patients with systemic metabolic disorders, such as diabetes or osteoporosis, those undergoing radiation therapy, and those who smoke, should follow a 2-staged approach for optimal implant outcome.

INTRODUCTION

The clinical effectiveness of the osseointegration concept introduced by Brånemark and colleagues[1] in the 1960s has revolutionized the clinical practice of dentistry. Dental implants are now the preferred line of treatment for the replacement of missing teeth. Additionally, implant-supported full-mouth prostheses are a good treatment option for patients who are completely edentulous, achieving a comprehensive and functional oral rehabilitation.[2] Although endosseous implants have a predictable outcome and long-term success, they sometimes fail. Several clinical studies have recognized risk factors that may lead to implant failure.[3,4] Implant failures are categorized as primary (early), when the body is unable to establish osseointegration, or secondary (late), when the body is unable to maintain the achieved osseointegration and a breakdown process results.[5] Implant failures also are classified on the basis of

Division of Periodontology, Department of Oral Health Practice, College of Dentistry, University of Kentucky, 800 Rose Street, Lexington, KY 40536-0297, USA
* Corresponding author.
E-mail addresses: malsa2@email.uky.edu; mvthom0@uky.edu

Dent Clin N Am 59 (2015) 1–23
http://dx.doi.org/10.1016/j.cden.2014.09.001
0011-8532/15/$ – see front matter © 2015 Elsevier Inc. All rights reserved.

dental.theclinics.com

the time of prosthesis placement; in this classification, early implant failure usually occurs before the prosthesis is placed, and late implant failure is associated with functional loading after the placement of the prosthesis. Because there are no known noninvasive methods for evaluating the extent of osseointegration, the factors associated with both early and late failures may coexist for a particular implant. Additionally, these factors can be difficult to interpret individually. In a retrospective study, Friberg and colleagues[6] followed 4641 Brånemark dental implants from stage 1 surgery to the completion of the prosthetic restoration. They found that maximal fixtures failed for completely edentulous maxillae with poor bone quality. They also found that some fixtures were not mobile at the abutment connections but were mobile just before the prosthesis was placed.[6] The reason that the fixture gave a false impression of initial stability was that, although the surgeon embedded the implants tightly into the bone, the bone in which the fixture was embedded was remodeled by resorption during the progression of the healing phase. Thus, implant mobility was evident, and the implant failed. Several local and systemic factors, such as lack of primary stability, surgical trauma, and existing periodontal infection, may play an important role in hindering the normal process of bone healing around implants and can subsequently lead to early implant failure. On the other hand, provisional overload and microbially induced peri-implant diseases are associated with late implant failure.

The process of osseointegration between the host's bone tissue and the implant is the key to the success of the implant. The term *osseointegration* has several definitions. Albrektsson and colleagues[7] defined it as "a direct structural and functional connection between bone and the surface of a load-bearing implant." Branemark[1] definition, which is based on macroscopic and microscopic biology from a medical point of view, is "close approximation of new and reformed bone and the fixture together with surface irregularities so that there is no interposition of connective or fibrous tissue at light microscopic level. Thus, a direct structural and functional connection, capable to carrying normal physiologic loads without extensive deformation and initiation of rejection."

OUTCOME OF THE DENTAL IMPLANT: SUCCESS OR FAILURE

Several reports have evaluated the successful outcome of dental implants. The term *success* means attainment of the desired aims. The criteria for successful implants proposed by Albrektsson and colleagues[8] were based on clinical and radiographic evidence of osseointegration, and this criterion is presently most widely accepted. Furthermore, several additions to the criteria of Albrektsson and colleagues[8] have been recently proposed for evaluating successful implants: these additions include clinical function, esthetics, patient satisfaction, radiographic evidence of minimal bone loss, stability of the prosthesis, absence of peri-implant soft tissue infection, and lack of implant mobility and pain.[8–10] If an implant does not meet all of the criteria for a successful implant, it is instead considered a surviving implant.

On the other hand, implant failure occurs when an implant fails to achieve its function. Usually, failure to attain osseointegration is considered an implant failure. A failed implant must usually be removed. Esposito and colleagues[11] established 4 categories of implant failure based on the osseointegration concept. The first category, biological failure, includes early or primary failure (before loading) and late or secondary failure (after loading). Early or primary failure occurs when osseointegration is not achieved during the initial normal bone-healing process. Late or secondary failure occurs when achieved osseointegration is not sustained. The second category, mechanical failure, is associated with fracture of implants or implant-related structures. The third category, iatrogenic failure, occurs when an implant violates important anatomic neurovascular structures and must be removed. The final category, adaption failure, involves patient-related factors, such as lack of satisfaction, poor esthetic qualities, and the patient's psychological state.

The most crucial finding related to implant failure is the presence of peri-implant radiolucency and implant mobility.[11] Loss of osseointegration is sometimes characterized by a fibrous connective tissue capsule, called fibro-osseous integration, which cannot withstand the normal physiologic load. Esposito and colleagues[11] stress the difference between failed and failing implants: a failing implant can be saved if it is detected early, whereas a failed implant cannot be saved and must be removed.

Some of the most common causes of implant failure at an early stage are surgical trauma (overheating, inexperienced surgeon), bacterial contamination (failure to maintain aseptic conditions during implant placement, poor oral hygiene status), delayed wound healing (host-related), and early loading of the implants. Esposito and colleagues[11] also reported that the epidemiology of early implant loss is associated with various implant systems, anatomic locations, and several other host-related factors. Reports in the dental literature suggest that the incidence of early implant failure ranges from 0.7% to 2.0%.[12–16] Implant failure is twice as common among completely edentulous patients as among partially edentulous patients. Both early and late implant failures appear to occur approximately 3 times more frequently in the maxilla than in the mandible.[11]

HISTOMORPHOLOGY OF IMPLANT FAILURE

To better understand the mechanism of failure of osseointegrated dental implants, Esposito and colleagues[17] performed histomorphologic analysis of the tissue surrounding 20 failed implants. Four of 20 implants were retrieved by a trephined bur, and the rest were gently unscrewed. Retrieved failed implants fell into 3 groups: group 1, implants failed before abutment connection; group 2, implants failed at the abutment connections; group 3, implants failed after abutment connection. No evidence of bacterial colonization was found in any specimen, but the presence of erythrocytes between implant and bone was a common finding. Failed implants in group 1 exhibited clinical symptoms of infection; the main histologic findings included well-vascularized connective tissue with a small number of inflammatory cells. Furthermore, bone tissue fragments were embedded in the connective tissue. This finding may indicate the situation in which the host cannot regenerate new bone because of surgical trauma. Failed implants in group 2 exhibited no clinical symptoms. There was no direct contact between bone and implant. Histologically, 2 patterns were evident, a finding indicating various mechanisms of failed osseointegration. In the first pattern, the implant was surrounded by dense connective tissue fibers with collagen fiber bundles and elongated fibroblasts as the major component. The second pattern consisted of several layers of nonkeratinized epithelial cells connected by desmosomes and the predominant infiltration of inflammatory cells, such as polymorphonuclear leukocytes, macrophages, and plasma cells. Failed implants in group 3, which were retrieved after abutment connections failed, exhibited variations with regard to the tissue surrounding the implants. In general, there was evidence of mineralized bone; however, it was separated from the implant connective tissue or a layer of nonmineralized bone. Taken together, the results of these histologic studies seem to provide in-depth knowledge about the mechanism of failing osseointegrated implants: these failures seem to be caused by a combination of traumatic and infective factors.[18]

FACTORS CONTRIBUTED TO IMPLANT FAILURE

In general, several factors can either directly or indirectly contribute to implant failure and can be broadly classified as internal or external factors (**Fig. 1**).

Internal Factors

This classification describes host-related systemic or local factors that may contribute to implant failures.

Host-related factors
Systemic factors

Gender and age It is unclear how a patient's gender and age can affect the success of oral implants. An experimental study involving rats demonstrated that the rate and amount of new bone formation surrounding hydroxyapatite-coated implants decrease as patients age.[19] Also, several studies have shown that women are more prone to implant failure than men.[20,21] Moy and colleagues[4] reported that the risk of implant failure was 2.55 times higher among menopausal women undergoing hormone replacement therapy than among younger women. Another study reported statistically lower implant success rates (78.1%, $P<.02$) for older patients (>60 years).[22] Although these factors may suggest that the risk of implant failure is higher for women than for men because of menopause and osteoporosis, some studies have shown that the rate of implant failure is higher among men because men tend to smoke more and to have poorer oral hygiene habits.[23–25] On the other hand, many reports have found no direct evidence indicating that patients' sex is a potential risk factor for implant failure.[26–28]

Smoking Clinical and scientific studies have stressed that smoking has a negative effect on the survival of implants. Smoking is considered an important risk factor for implant failure and is covered in more detail in the article discussing systemic and environmental risk factors for dental implant failure.

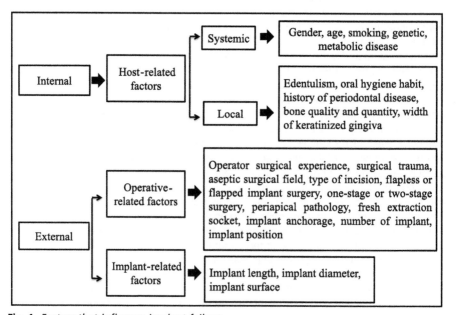

Fig. 1. Factors that influence implant failure.

Genetics Although several studies have assessed the genetic polymorphism of the host, it is unclear whether genetic factors are directly related to a patient's susceptibility to implant failure. Genetics is covered in more detail in systemic and environmental risk factors for dental implant failure.

Metabolic disease Metabolic disease can directly influence the healing process by affecting bone metabolism (bone remodeling). For patients with systemic conditions, such as diabetes, osteoporosis, hyperparathyroidism, or a history of radiation therapy, clinicians should follow the conventional 2-staged implant system, which provides sufficient time for tissue healing before implant loading occurs. This topic is covered in more detail in systemic and environmental risk factors for dental implant failure.

Local factors

Edentulism As the patient's age increases, the patient's need for periodontal and prosthetic rehabilitation also increases. Furthermore, several studies have reported higher success rates for implant-supported overdentures (>90%) and an improved quality of life among completely edentulous patients.[29–31] The cost associated with implant-stabilized prostheses sometimes is lower than that associated with alternative treatment options, such as fixed crowns or bridge prostheses. Because the demand for implant-supported overdentures is increasing, it is important that clinicians discuss all of the treatment options available to elderly patients. A common finding among aging patients is an atrophic alveolar ridge, which may limit treatment planning by requiring the insertion of shorter dental implants or the incorporation of procedures such as guided bone regeneration and sinus lift. Several studies have shown that the likelihood of success is lower for short dental implants than for regular dental implants.[32] A morphometric study involving dry edentulous and dentulous mandibles of adult humans found that the presence of some natural teeth significantly influences the dimensions and the anatomy of the mandible.[33] For the reasons discussed previously, the possibility exists that implant outcome also may depend on the presence or absence of dentition. Esposito and colleagues[34] reported that the implant failure rate for subjects with partially edentulous ridges was approximately half that for subjects with completely edentulous ridges. Hultin and colleagues[35] reported that implant failure was more common among completely edentulous patients with implant-supported fixtures than among partially edentulous patients with implants and teeth in the same jaw. There was no significant difference between the survival rates of implants placed in edentulous or partially edentulous jaws.[36] Recently published reports offer limited information about patients' edentulous status as a factor determining implant success. Future longitudinal studies should evaluate the association between implant success and patients' edentulous status.

Oral hygiene status Increased formation of oral biofilm can be expected when a patient has poor oral hygiene. Unlike the natural tooth, dental implants have no periodontal ligament between their surface and the alveolar bone. Thus, microbial plaque can adhere more easily to the rough surface of the implant and can elicit an inflammatory process. If the inflammatory process around the implant is not controlled, it can lead to progressive bone loss and, ultimately, to implant failure. Lindquist and colleagues[37] followed patients with implant-supported fixed mandibular prostheses for 6 years and found that patients with poor oral hygiene and parafunctional habits (jaw clenching) experienced substantial bone loss. A 10-year longitudinal study found that patients who smoked and had poor oral hygiene exhibited significantly ($P<.001$) more marginal bone loss than did patients who did not smoke.[38] Likewise, Kourtis and colleagues[39] found that the implant failure rate is higher among patients with unsatisfactory oral hygiene than among those with good oral hygiene (**Fig. 2**).

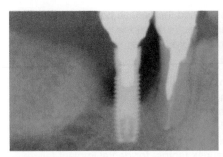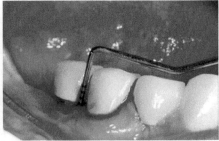

Fig. 2. Radiographic and clinical presentation of peri-implantitis in a patient with poor oral hygiene practices. Note the radiographic bone loss, deep probing depth, bleeding on probing, and gingival inflammation around the implant.

History of periodontal disease Like periodontitis, peri-implant infection may take years to progress. Therefore, it is not unlikely that peri-implant disease and periodontal disease share common risk factors. The dental literature provides sufficient evidence to indicate that patients with a history of periodontal disease (chronic and aggressive periodontitis) may have an increased susceptibility to peri-implant diseases because of the host's immune response.[40–43]

Schou and colleagues[42] reported that the incidence of peri-implant marginal bone loss and peri-implantitis is significantly higher among patients who have already lost teeth because of periodontitis. Additionally, the survival of the suprastructure, bone tissue, and implant was not different in patients with periodontitis and healthy subjects. A recent retrospective study evaluated the outcome of peri-implantitis when patients with severe periodontitis were treated with flap surgery with osteoplasty (47% of cases) or with a few regenerative procedures (20% of cases). Poor treatment outcome was reported for patients with severe periodontitis; this finding suggests the importance of good periodontal and oral health for the success of peri-implant therapy.[44] In contrast, Karoussis and colleagues[45] reported no statistically significant difference in implant outcome between patients with a history of chronic periodontitis and periodontally healthy subjects. However, those researchers also found that, compared with patients with chronic periodontitis, periodontally healthy subjects exhibited shallower probing pockets, less peri-implant marginal bone loss, and fewer incidences of peri-implantitis.

Several reports have suggested that the implant survival rate is poorer and that attachment loss and bone loss are greater among patients with generalized aggressive periodontitis (GAP) than among patients with chronic periodontitis or healthy patients.[46,47] A recent systematic review and meta-analysis found that the placement of oral implants is a good treatment option for a patient with history of GAP and that the survival outcome is similar for healthy patients and for patients with chronic periodontitis. However, the study also found that the failure rate for dental implants is significantly higher (risk ratio, 4) for patients with GAP than for healthy patients or for those with chronic periodontitis (risk ratio, 3.97) **(Fig. 3)**.[48]

Bone quality and quantity Published studies have found that failure rates are much higher when the quality and quantity of bone are insufficient at the implant site.[49,50] Attaining primary stability is a prerequisite for successful osseointegration, and accomplishing primary stability requires adequate bone quantity and density. Lekholm and Zarb[51] developed 4 categories classifying the quantity and quality (shape) of the jawbone to assist in the treatment planning of oral implants: Type I, homogeneous

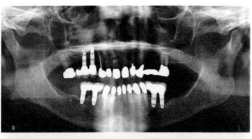

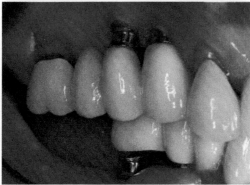

Fig. 3. Radiographic and clinical presentation of multiple failing implants in a patient with a history of periodontal disease.

compact bone; Type II, a dense core of trabecular bone surrounded by a layer of thick compact bone; Type III, a dense core of trabecular bone of favorable strength surrounded by a layer of thin cortical bone; and Type IV, a very thin layer of cortical bone with low-density trabecular bone in the center. The investigators also categorized bone quantity (shape): Type A, alveolar bone that is not resorbed; Type B, alveolar bone with some resorption; Type C, complete resorption of the basal bone; Type D, some resorption of the basal bone; and Type E, severe resorption of the basal bone. Various areas of the jawbone have various levels of bone quality. In general, the cortical thickness and density of the mandibular bone are higher than those of the maxillary bone.[34] The posterior segments of both jaws exhibit a marked reduction in cortical bone and increased porosity of the trabecular bone. As a result, implant success rates are higher for mandibular implants, and failure rates are higher in the posterior regions of the jaws.[6,52,53] Type 3 or 4 bone quality in the jawbone is associated with high implant failure rates (**Fig. 4**).[54–56] Poor bone quantity (inadequate bone height or width) can ultimately lead to the loss of osseointegration because of the limited availability of bone for implant placement. Studies have reported that failure rates are higher for implants placed in Type IV bone.[57] Lindh and colleagues[50] emphasized that the term *bone quality* is not synonymous with the term *bone density*. Additionally, these terms refer to different entities: bone quality encompasses not only the mineral content (matrix property and bone density) of the bone but also its structural component (skeletal size, architecture, and 3-dimensional orientation of the trabecular).[50] Furthermore, advanced resorption of the residual ridge of both the maxilla and the mandibular alveolus precludes the placement of longer implants with greater stability because of the proximity of the anatomic structures (maxillary sinus or nasal cavity and mandibular nerve canal). Thus, achieving primary stabilization and a successful outcome for oral implants placed in the jawbone depends primarily on the quality and quantity of bone.

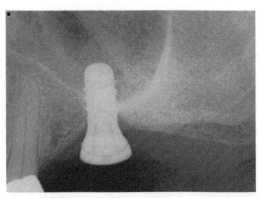

Fig. 4. Early implant failure because of poor quality of bone (Type IV) in the posterior maxillary region. Procedure to lift the floor of maxillary sinus and to condense the bone was not performed properly.

Width of keratinized gingiva The width of the attached gingiva varies from patient to patient and can be different for different teeth in the same patient. The effect of the presence or absence of adequate keratinized gingiva around dental implants on the success or failure of an implant is a controversial topic. Clinical studies have found that the lack of keratinized[58] or attached mucosa[59] does not compromise the health of peri-implant soft or hard tissues. On the other hand, one study has shown that dental implants that lack adequate keratinized or attached mucosa exhibit more plaque accumulation and mucosal inflammation than implants with adequate keratinized or attached mucosa. However, this study found no correlation between the amount of attached mucosa and implant survival.[60] The presence of keratinized mucosa is strongly correlated with optimal mucosal health and can help prevent infection around implants. Furthermore, a lack of keratinized mucosa is associated with crestal bone loss of 2 mm or more.[61] Therefore, many clinicians believe that the creation of keratinized peri-implant mucosa with sufficient width and thickness is required for preventing implant failure (**Fig. 5**).

External Factors

Operative factors
Factors related to surgery

Surgical experience The skill and experience of the surgeon are important factors in the successful outcome of dental implants. Andersson and colleagues[62] reported that general practitioners with 8 days of training achieved clinical results similar to those achieved at a specialty clinic for single-tooth implant placement. On the other hand, Zoghbi and colleagues[63] reported that the experience of the surgeon exerted a positive influence on osseointegration of the dental implants. In that study, surgical experience was defined as the number of implants placed: less-experienced professionals had placed no more than 50 dental implants; more-experienced professionals had placed more than 50. More-experienced professionals achieved a higher implant osseointegration rate (94.4%) than did less-experienced professionals (84.0%). Likewise, Lambert and colleagues[64] reported that implant failure rates were lower when the implants were placed by an experienced surgeon. As surgical experience increases, the surgeon exhibits better judgment in selecting patients and sites for implants.[34] On the other hand, another study has reported no significant difference between the implant survival rate and the level of the surgeon's residency training program[65] or the clinician's experience.[66] This discrepancy in the findings can be

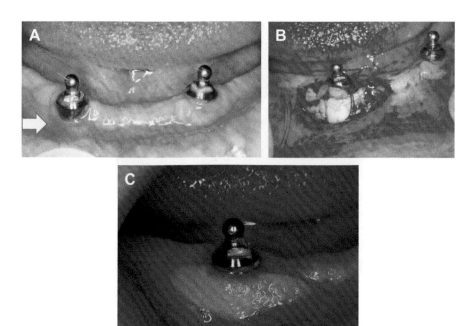

Fig. 5. (*A*) Arrow showing lack of keratinized and attached mucosal tissue around dental implant. Mucosal tissue is mobile and retractable leading to the introduction of plaque into the implant pocket. (*B*) Soft tissue augmentation was performed. (*C*) Wide zone of attached and keratinized gingiva around implant provides better gingival seal around the implant.

attributed to differences in the definition of experience. Using levels of training (years) as a definition of experience cannot be considered reliable because residents in a training program can place more or fewer implants over a period of time, and results can differ. Thus, although the surgeon's skill, judgment, and experience are crucial factors in the successful osseointegration of implants, additional studies are necessary so that we can better understand the role of surgical experience, particularly when practitioners participate in a university training program.

Surgical trauma For optimal implant outcome, surgical trauma should be minimized. Bone is viable and is sensitive to temperature. Overheating the bone during preparation of the implant osteotomy site can lead to necrosis of the bone tissue surrounding the dental implant. Furthermore, if bone drilling is performed without adequate cooling, bone damage is increased because of the generation of heat.[67] A temperature higher than 47°C for 1 minute can cause irreversible damage to bone tissue,[68] and Yacker and Klein[69] reported that a bur temperature higher than 47°C was reached within seconds during osteotomy preparation without irrigation (**Figs. 6** and **7**). It can be argued that the experience of the surgeon may play an important role and that as experience increases, less surgical trauma can be expected. Furthermore, a lack of osseointegration, in the form of the presence of a soft tissue interface between the bone and the implant, occasionally occurs in association with poor surgical technique. One study found that a critical gap of zero in the interface between the bone and the implant is vital for achieving direct bone apposition on the implant surface; it also found that bone apposition was better with screw-shaped implants than with cylindrical implants.[70]

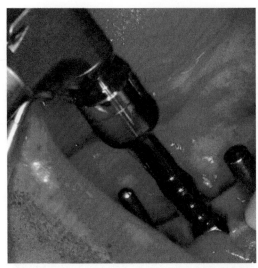

Fig. 6. Copious external irrigation of implant drill during osteotomy preparation of an implant site.

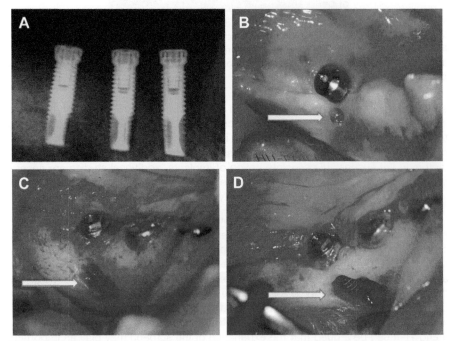

Fig. 7. Radiographic and clinical sign of early implant failure. The presumptive etiology was overheating the bone during the preparation of the osteotomy by drilling in the dense mandibular bone using dull twist drills. (*A*) Bone loss could not be clearly visualized on the periapical radiograph because it was on the lingual aspect of the implant. (*B*) Arrow showing a small opening through the mucosal tissue on the lingual aspect of the implant with no sign of suppuration. (*C*) Arrow showing the bone fenestration after the reflection of periosteal flap. (*D*) Arrow showing the complete removal of the granulation tissue. The implant was salvaged.

Aseptic environment If a strict antiseptic protocol is followed during surgical implant placement, minimal bacterial contamination can be expected, and lower implant failure rates can be expected (**Fig. 8**).

Incision technique Crestal or vestibular incisions are placed on the ridge during implant placement. Currently, the location and type of incision seem to exert no influence on the successful outcome of implants. Crestal incisions are preferable for wide edentulous ridges. Special attention should be given to releasing the periosteum with a full-thickness flap. This technique not only will achieve good surgical exposure but also will allow observation of the underlying anatomic features, such as nerve structures, tooth root anatomy, and bone defects. There is no difference in implant failure rates for implants placed with a crestal incision or with a mucobuccal fold incision.[71,72]

Flapless implant surgery Flapless implant surgery allows the preparation of an implant osteotomy without the elevation of a mucoperiosteal flap. The advantages of this surgical procedure include preservation of the blood supply, protection of the soft and hard tissues, shorter surgical times, less postoperative pain, and increased patient satisfaction. Published reports indicate that patients who undergo flapless surgical implant procedures experience a significant reduction in postoperative pain and swelling[73] and in the use of analgesics.[74] Despite the obvious benefits, the primary disadvantage of this technique is the lack of direct access to the underlying bone and the possibility of perforation of the buccal or lingual bone that leads to invasion of anatomic structures. Recent advances in dental radiographic imaging, such as computed tomography, and newer software that helps with 3-dimensional evaluation and positioning of dental implants have been of great assistance in flapless surgical implant procedures.[75] Furthermore, the use of surgical guides can help the clinician place dental implants without the fear of overpenetration or perforation into the nerve

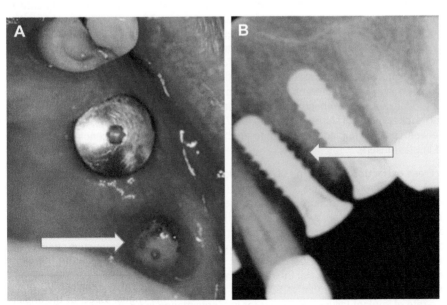

Fig. 8. (*A*) Arrow showing a clinical sign of early implant failure because of bacterial infection. (*B*) Arrow showing a radiographic sign of early implant failure because of bacterial infection.

canals. Brodala[76] compared the clinical outcome of dental implants placed by flapless techniques and concluded that this procedure yields higher implant survival rates. However, these results were based on short-term data. With the combination of advanced dental radiographic imaging studies and the surgeon's experience, the flapless surgical implant technique is considered an efficient treatment method.

One-stage (nonsubmerged) implants and 2-stage (submerged) implants The nonsubmerged implant approach consists of placing an implant and an abutment at the same time during the first surgical procedure. In contrast, the submerged implant insertion approach consists of placing an implant at the level of the bone or lower and performing a second surgical procedure to expose the implant and place the abutment. The nonsubmerged implant-insertion technique offers several advantages: reduced treatment time and cost, preservation of crestal bone because of the absence of a microgap,[77] and immediate loading of the implant with provisional restorations. Because of these clinical advantages, the nonsubmerged approach has become increasingly common in implant dentistry. Several studies have shown that the risk of implant failure is lower with the submerged technique (2-stage) than with the nonsubmerged technique.[78–80] The reason for the higher success rate with the submerged implant technique could be because of the minimal risk of bacterial infection.

Periapical pathology Placing immediate implants unquestionably has several advantages; however, the reports about successful placement of implants in an extraction socket with periapical pathology are inconsistent. Del Fabbro and colleagues[81] evaluated the clinical outcome of surgical implants placed immediately into extraction sockets with chronic periapical pathology in 30 subjects. After extraction, thorough debridement with plasma rich in growth factors (PRGF) was performed, and the implant surface was bioactivated by humidification with liquid PRGFs before placement. Of the total of 61 implants placed, only 1 failed. The investigators reported an overall implant success and survival rate of 98.4% and concluded that it is safe to place implants in sockets with periapical pathology. Other studies have reported similar results.[82,83] Lefever and colleagues[84] reported that there is a significant risk of periapical lesions when implants are placed adjacent to teeth with endodontic pathology (**Fig. 9**). Likewise, a recent review found that placing dental implants in extraction sockets with chronic periapical infection is a safe and viable option. The review found no significant difference in success rates between implants placed into fresh extraction sockets with chronic periapical infection (97.5%) and implants placed into sockets without signs of infection (98.7%). However, there is a positive correlation between placing implants adjacent to teeth with periapical radiolucencies and the risk of implant failure.[85]

Fresh extraction socket The alveolar ridge undergoes substantial changes (resorption) immediately after tooth extraction. A protocol for avoiding substantial bone resorption in the extraction socket proposes immediate implant placement (placing the implant in a fresh extraction socket). However, the question of whether the outcome of the dental implant differs when it is placed in a completely healed socket or a fresh extraction socket remains unanswered. A recent animal study performed histologic analyses to compare the effect of immediate implant placement in healed and fresh extraction sockets; the results showed that placing implants in fresh extraction sockets can jeopardize vertical bone remodeling.[86] Another study reported that the rate of implant failure was higher for implants placed in fresh extraction sockets.[87] However, another study found that placing implants in fresh extraction sockets can be an effective treatment.[88]

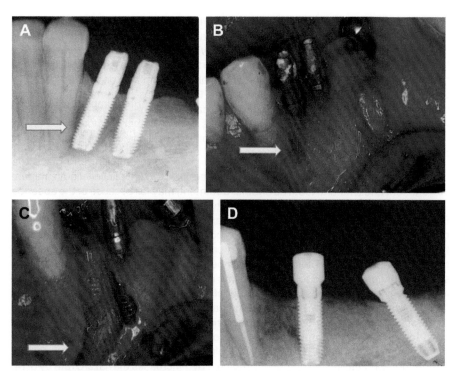

Fig. 9. (*A*) Radiographic sign of bone loss (*arrow*) around the apex of the mesial implant. Canine is tested nonvital. (*B*) Intraoperative view (*arrow*) after flap reflection showing bone fenestration between implant and canine. (*C*) Intraoperative view (*arrow*) after the removal of infected implant showing the extent of bone loss to the apex of the canine. (*D*) Guided bone regeneration of the implant site and endodontic treatment of the canine were performed.

In conclusion, after extraction, thorough curettage of the extraction socket is recommended. Depending on whether primary stability is attained, the appropriate implant placement procedure can be selected.

Implant anchorage Studies have shown that the primary stability and success of implants are higher when implants are supported by cortical bone.[89] Bicortical anchorage consists of supporting the implant not only with crestal cortical bone (the cervical part of the implant) but also with cancellous bone on the lateral or apical side (the inferior part of the implant). In the maxilla, bicortical anchorage is associated with engagement of the implant with the anterior or inferior border of the maxillary sinus or nasal cavity. On the other hand, monocortical anchorage is associated with support of the implant by only crestal cortical bone. Studies have suggested that bicortical anchorage can help improve the primary stability of the implant and can provide a better distribution of forces around the apex of the implant. One study found that the removal torque for bicortical implants is 2 times higher after 6 weeks and 3 times higher after 12 weeks than that for monocortical implants.[90] Several investigators have questioned the success of bicortical anchorage, because it can increase the risk of infection in the sinus. In contrast, other studies have recommended the use of bicortical implant anchorage, which yields a good implant success rate.[91,92] Ivanoff and colleagues[93] evaluated the implant survival rates and the marginal bone loss in the maxilla associated with implants placed with either monocortical (110 implants) or bicortical (97 implants) anchorage with a follow-up period of 15 years. The study found that implants with bicortical anchorage fail nearly 4 times more often than implants with monocortical anchorage. An in vitro study by Xiao and colleagues[94] found that the implant stability quotient of bicortical anchorage was higher than that of monocortical anchorage. Furthermore, the stability of implants decreased gradually under higher loading forces when immediate loading was performed for implants placed with bicortical anchorage (lateral cortical anchorage) than for those placed with monocortical anchorage. These results indicate that, although bicortical anchorage is associated with some complications, it results in good primary stability and better distribution of loading forces.

Number of implants placed Implant-supported fixed bridges (involving an implant as abutment and a natural tooth as another abutment) may fail because of the absence of good distribution of the occlusal forces between the implants and the natural teeth. Rangert and colleagues[95] reported that better stress distribution can be achieved by placing dental implants in a tripod fashion: positioning the implant either buccally or lingually instead of in a straight line, which can increase the susceptibility of the implants to bending forces. Therefore, the number of implants used in a given edentulous space should be increased to allow adequate distribution of forces (**Fig. 10**). However, it is possible that the increase in the number of implants can also increase the chances of complications, probably because of increased surgical time, increased trauma to the tissue, longer healing times, increased risk of injury to vital structures, and the need for a larger blood supply. Naert and colleagues[96] reported that the higher the number of implants used per patient, the higher the hazard risk of implant failure. Furthermore, increasing the number of implants by 1 increases the hazard rate by 0.14.

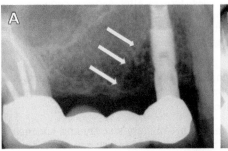
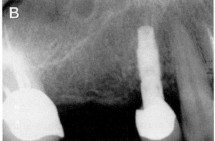
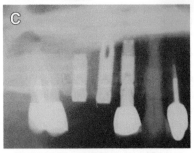

Fig. 10. (A) Arrows showing early radiographic sign of failing implant. Decreased bone density around implant because of long-span bridge and absence of good distribution of the occlusal forces between the implant and the natural tooth. (B) Radiographic sign of improved bone density around implant after the removal of long-span bridge. (C) Two more implants were placed to better distribute the occlusal forces.

Implant position Using conventional complete dentures to rehabilitate older patients with complete edentulism accompanied by resorbed or atrophic ridges is usually unsatisfying, probably because of the instability of the dentures during eating, biting, and speaking. Furthermore, atrophic edentulous ridges also are associated with anatomic restrictions that impede the placement of conventional endosseous dental implants. Some of these restrictions are poor bone volume, poor bone quality, and the proximity of the mental foramen or the maxillary sinuses. Placing oral implants under such conditions requires a long bilateral cantilever (20 mm) for the primary purpose of efficient masticatory function. Although several treatment options have been proposed to overcome such anatomic complications, such as placement of shorter implants, alveolar ridge augmentation, maxillary sinus lifts, and mandibular nerve transposition, these procedures require longer treatment times, higher costs, and more postoperative discomfort. An alternative treatment for overcoming these procedures is the placement of tilted implants. Tilting the posterior dental implants has several advantages: it increases primary stability, allows for the use of longer implants and therefore increases the surface area between the bone and the implant, reduces the length of the cantilever bridge, and improves implant anchorage. Krekmanov and colleagues[97] investigated the outcome of tilted implants in both atrophic edentulous arches. Mandibular implants were placed close to the mental foramina where the tilt was approximately 25 to 35° posteriorly (25 patients; 36 mandibular implants), and implants in the maxillary arch were placed close to and parallel to the sinus walls and were titled anteriorly or posteriorly by approximately 30 to 35° (22 patients; 30 maxillary implants). The investigators found that patients gained 6.5 mm of prosthetic support in the mandible and 9.3 mm of prosthetic support in the maxilla because of the placement of tilted implants.[97] Agliardi and colleagues[98] evaluated the long-term outcome of immediately loaded implant-supported full prostheses in 24 patients with atrophic mandibular ridges. The implants were compared on the basis of axial and tilted angulations. No significant difference was found between axial and tilted implants, and both exhibited good survival outcomes (after 1 year of follow-up). Kim and colleagues[99] fabricated 2 photoelastic models simulating human edentulous mandibles and used photoelastic stress analysis to compare the stress distribution at the bone-implant interface between tilted (30°) and axial implants supported by fixed mandibular prostheses. The investigators reported that tilting mandibular implants by approximately 30° reduced the cantilever by 5 mm. Furthermore, in comparison to axial implants, distal tilted implants resulted in a decrease of 17% in the stress concentration at the distal crestal bone.

Factors related to implants

Implant length and diameter Published reports indicate that the success rates for short implants (<10 mm) are lower than those for longer implants (>10 mm).[100] The advantages of longer implants include increased contact between the bone and the implant, increased initial stability, and greater resistance for withstanding occlusal forces.[32,96,101] Naert and colleagues[96] reported that shorter implants, a larger number of implants per patient, and a low number of implants per prosthesis were associated with a higher risk of implant failure. A decrease of 1 mm in the length of the implant increases the risk of implant failure by 0.16. The use of several wide-diameter implants in posterior sites has been recommended for overcoming the failure rate and increasing the surface area contact between the bone and the implant. Studies have shown that the rate of implant failure is significantly higher for implants with a smaller diameter than for implants with a wider diameter (a higher survival rate for implants 4 mm or more in diameter than for implants 3 mm or more diameter).[32,100] On the other hand, no statistically significant difference in implant failure rates has been reported between narrow and wide implants.[102]

Implant surface characteristics The primary goal of modern implantology is to achieve optimal and satisfactory osseointegration as a result of which an early loading can be allowed. The implant surface characteristics can plan an important role to regulate effective peri-implant bone healing. The different surface characteristics in which dental implants are available include smooth machined surfaces, roughened surfaces produced by coatings, blasting by various substances, acid treatments, or combinations of various treatments. Alteration of surface characteristics of an implant can help improve primary stability.[103] The 3 types of surface roughness on implants includes the following: minimally rough with Sa 0.5 μm, moderate roughness with Sa 1 to 2 μm, and rough, where Sa is greater than 2 μm.[104–106] Cochran[107] reported rough-surfaced implants had significantly higher success rates compared with implants with more smooth surfaces. Teughels and colleagues[108] reported that increased surface roughness facilitates microbial retention and increases the risk of implant failure due to peri-implantitis. Astrand and colleagues[109] reported increased frequency of peri-implantitis with straumann implants (rough surface) in comparison with Branemark implants (smooth surfaced). In conclusion, a clinician must also consider the biomechanics of the implant system in addition to clinical findings, such as bone quality and quantity, for a patient requiring dental implants.

Factors Related to Occlusion

Excessive occlusal forces

Patients who generate abnormal or excessive occlusal forces (for example, those with parafunctional habits such as bruxism) are usually not appropriate candidates for immediate implant loading, because such excessive forces can lead to failure of osseointegration and can cause progressive crestal bone resorption during immediate loading. During treatment planning, these patients should be thoroughly informed about the potential risks associated with the procedure.

SUMMARY

With the success of dental implant treatment, new treatment protocols have been proposed. Immediate implant loading protocols provide patients with satisfactory results by reducing the time interval between implant surgery and prosthesis delivery. However, it is important that the practitioner carefully select the patients before suggesting dental implant treatment. Although the aforementioned factors may influence implant failure, prosthetic design also can play an important role in affecting the implant outcome; this topic is not covered in this review. The following is a list of some guidelines that can help practitioners prevent implant failure.

a. Clinicians should critically evaluate the patient's oral hygiene, compliance, motivation, and risk factors before suggesting dental implant treatment.
b. Achieving primary stability is important for successful implant placement.
c. Host-related factors, operative-related factors, and implant-related factors may influence the outcome of implant treatment and should be thoroughly evaluated during treatment planning.
d. Practitioners treating patients with systemic metabolic disorders, such as diabetes or osteoporosis, those undergoing radiation therapy, and those who smoke, should follow a 2-staged approach for optimal implant outcome. Further studies are needed for evaluating the response of these patients to immediate implant loading.

Additional clinical and histologic studies are needed for the evaluation of other etiologic factors that may influence implant failure.

REFERENCES

1. Branemark PI, Adell R, Breine U, et al. Intra-osseous anchorage of dental prostheses. I. Experimental studies. Scand J Plast Reconstr Surg 1969;3(2): 81–100.
2. Malo P, Nobre Mde A, Petersson U, et al. A pilot study of complete edentulous rehabilitation with immediate function using a new implant design: case series. Clin Implant Dent Relat Res 2006;8(4):223–32.
3. Ekfeldt A, Christiansson U, Eriksson T, et al. A retrospective analysis of factors associated with multiple implant failures in maxillae. Clin Oral Implants Res 2001;12(5):462–7.
4. Moy PK, Medina D, Shetty V, et al. Dental implant failure rates and associated risk factors. Int J Oral Maxillofac Implants 2005;20(4):569–77.
5. Heydenrijk K, Meijer HJ, van der Reijden WA, et al. Microbiota around root-form endosseous implants: a review of the literature. Int J Oral Maxillofac Implants 2002;17(6):829–38.
6. Friberg B, Jemt T, Lekholm U. Early failures in 4,641 consecutively placed Branemark dental implants: a study from stage 1 surgery to the connection of completed prostheses. Int J Oral Maxillofac Implants 1991;6(2):142–6.
7. Albrektsson T, Branemark PI, Hansson HA, et al. Osseointegrated titanium implants. Requirements for ensuring a long-lasting, direct bone-to-implant anchorage in man. Acta Orthop Scand 1981;52(2):155–70.
8. Albrektsson T, Zarb G, Worthington P, et al. The long-term efficacy of currently used dental implants: a review and proposed criteria of success. Int J Oral Maxillofac Implants 1986;1(1):11–25.
9. Buser D, Weber HP, Lang NP. Tissue integration of non-submerged implants. 1-year results of a prospective study with 100 ITI hollow-cylinder and hollow-screw implants. Clin Oral Implants Res 1990;1(1):33–40.
10. Smith DE, Zarb GA. Criteria for success of osseointegrated endosseous implants. J Prosthet Dent 1989;62(5):567–72.
11. Esposito M, Hirsch JM, Lekholm U, et al. Biological factors contributing to failures of osseointegrated oral implants. (I). Success criteria and epidemiology. Eur J Oral Sci 1998;106(1):527–51.
12. Alsaadi G, Quirynen M, Komarek A, et al. Impact of local and systemic factors on the incidence of oral implant failures, up to abutment connection. J Clin Periodontol 2007;34(7):610–7.
13. Koldsland OC, Scheie AA, Aass AM. Prevalence of implant loss and the influence of associated factors. J Periodontol 2009;80(7):1069–75.
14. Huynh-Ba G, Friedberg JR, Vogiatzi D, et al. Implant failure predictors in the posterior maxilla: a retrospective study of 273 consecutive implants. J Periodontol 2008;79(12):2256–61.
15. Baqain ZH, Moqbel WY, Sawair FA. Early dental implant failure: risk factors. Br J Oral Maxillofac Surg 2012;50(3):239–43.
16. Busenlechner D, Furhauser R, Haas R, et al. Long-term implant success at the Academy for Oral Implantology: 8-year follow-up and risk factor analysis. J Periodontal Implant Sci 2014;44(3):102–8.
17. Esposito M, Thomsen P, Ericson LE, et al. Histopathologic observations on early oral implant failures. Int J Oral Maxillofac Implants 1999;14(6):798–810.

18. Piattelli A, Scarano A, Piattelli M. Microscopical aspects of failure in osseointe-grated dental implants: a report of five cases. Biomaterials 1996;17(12):1235–41.
19. Shirota T, Ohno K, Suzuki K, et al. The effect of aging on the healing of hydrox-ylapatite implants. J Oral Maxillofac Surg 1993;51(1):51–6.
20. Manor Y, Oubaid S, Mardinger O, et al. Characteristics of early versus late implant failure: a retrospective study. J Oral Maxillofac Surg 2009;67(12):2649–52.
21. Babbush CA, Shimura M. Five-year statistical and clinical observations with the IMZ two-stage osteointegrated implant system. Int J Oral Maxillofac Implants 1993;8(3):245–53.
22. Brocard D, Barthet P, Baysse E, et al. A multicenter report on 1,022 consecu-tively placed ITI implants: a 7-year longitudinal study. Int J Oral Maxillofac Im-plants 2000;15(5):691–700.
23. Wagenberg B, Froum SJ. A retrospective study of 1925 consecutively placed immediate implants from 1988 to 2004. Int J Oral Maxillofac Implants 2006;21(1):71–80.
24. Schwartz-Arad D, Grossman Y, Chaushu G. The clinical effectiveness of implants placed immediately into fresh extraction sites of molar teeth. J Periodontol 2000;71(5):839–44.
25. van Steenberghe D, Lekholm U, Bolender C, et al. Applicability of osseointegrated oral implants in the rehabilitation of partial edentulism: a prospective multicenter study on 558 fixtures. Int J Oral Maxillofac Implants 1990;5(3):272–81.
26. Penarrocha M, Guarinos J, Sanchis JM, et al. A retrospective study (1994-1999) of 441 ITI(r) implants in 114 patients followed-up during an average of 2.3 years. Med Oral 2002;7(2):144–55 [in English, Spanish].
27. Balshi SF, Wolfinger GJ, Balshi TJ. A retrospective analysis of 44 implants with no rotational primary stability used for fixed prosthesis anchorage. Int J Oral Maxillofac Implants 2007;22(3):467–71.
28. Snauwaert K, Duyck J, van Steenberghe D, et al. Time dependent failure rate and marginal bone loss of implant supported prostheses: a 15-year follow-up study. Clin Oral Investig 2000;4(1):13–20.
29. Pera P, Bassi F, Schierano G, et al. Implant anchored complete mandibular den-ture: evaluation of masticatory efficiency, oral function and degree of satisfac-tion. J Oral Rehabil 1998;25(6):462–7.
30. Cibirka RM, Razzoog M, Lang BR. Critical evaluation of patient responses to dental implant therapy. J Prosthet Dent 1997;78(6):574–81.
31. Mericske-Stern R, Zarb GA. Overdentures: an alternative implant methodology for edentulous patients. Int J Prosthodont 1993;6(2):203–8.
32. Winkler S, Morris HF, Ochi S. Implant survival to 36 months as related to length and diameter. Ann Periodontol 2000;5(1):22–31.
33. Chrcanovic BR, Abreu MH, Custodio AL. Morphological variation in dentate and edentulous human mandibles. Surg Radiol Anat 2011;33(3):203–13.
34. Esposito M, Hirsch JM, Lekholm U, et al. Biological factors contributing to fail-ures of osseointegrated oral implants. (II). Etiopathogenesis. Eur J Oral Sci 1998;106(3):721–64.
35. Hultin M, Fischer J, Gustafsson A, et al. Factors affecting late fixture loss and marginal bone loss around teeth and dental implants. Clin Implant Dent Relat Res 2000;2(4):203–8.
36. Friberg B, Sennerby L, Grondahl K, et al. On cutting torque measurements dur-ing implant placement: a 3-year clinical prospective study. Clin Implant Dent Re-lat Res 1999;1(2):75–83.

37. Lindquist LW, Rockler B, Carlsson GE. Bone resorption around fixtures in edentulous patients treated with mandibular fixed tissue-integrated prostheses. J Prosthet Dent 1988;59(1):59–63.
38. Lindquist LW, Carlsson GE, Jemt T. Association between marginal bone loss around osseointegrated mandibular implants and smoking habits: a 10-year follow-up study. J Dent Res 1997;76(10):1667–74.
39. Kourtis SG, Sotiriadou S, Voliotis S, et al. Private practice results of dental implants. Part I: survival and evaluation of risk factors–Part II: surgical and prosthetic complications. Implant Dent 2004;13(4):373–85.
40. Van der Weijden GA, van Bemmel KM, Renvert S. Implant therapy in partially edentulous, periodontally compromised patients: a review. J Clin Periodontol 2005;32(5):506–11.
41. Renvert S, Persson GR. Periodontitis as a potential risk factor for peri-implantitis. J Clin Periodontol 2009;36(Suppl 10):9–14.
42. Schou S, Holmstrup P, Worthington HV, et al. Outcome of implant therapy in patients with previous tooth loss due to periodontitis. Clin Oral Implants Res 2006; 17(Suppl 2):104–23.
43. Roos-Jansaker AM, Renvert H, Lindahl C, et al. Nine- to fourteen-year follow-up of implant treatment. Part III: factors associated with peri-implant lesions. J Clin Periodontol 2006;33(4):296–301.
44. Lagervall M, Jansson LE. Treatment outcome in patients with peri-implantitis in a periodontal clinic: a retrospective study. J Periodontol 2013;84(10):1365–73.
45. Karoussis IK, Kotsovilis S, Fourmousis I. A comprehensive and critical review of dental implant prognosis in periodontally compromised partially edentulous patients. Clin Oral Implants Res 2007;18(6):669–79.
46. Mengel R, Behle M, Flores-de-Jacoby L. Osseointegrated implants in subjects treated for generalized aggressive periodontitis: 10-year results of a prospective, long-term cohort study. J Periodontol 2007;78(12):2229–37.
47. De Boever AL, Quirynen M, Coucke W, et al. Clinical and radiographic study of implant treatment outcome in periodontally susceptible and non-susceptible patients: a prospective long-term study. Clin Oral Implants Res 2009;20(12): 1341–50.
48. Monje A, Alcoforado G, Padial-Molina M, et al. Generalized aggressive periodontitis as a risk factor for dental implant failure: a systematic-review and meta-analysis. J Periodontol 2014;16:1–17.
49. Drage NA, Palmer RM, Blake G, et al. A comparison of bone mineral density in the spine, hip and jaws of edentulous subjects. Clin Oral Implants Res 2007; 18(4):496–500.
50. Lindh C, Obrant K, Petersson A. Maxillary bone mineral density and its relationship to the bone mineral density of the lumbar spine and hip. Oral Surg Oral Med Oral Pathol Oral Radiol Endod 2004;98(1):102–9.
51. Lekholm U, Zarb GA. Patient selection and preparation. In: Branemark PI, Zarb GA, Albrektsson T, editors. Tissue integrated prostheses: osseointegration in clinical dentistry. Chicago: Quintessence Publishing Company; 1985. p. 199–209.
52. Friberg B, Nilson H, Olsson M, et al. Mk II: the self-tapping Branemark implant: 5-year results of a prospective 3-center study. Clin Oral Implants Res 1997;8(4): 279–85.
53. Buser D, Mericske-Stern R, Bernard JP, et al. Long-term evaluation of non-submerged ITI implants. Part 1: 8-year life table analysis of a prospective multi-center study with 2359 implants. Clin Oral Implants Res 1997;8(3):161–72.

54. Holahan CM, Wiens JL, Weaver A, et al. Relationship between systemic bone mineral density and local bone quality as effectors of dental implant survival. Clin Implant Dent Relat Res 2011;13(1):29–33.

55. Rocci A, Martignoni M, Gottlow J. Immediate loading in the maxilla using flapless surgery, implants placed in predetermined positions, and prefabricated provisional restorations: a retrospective 3-year clinical study. Clin Implant Dent Relat Res 2003;5(Suppl 1):29–36.

56. Jemt T, Lekholm U. Implant treatment in edentulous maxillae: a 5-year follow-up report on patients with different degrees of jaw resorption. Int J Oral Maxillofac Implants 1995;10(3):303–11.

57. Jaffin RA, Berman CL. The excessive loss of Branemark fixtures in type IV bone: a 5-year analysis. J Periodontol 1991;62(1):2–4.

58. Zitzmann NU, Scharer P, Marinello CP. Long-term results of implants treated with guided bone regeneration: a 5-year prospective study. Int J Oral Maxillofac Implants 2001;16(3):355–66.

59. Wennstrom JL, Bengazi F, Lekholm U. The influence of the masticatory mucosa on the peri-implant soft tissue condition. Clin Oral Implants Res 1994;5(1):1–8.

60. Chung DM, Oh TJ, Shotwell JL, et al. Significance of keratinized mucosa in maintenance of dental implants with different surfaces. J Periodontol 2006; 77(8):1410–20.

61. Block MS, Kent JN. Factors associated with soft- and hard-tissue compromise of endosseous implants. J Oral Maxillofac Surg 1990;48(11):1153–60.

62. Andersson B, Odman P, Lindvall AM, et al. Surgical and prosthodontic training of general practitioners for single tooth implants: a study of treatments performed at four general practitioners' offices and at a specialist clinic after 2 years. J Oral Rehabil 1995;22(8):543–8.

63. Zoghbi SA, de Lima LA, Saraiva L, et al. Surgical experience influences 2-stage implant osseointegration. J Oral Maxillofac Surg 2011;69(11):2771–6.

64. Lambert PM, Morris HF, Ochi S. Positive effect of surgical experience with implants on second-stage implant survival. J Oral Maxillofac Surg 1997;55(12 Suppl 5):12–8.

65. Melo MD, Shafie H, Obeid G. Implant survival rates for oral and maxillofacial surgery residents: a retrospective clinical review with analysis of resident level of training on implant survival. J Oral Maxillofac Surg 2006;64(8):1185–9.

66. Kohavi D, Azran G, Shapira L, et al. Retrospective clinical review of dental implants placed in a university training program. J Oral Implantol 2004;30(1): 23–9.

67. Eriksson RA, Albrektsson T, Magnusson B. Assessment of bone viability after heat trauma. A histological, histochemical and vital microscopic study in the rabbit. Scand J Plast Reconstr Surg 1984;18(3):261–8.

68. Eriksson AR, Albrektsson T. Temperature threshold levels for heat-induced bone tissue injury: a vital-microscopic study in the rabbit. J Prosthet Dent 1983;50(1): 101–7.

69. Yacker MJ, Klein M. The effect of irrigation on osteotomy depth and bur diameter. Int J Oral Maxillofac Implants 1996;11(5):634–8.

70. Carlsson L, Rostlund T, Albrektsson B, et al. Implant fixation improved by close fit. Cylindrical implant-bone interface studied in rabbits. Acta Orthop Scand 1988;59(3):272–5.

71. Scharf DR, Tarnow DP. The effect of crestal versus mucobuccal incisions on the success rate of implant osseointegration. Int J Oral Maxillofac Implants 1993; 8(2):187–90.

72. Casino AJ, Harrison P, Tarnow DP, et al. The influence of type of incision on the success rate of implant integration at stage II uncovering surgery. J Oral Maxillofac Surg 1997;55(12 Suppl 5):31–7.

73. Nkenke E, Eitner S, Radespiel-Troger M, et al. Patient-centred outcomes comparing transmucosal implant placement with an open approach in the maxilla: a prospective, non-randomized pilot study. Clin Oral Implants Res 2007;18(2): 197–203.

74. Fortin T, Bosson JL, Isidori M, et al. Effect of flapless surgery on pain experienced in implant placement using an image-guided system. Int J Oral Maxillofac Implants 2006;21(2):298–304.

75. Ozan O, Turkyilmaz I, Yilmaz B. A preliminary report of patients treated with early loaded implants using computerized tomography-guided surgical stents: flapless versus conventional flapped surgery. J Oral Rehabil 2007;34(11): 835–40.

76. Brodala N. Flapless surgery and its effect on dental implant outcomes. Int J Oral Maxillofac Implants 2009;24(Suppl):118–25.

77. Prasad DK, Shetty M, Bansal N, et al. Crestal bone preservation: a review of different approaches for successful implant therapy. Indian J Dent Res 2011; 22(2):317–23.

78. Engquist B, Astrand P, Anzen B, et al. Simplified methods of implant treatment in the edentulous lower jaw: a 3-year follow-up report of a controlled prospective study of one-stage versus two-stage surgery and early loading. Clin Implant Dent Relat Res 2005;7(2):95–104.

79. Becktor JP, Isaksson S, Billstrom C. A prospective multicenter study using two different surgical approaches in the mandible with turned Branemark implants: conventional loading using fixed prostheses. Clin Implant Dent Relat Res 2007; 9(4):179–85.

80. Baelum V, Ellegaard B. Implant survival in periodontally compromised patients. J Periodontol 2004;75(10):1404–12.

81. Del Fabbro M, Boggian C, Taschieri S. Immediate implant placement into fresh extraction sites with chronic periapical pathologic features combined with plasma rich in growth factors: preliminary results of single-cohort study. J Oral Maxillofac Surg 2009;67(11):2476–84.

82. Crespi R, Cappare P, Gherlone E. Fresh-socket implants in periapical infected sites in humans. J Periodontol 2010;81(3):378–83.

83. Waasdorp JA, Evian CI, Mandracchia M. Immediate placement of implants into infected sites: a systematic review of the literature. J Periodontol 2010;81(6): 801–8.

84. Lefever D, Van Assche N, Temmerman A, et al. Aetiology, microbiology and therapy of periapical lesions around oral implants: a retrospective analysis. J Clin Periodontol 2013;40(3):296–302.

85. Bell CL, Diehl D, Bell BM, et al. The immediate placement of dental implants into extraction sites with periapical lesions: a retrospective chart review. J Oral Maxillofac Surg 2011;69(6):1623–7.

86. Discepoli N, Vignoletti F, Laino L, et al. Fresh extraction socket: spontaneous healing vs. immediate implant placement. Clin Oral Implants Res 2014. [Epub ahead of print].

87. Deng F, Zhang H, Zhang H, et al. A comparison of clinical outcomes for implants placed in fresh extraction sockets versus healed sites in periodontally compromised patients: a 1-year follow-up report. Int J Oral Maxillofac Implants 2010; 25(5):1036–40.

88. Barone A, Toti P, Quaranta A, et al. The clinical outcomes of immediate versus delayed restoration procedures on immediate implants: a comparative cohort study for single-tooth replacement. Clin Implant Dent Relat Res 2014. [Epub ahead of print].

89. Tawse-Smith A, Perio C, Payne AG, et al. One-stage operative procedure using two different implant systems: a prospective study on implant overdentures in the edentulous mandible. Clin Implant Dent Relat Res 2001;3(4):185–93.

90. Ivanoff CJ, Sennerby L, Lekholm U. Influence of mono- and bicortical anchorage on the integration of titanium implants. A study in the rabbit tibia. Int J Oral Maxillofac Surg 1996;25(3):229–35.

91. Jensen J, Sindet-Pedersen S, Oliver AJ. Varying treatment strategies for reconstruction of maxillary atrophy with implants: results in 98 patients. J Oral Maxillofac Surg 1994;52(3):210–6 [discussion: 216–8].

92. Branemark PI, Adell R, Albrektsson T, et al. An experimental and clinical study of osseointegrated implants penetrating the nasal cavity and maxillary sinus. J Oral Maxillofac Surg 1984;42(8):497–505.

93. Ivanoff CJ, Grondahl K, Bergstrom C, et al. Influence of bicortical or monocortical anchorage on maxillary implant stability: a 15-year retrospective study of Branemark System implants. Int J Oral Maxillofac Implants 2000;15(1):103–10.

94. Xiao JR, Li YQ, Guan SM, et al. Effects of lateral cortical anchorage on the primary stability of implants subjected to controlled loads: an in vitro study. Br J Oral Maxillofac Surg 2012;50(2):161–5.

95. Rangert B, Jemt T, Jorneus L. Forces and moments on Branemark implants. Int J Oral Maxillofac Implants 1989;4(3):241–7.

96. Naert I, Koutsikakis G, Duyck J, et al. Biologic outcome of implant-supported restorations in the treatment of partial edentulism. Part I: a longitudinal clinical evaluation. Clin Oral Implants Res 2002;13(4):381–9.

97. Krekmanov L, Kahn M, Rangert B, et al. Tilting of posterior mandibular and maxillary implants for improved prosthesis support. Int J Oral Maxillofac Implants 2000;15(3):405–14.

98. Agliardi E, Clerico M, Ciancio P, et al. Immediate loading of full-arch fixed prostheses supported by axial and tilted implants for the treatment of edentulous atrophic mandibles. Quintessence Int 2010;41(4):285–93.

99. Kim KS, Kim YL, Bae JM, et al. Biomechanical comparison of axial and tilted implants for mandibular full-arch fixed prostheses. Int J Oral Maxillofac Implants 2011;26(5):976–84.

100. Olate S, Lyrio MC, de Moraes M, et al. Influence of diameter and length of implant on early dental implant failure. J Oral Maxillofac Surg 2010;68(2):414–9.

101. Sennerby L, Roos J. Surgical determinants of clinical success of osseointegrated oral implants: a review of the literature. Int J Prosthodont 1998;11(5):408–20.

102. Haas R, Mensdorff-Pouilly N, Mailath G, et al. Survival of 1,920 IMZ implants followed for up to 100 months. Int J Oral Maxillofac Implants 1996;11(5):581–8.

103. Simon Z, Watson PA. Biomimetic dental implants–new ways to enhance osseointegration. J Can Dent Assoc 2002;68(5):286–8.

104. Wennerberg A, Albrektsson T, Andersson B. Bone tissue response to commercially pure titanium implants blasted with fine and coarse particles of aluminum oxide. Int J Oral Maxillofac Implants 1996;11(1):38–45.

105. Wennerberg A, Albrektsson T, Andersson B, et al. A histomorphometric and removal torque study of screw-shaped titanium implants with three different surface topographies. Clin Oral Implants Res 1995;6(1):24–30.

106. Wennerberg A, Hallgren C, Johansson C, et al. A histomorphometric evaluation of screw-shaped implants each prepared with two surface roughnesses. Clin Oral Implants Res 1998;9(1):11–9.

107. Cochran DL. A comparison of endosseous dental implant surfaces. J Periodontol 1999;70(12):1523–39.

108. Teughels W, Van Assche N, Sliepen I, et al. Effect of material characteristics and/or surface topography on biofilm development. Clin Oral Implants Res 2006; 17(Suppl 2):68–81.

109. Astrand P, Engquist B, Anzen B, et al. A three-year follow-up report of a comparative study of ITI dental implants and Branemark system implants in the treatment of the partially edentulous maxilla. Clin Implant Dent Relat Res 2004; 6(3):130–41.

Key Systemic and Environmental Risk Factors for Implant Failure

Dolphus R. Dawson III, DMD, MS, MPH*, Samuel Jasper, DDS, MS

KEYWORDS

- Risk factors • Dental implant failure • Systemic disease • Peri-implantitis • Smoking
- Marginal bone loss

KEY POINTS

- Dental implant failure is related to several risk factors, including systemic disease, periodontal disease, and environmental factors.
- Poorly controlled disease may contribute to perimucositis and peri-implantitis, potentially leading to implant complications, including failure.
- Although few risk factors are absolute contraindications to implant placement, further research is needed to determine which combination(s) of factors predisposes patients to perimucositis and peri-implantitis, important precursors to implant failure.

INTRODUCTION

Many studies have demonstrated the long-term success of dental implants in replacing teeth missing because of caries or periodontal disease. A significant number of published articles detail the success of various types of implants placed in specific situations, such as those placed in bone-augmented sites. Implant failure has long been understood as the complete loss of the dental implant, but it is becoming apparent that an increasing number of implants are associated with perimucositis or peri-implantitis. Published reports indicate that peri-implantitis affects approximately 10% of implants and 20% of patients[1]; however, the incidence is higher in some reports, depending on the thresholds used to define the condition.[2] Despite the variability in definitions and the wide array of designs of the studies assessing the success or failure of implants, it is reasonable to assume that we will continue to see an increase in the prevalence of inflammatory processes that affect implants and that

Division of Periodontology, Department of Oral Health Practice, College of Dentistry, University of Kentucky, 800 Rose Street, Lexington, KY 40536, USA
* Corresponding author. Division of Periodontology, Department of Oral Health Practice, College of Dentistry, University of Kentucky, 800 Rose Street, D-444 Dental Sciences Building, Lexington, KY 40536.
E-mail address: dolph.dawson@uky.edu

Dent Clin N Am 59 (2015) 25–39
http://dx.doi.org/10.1016/j.cden.2014.09.002
0011-8532/15/$ – see front matter © 2015 Elsevier Inc. All rights reserved.

may lead to destruction of connective tissue or bone. This article reviews key systemic, periodontal, and environmental risk factors associated with implant failure, as well as perimucositis and peri-implantitis.

MICROBIOLOGY OF PERI-IMPLANTITIS AND PERIMUCOSITIS AND COMPARISON WITH PERIODONTITIS

The primary etiologic factor for peri-implant mucositis is the oral biofilm. This initial challenge to the host defense mirrors the challenge that affects the natural dentition. The initial adherence of bacteria to the implant surface can vary with the type of surface topography. Implants with rough surfaces enhance the initial bacterial colonization.[3,4] In general, sites affected by periodontitis and peri-implantitis contain more gram-negative bacteria than healthy sites.[5] The types of bacteria associated with healthy implants and failing implants are similar to those associated with healthy and diseased teeth, but there are also some important differences. Kumar and colleagues[6] used 16S pyrosequencing to analyze subgingival and submucosal plaque samples from subjects with healthy implants and from subjects with periodontitis and peri-implantitis. They found that peri-implant biofilms differed between the 2 groups: There was less diversity in the type of bacteria, but, with increasing disease, the numbers of *Prevotella* and *Leptotrichia* were lower and the numbers of *Campylobacter, Actinomyces,* and *Peptococcus* were higher. Cortelli and colleagues[7] found that the frequency of *Porphymonas gingivalis* was higher in cases of peri-implantitis than in cases of perimucositis and that the levels of *P gingivalis and Aggregatibacter actinomycetemcomitans* were similar in periodontitis and peri-implantitis. The levels of *Campylobacter rectus* and *Tannerella forsythia* were higher in healthy gingiva than in gingiva affected by peri-implant mucositis. On the other hand, a study by Koyanagi and colleagues[8] found more bacterial diversity in peri-implantitis sites than in periodontitis sites (198 taxa in peri-implantitis, 148 taxa in periodontitis). *Fusiform bacterium* and *Streptococcus* species were common in association with both peri-implantitis and periodontitis, whereas *Parvimonas micra* were seen only in association with peri-implantitis. Dabdoub and colleagues[9] conducted a patient-specific analysis of peri-implant and periodontal microbiomes associated with implants adjacent to teeth and found significant differences in both the populations and the levels of participant microbes, concluding that the proximity of an implant to a tooth does not account for the bacterial species seen in peri-implant tissues.

The microbial community may have shared attributes and, as discussed, some differences when both natural dentition and implants are present, but what are the microbial characteristics of implants when no natural teeth are present? A study by Kocar and colleagues[10] evaluated partially edentulous patients and found the frequency of 4 of the periodontopathogens assessed (*P gingivalis, T forsythia, T denticola,* and *A actinomycetemcomitans)* was higher in pockets 4 mm or deeper than in shallow pockets ($\leq$4 mm), but was not different from the frequency of these pathogens in association with implants adjacent to natural teeth. However, none of these bacteria were found in the implant sites of completely edentulous patients. Additional studies are needed to assess the progression of peri-implantitis and the microbial ecology in edentulous patients.

Reported risk factors for perimucositis and peri-implantitis include a history of previous periodontal disease.[2] Presumably, if the periodontopathogens that exist in the peri-implant pocket are similar to those that exist in the natural dentition, then the host response and the subsequent soft tissue and hard tissue destruction would be similar to those for a natural tooth. In comparing the various levels of severity of periodontitis, Aloufi and colleagues[11] found that the rate of loss of clinical attachment around implants was higher when severe periodontitis was present. Another study compared patients with or without residual periodontal pockets 6 mm or deeper and found that for patients with these pockets the prevalence of probing pockets 5 mm or deeper, bleeding on probing, and bone loss was higher than for patients with no residual periodontal pockets.[12] The authors surmised that the maintenance of periodontal health is more important than a past history of periodontitis and is a crucial determinant of the risk of peri-implantitis. The result of a recent retrospective study of treatment outcomes of peri-implantitis supported the importance of maintaining periodontal health: The effectiveness of peri-implant therapy by various surgical methods was lower in association with a diagnosis of generalized or localized severe periodontitis.[13] Other studies have also suggested that the development of peri-implantitis or the loss of implants is more likely for patients in whom reinfections of treated periodontal sites occur during maintenance therapy than for patients with periodontal stablity.[14]

Although a number of studies have focused on the relationship between microbial ecology and the pockets associated with perimucositis or peri-implantitis, fewer studies have investigated the significance of adjacent periapical infections. Lefever and colleagues[15] conducted a retrospective analysis of implants adjacent to teeth with endodontic pathology and found that the likelihood of the development of periapical lesions was 7.2 times higher for an implant placed next to a tooth that already has such a lesion than for an implant placed next to teeth without periapical lesions. The most prominent species found in these lesions was *P gingivalis*.

SMOKING

The list of risk or potential risk factors for peri-implantitis or implant failure is extensive. It includes systemic disease, genetic traits, chronic drug or alcohol consumption, smoking, periodontal disease, radiotherapy, diabetes, osteoporosis, dental plaque, and poor oral hygiene.[1,16,17] Smoking and its relationship to periodontitis has received a great deal of attention in the periodontal literature.[18,19] It is well known that patients who smoke have more periodontal destruction than nonsmokers.[18–20] According to the result of a study by Karbach and colleagues,[21] smoking was also the most important risk factor for the formation of peri-implant mucositis. As the number of dental implant placements continues to increase and patients' requests for implants become more commonplace, many dentists wonder whether their placement in smokers presents any risks for unsuccessful restoration of the dentition.

The accuracy of implant placement is crucial to implant success, especially when the alveolar ridge is narrow. D'haese and De Bruyn[22] found small deviations between the planned location and the actual placement site of implants for smokers, but not for nonsmokers. The authors speculated that, because mucosal tissues are thicker in smokers than in nonsmokers, there was a decrease in the stability of the surgical guide or the scanning prosthesis, and that this instability caused alterations in the final placement of implants.[22]

Many edentulous patients seek implant placement to allow the construction of a stable mandibular denture. One study compared 36 patients treated with 2 implants and ball attachments, 37 patients treated with 2 implants and a bar, and 37 patients treated with 4 implants and a triple bar attachment in the mandibular arch. The mean evaluation time for this group of patients was 8.3 years. The group with 4 implants lost significantly more bone than the groups with 2 implants. Marginal bone loss in smokers was almost twice that observed in nonsmokers, irrespective of the treatment modality.[23] Smoking may affect the implants anchoring a fixed dental prosthesis. Wahlström and colleagues[24] used clinical and radiographic examinations to study fixed dental prostheses in 46 patients. All fixed dental prostheses had been in function for at least 3 years. The authors found that smokers had fewer teeth, more periodontal pockets 4 mm or deeper, and a greater tendency toward increased marginal bone loss than nonsmokers. Increases in the loss of osseous support could lead to increases in implant failure and the loss of anchorage for a removable or fixed prosthesis.

The location of implants in the oral cavity may influence the overall success rate of these implants if a variation in bone loss is present. A comparison of the maxillary arches of smokers and nonsmokers showed that smokers lost slightly more than twice as much bone, whereas smokers and nonsmokers lost approximately the same amount of bone around mandibular implants.[25] A radiographic evaluation of maxillary implants by Haas and his group showed that smokers experienced more bone resorption than nonsmokers. The analysis revealed no difference between smokers and nonsmokers in bone loss in the mandibular arch.[26]

Kourtis and colleagues[27] also found that the rate of implant failure was higher for smokers than for nonsmokers. They speculated that the higher failure rate may have been owing to smokers' reduced healing capability.

A wide choice of implant surfaces is available to the practitioner, and the selection of the proper surface may make a difference in the overall failure rate. Sayardoust's group compared turned and oxidized implants 5 years after placement in smokers and never smokers. Smokers with turned implants lost almost twice as much bone as never smokers with turned implants, whereas the failure rate for oxidized implants was almost equal for smokers and never smokers.[28] Aalam and Nowzari[29] compared (1) surfaces roughened by anodic oxidation (TiUnite dental implants), (2) dual acid-etched surfaces (Osseotite dental implants), and (3) machined implants (Brånemark dental implants). Smoking had no impact on the success rates of these 3 implant types.[29] Balshe and coworkers[30] found no significant failure rate for smokers with rough surface implants, whereas the failure rate was significant for smokers with smooth surface implants. In this study, the largest number of failures was associated with smooth surface implants placed in the posterior maxilla. In a meta-analysis, Strietzel and his associates[31] found that the enhanced risk of implant failure was higher for smokers than for nonsmokers. Their systematic review found that the risk of biologic complications was greater in smokers than in nonsmokers. The authors found 5 published studies that reported no impact of surface types on implant prognosis, but these studies investigated only implants with particle-blasted, acid-etched, or anodic oxidized surfaces.[31] The characteristics of implants may affect their survival rate. Surface characteristics combined with length, width, and support of a fixed prosthesis may produce differing responses in the surrounding bone. A study of 339 implants placed over a 21-year period found that annual bone loss was higher in association with implants that were shorter or wider, that supported a fixed prosthesis, or that were placed in smokers. Smokers had almost 3 times more annual bone loss than nonsmokers. The most important factor to consider for maintaining implants was implant length: Better results were achieved with longer implants.[32]

Smoking may influence the healing of tissues after implant placement. D'Avila and associates[33] studied the surfaces of implants placed 2 months earlier in the posterior maxilla (type IV bone) of smokers. Their histometric evaluation showed that bone-to-implant contact was twice as high for sandblasted, acid-etched implants than for machined implants.[33] Many patients require only a single implant between 2 natural teeth.

One study performed clinical and radiographic evaluation of implants placed between 2 natural teeth at least 5 years earlier in former smokers, smokers, and nonsmokers. Although the authors concluded that smoking was not related to the rate of implant survival, current smokers experienced more marginal bone loss than former smokers or nonsmokers, and nonsmokers lost less marginal bone than any other group.[34] Leonhardt and colleagues[35] used surgery and antimicrobial therapy to treat peri-implantitis and followed these patients for 5 years after treatment. They concluded that treatment outcome was less favorable for smokers with severe peri-implantitis than for nonsmokers. Orthodontists use miniscrews to assist them in achieving patient treatment goals. Anything that has a negative effect on miniscrew anchorage would be detrimental to treatment outcome. Bayat and Bauss[36] considered patients' daily amount of smoking, defining light smokers as those who smoked fewer than 10 cigarettes per day and heavy smokers as those who smoked more than 10 cigarettes per day. The failure rate of miniscrews was higher for heavy smokers than for either light smokers or nonsmokers. The authors found no differences in miniscrew failures between light smokers and nonsmokers.[36]

Patients testing positive for the interleukin (IL)-1 genotype have been found to be more susceptible to periodontal disease.[20] Jansson and colleagues[37] evaluated Brånemark implants that had been placed over a 10-year period. IL-1–positive patients in general were not more prone to implant failure, but failure rates were higher for smokers who IL-1 positive. Gruica and associates[38] found that 64 of the 180 patients in their study were IL-1 positive. There was no significant correlation between the nonsmoking IL-1–positive patients and implant complications. However, the rates of complications and implant failures were higher in IL-1–positive smokers.[38]

Dental practitioners always promote the practice of good oral hygiene in their practices. Oral hygiene may be a factor in increasing the success rate of implants placed in smokers. One study evaluated fixed implant-supported prosthetics in the mandibular arches of 45 patients over a 10-year period. They found good results for both smokers and nonsmokers. Marginal bone loss was higher for smokers than for nonsmokers and was even higher for smokers with poor oral hygiene.[39]

Because many research articles have reported smoking's negative impact on dental implants, should practitioners recommend implants for patients who smoke? A literature review by Takamiya and colleagues[40] found that even though many negative factors were associated with smoking and dental implants, smoking was not an absolute contraindication to implant placement. The authors noted that smokers should be advised that their risk of implant failure is greater than that for nonsmokers. Heinikainen and associates[41] sent 10 cases with various characteristics to 400 general practitioners and 47 dental teachers in Finland. They were asked if they would or would not recommend implants for each case. Approximately 50% of general practitioners but only 15% of dental teachers replied that they would recommend implants for smoking patients.[41]

Smoking cessation therapy could be a positive factor in implant therapy. Yilmazel Ucar and colleagues[42] used varenicline, bupropion, and nicotine replacement therapy in a smoking cessation clinic. The highest success rate was 52.8% in the nicotine replacement group. The overall success rate was 35% and the overall relapse rate was 21.6%. Yasin's group[43] uses behavioral therapy and free nicotine replacement to treat 185 smokers for 8 weeks. Six months after therapy, only 15% of the patients were still not smoking.[43]

Research results show that the decision to place implants in smokers may not be clear cut. Ideally, it would be better for smokers to enter a smoking cessation program and to quit smoking before implant placement. Smoking has a negative impact on implant survival for patients with machined-surface implants, fixed prosthetics, marginal bone loss, bone-to-implant contact area, and IL-1 genotype. There is lack of agreement among dentists about whether implants should be recommended to their patients who smoke. Smoking cessation programs seem to be the ideal solution, but study results are not encouraging. Dentists who consider the use of implants for smokers must clearly explain the increased risk of implant failure to every patient.

SYSTEMIC RISK FACTORS
Diabetes

A substantial amount of literature has examined the relationship between diabetes and periodontitis.[44,45] A number of these studies have supported a bidirectional relationship in which improving the overall status of one disease may improve the status of the other. The hyperglycemic state of diabetes, if left unchecked, results in shifts in the advanced glycation end product/receptor for AGE (AGE/RAGE) axis and the receptor activator of nuclear factor-κB ligand and osteoprotegerin (RANKL/OPG) axis and can lead to overall immune and cytokine imbalance, as well as cellular stress. This imbalance can contribute to periodontal pathogenesis by enhancing tissue destruction and can also result in impaired healing. There seems to be a dose-dependent relationship between severity of periodontitis and diabetes, and evidence indicates that periodontitis control can improve diabetes control.[46,47] Likewise, patients with poorly controlled diabetes tend to have an increased likelihood of and severity of periodontal disease.[48,49]

As with periodontal therapy, it is believed that good control of diabetes (hemoglobin A1c $\leq$ 7) can contribute to successful implant therapy.[50] A review by Bornstein and colleagues[51] found that the rate of implant failure was higher among diabetic patients and that these patients experienced earlier implant failure than patients without diabetes. Given the importance of controlling periodontal inflammation relative to diabetes, it may be worthwhile to consider the relationship between peri-implant tissues and diabetes. Several animal studies have examined osseointegration in terms of bone quality or timing of failure, as well as other clinical parameters. A study using a diabetes-induced pig model found that diabetic pigs had less bone-to-implant contact than nondiabetic pigs.[52] Rats injected with AGEs exhibited a slower rate of osseointegration, and the injections had a negative effect on implant stability.[53] Another study using diabetic rats found decreased bone density around osseointegrated implants.[54] A study followed several clinical parameters over a period of 3 years in patients with various levels of diabetic control as measured by hemoglobin A1c levels.[55] Within the 4 levels of diabetic control defined by the study, the highest level (hemoglobin A1c $\geq$ 10.1) was associated with the greatest level of bleeding on probing and a greater bleeding level over the course of 3 years. On the other hand, a recent review of glycemic control and implant therapy failed to find a relationship between levels of glycemic control and implant failure.[56]

Although some studies have investigated the level of inflammatory cytokines relative to diabetes and periodontitis, there is a paucity of information about inflammatory biomarkers in the perimucosal tissues of diabetic patients. An animal model using rates with type 2 diabetes to study proinflammatory markers and growth factors related to healing of bone after implant placement found delayed osteoblast differentiation and decreased levels of IL-1β, tumor necrosis factor (TNF)-α, and macrophages.[57] A study by Venza and colleagues[58] evaluated proinflammatory gene expression in patients with or without diabetes and found that levels of TNF-α, CCR5, and CXR3 were higher in sites with peri-implantitis ($P<.01$) in patients without diabetes or with well-controlled diabetes. The levels of TNF-α, CCR5, and CXR3 were higher in chronic periodontitis sites in poorly controlled diabetics. Further work is needed to clarify the proinflammatory and anti-inflammatory responses in peri-implant tissues in diabetic patients.

Obesity/Hyperlipidemia

A number of reviews indicate positive correlations between obesity or hyperlipidemia and periodontitis,[59–61] particularly as it relates to metabolic syndrome. Currently, there is a lack of information about how hyperlipidemia may affect the risk of implant failure or peri-implant inflammation.

Impaired Organ Function

The number of published studies reporting the risk of implant failure associated with impaired organ function is limited. Studies focused on the success of implants in patients who have received organ transplants (ie, heart, liver) have found that the clinical parameters and radiographs of dental implants for those patients do not differ from those of healthy patients.[62–64] Because these studies have involved patients who are immunocompromised because of organ transplant, further studies are needed to determine failing organs contribute to the risk of implant failure or peri-implantitis.

Osteoporosis

Osteoporosis results in a decrease in bone density and has been considered a relative contraindication to implant placement. A significant number of more recent studies have focused on the treatment of osteoporosis with bisphosphonates, a topic that is reviewed elsewhere in this article. Recent reviews have indicated that there is no absolute contraindication to implants in patients with osteoporosis.[65,66] A retrospective study of 3224 implants placed in 746 women 50 years of age or older evaluated bone mineral densities on a subset of 192 women with 646 implants with a diagnosis of either osteoporosis, osteopenia or no osteoporosis or osteopenia and found that a neither a diagnosis of osteoporosis nor osteopenia conferred a greater risk of implant failure.[67] In this study, the risk of implant failure was 2.6 times higher for smokers than for nonsmokers.

Hormonal Disturbances

A recent review by Fu and colleagues[68] reported the influence of glucocorticosteroids, nonsteroidal anti-inflammatory drugs, and statins on implant healing. In general, nonsteroidal anti-inflammatory drugs had a deleterious effect on bone-to-implant contact and bone density after implant placement, whereas statins seemed to have a positive effect on bone formation. Several animal studies investigating the local application of growth hormones have found a positive effect on bone formation and a loss of bone density when estrogen levels are low.[69–73] A study by Moy and colleagues[74] found that women aged 60 to 79 had a higher rate of implant failure than those 40 or younger. In this study, however, women on postmenopausal estrogen therapy had an increased risk of 2.55 times that of those postmenopausal women not on hormone replacement therapy.

Medications

Aside from bisphosphonates, no specific medication seems to be directly associated with implant failure in humans. A study investigating implants in medically treated hypothyroid patients found more bone loss and a less favorable soft tissue response after stage one surgery 1 year after implant placement but no increased risk of failure.[75] In an animal study, the administration of cyclosporine to rabbits was associated with negative bone quantity as determined by subtractive radiography.[76] Further studies are needed to delineate the direct effects of medications on the risk of implant failure and on peri-implant tissues.

Bisphosphonates

Many patients commonly take bisphosphonates for the treatment of osteoporosis or during cancer therapy. Osteonecrosis of the jaws has been listed as a complication that may occur in some patients treated with bisphosphonates.[77] Bisphosphonate-related osteonecrosis of the jaws (BRONJ), also called bisphosphonate-induced osteonecrosis of the jaws, can occur in patients taking an oral or intravenous bisphosphonate.[77] Dentoalveolar trauma, such as dental extraction, seems to trigger BRONJ.[77,78] The placement of dental implants in patients undergoing bisphosphonate therapy requires careful evaluation. The effect of bisphosphonates on the osseointegration of dental implants is unclear.[79] Shabestari's group[79] placed 46 ITI implants in 21 osteoporotic female patients taking oral bisphosphonates. No implant mobility was recorded, and no cases of peri-implantitis were found by examination at the end of the study period. There was no effect of implant location, type of prosthesis, opposing dentition, or the time at which implant therapy began on successful osseointegration.[79] A study by Zahid and colleagues[80] involved 227 patients and recorded surgical complications, number of exposed implant threads, implant failure, age, gender, smoking status, systemic conditions, and medications. Of 51 implants placed in 26 patients taking bisphosphonates, 3 failed, for a success rate of 94%. No variable other than bisphosphonate therapy was associated with either implant failure or thread exposure.

Animal studies have been used to gain information difficult to obtain from human subjects. Abtahi and associates[81] placed titanium implants in rats being treated with systemic bisphosphonates and also placed implants coated with bisphosphonates in rats not taking systemic bisphosphonates. Changes similar to those seen in osteonecrosis of the jaw were evident in the systemically treated rats, but no such changes were seen in the rats with coated implants, except for an increase in implant removal torque.[81] Shibutani's group[82] used ligatures to induce peri-implantitis in 10 beagle dogs. Induction began 6 months after implant placement. A bisphosphonate (pamidronate) was injected into 5 of the dogs every 3 days for 12 weeks after the ligatures were placed. Bone loss was significantly greater in the control dogs than in dogs treated with pamidronate.[82]

Kumar and Honne[83] evaluated published studies that compared implant survival in users and nonusers of bisphosphonates. Five articles met their inclusion criteria. Only 1 article stated that implant failure was higher for patients taking bisphosphonates. The range of survival rates for dental implants was approximately equal for short-term users and nonusers of bisphosphonate.[83] Lazarovici and colleagues[84] followed 145 patients with BRONJ, 27 of whom developed BRONJ associated with dental implants. The mean time to the development of BRONJ was 16.2 months for patients who had been taking bisphosphonate therapy before implant placement.

Although much has been discovered about the effects of bisphosphonates, considerably more research is necessary for providing a clear picture for practitioners. Some studies have shown no effects, whereas others have shown both positive and negative effects. A complicating factor is time. A number of studies have found a significant time lag between implant placement and evidence of alterations in osseous structure. Until more answers are forthcoming, great care and caution would be prudent when dentists are considering the placement of implant fixtures in patients taking bisphosphonates.

Irradiation

Radiation therapy is often prescribed for the treatment of head and neck cancer. Adverse effects can include xerostomia and altered function of the irradiated area. A recent systematic review of irradiation and dental implants by Chambrone and colleagues[85] evaluated the number and percentage of implants lost, with the exclusion of implants placed only in grafted areas. The risk of implant loss was 174% higher for implants placed in irradiated bone than for those placed in nonirradiated bone. The risk of loss of maxillary implants was 496% higher than the risk of loss of mandibular implants. The authors found no indication that hyperbaric oxygen therapy affected implant loss.

A retrospective study evaluated the survival of 225 implants in 30 patients who received irradiation therapy and found a 5-year success rate of 92.6%.[86] A dose–response relationship has been observed between increases in implant failure and high-dose irradiation; some authors recommend 55 Gy as a cutoff for high-dose therapy.[87] Others have noted continued implant loss over a long period of time after irradiation,[51] up to 25 years in 1 study.[88] Another study by Buddula and colleagues[89] found that the success rates for implants placed in irradiated patients decreased over time (98.9% at 1 year, 89.9% at 5 years, and 72.3% at 10 years) and that the success rate for maxillary implants are lower than those for mandibular implants.

Genetics

Genetic polymorphisms have been studied to assess their potential role in predisposition to implant failure or peri-implantitis. A number of the genes investigated parallel those that have been evaluated for periodontitis and focus on inflammation and bone turnover. A recent study examined IL-1β and TNF-α genotyping and to placement of titanium implants and reported that implant loss was significantly related to increasing number of risk genotypes of Il-1β and TNF-α.[90] An examination of IL-1 gene clusters by Vaz and colleagues[91] in 155 Portuguese patients with 100 successful implants and 55 unsuccessful implants (defined by the authors as "implant loss or mobility, pain on palpation, percussion or function; recurrent infection [fistula or suppuration], perimucositis, peri-implantitis, and vestibular metal exposing during or after the abutment connection"). They concluded that successful implants were associated with a negative genetic test and that unsuccessful implants were associated with a positive genetic test. An earlier review by Huynh-Ba and colleagues[92] examined 44 studies, 2 of which were longitudinal; the authors did not find enough evidence to support or refute the contribution of the IL-1geneotype to implant failure and did not support systematic genetic testing. Casado and colleagues[93] examined susceptibility to IL-6 G174 C and peri-implant disease in a Brazilian population and found that, at a minimum, the IL-6 genotype was 1.53 times more likely to convey peri-implant disease if the individuals had the GC genotype and allele G. Another recent study by Pigossi and colleagues[94] examined 3 single nucleotide polymorphisms for IL-10 and found no association with implant failure.

COMBINED RISK FACTORS

Although some systemic diseases, such as cardiovascular disease, taken as a singular entity, may not represent a risk for implant failure,[95] a combination of risk factors may present a risk. A large study by Moy and colleagues,[74] in which 4680 implants were placed in 1140 patients by the same surgeon over a 21-year period, investigated potential risk factors for implant failure. The study performed stepwise linear regression analysis of a number of variables and concluded that diabetes, smoking, and head and neck irradiation were significant predictors of implant failure. Interestingly, a life table analysis showed more implant failure in medically healthy subjects than in medically compromised subjects. The authors concluded that these 3 variables were not absolute contraindications to implant placement. A recent meta-analysis of 51 studies involving more than 40,000 implants evaluated the association between implant failure and smoking, radiotherapy, diabetes, and osteoporosis.[16] The study found a positive association of smoking and radiotherapy with dental implant failure in the model, but not the other factors.

SUMMARY

The array of potential risk factors for implant failure includes systemic, local, prosthetic, environmental, and genetic factors: This article has focused on key factors such as systemic disease, microbiology, periodontitis, smoking, medications (particularly bisphosphonates), genetics, and combinations of factors. Although the results of published studies indicate that there are few absolute contraindications to implant placement, smoking is a significant risk factor for implant failure, particularly at higher exposure levels. In general, poorly controlled diseases, including uncontrolled periodontitis, may also contribute to perimucositis and peri-implantitis. There are similarities between peri-implant and periodontal microbial communities, but recent studies indicate that there are also differences. The results of these studies suggest that, although the inflammatory process seems to be similar, the putative pathogens may not be the same. Future research must clarify combination(s) of factors that predisposes patients to perimucositis and peri-implantitis, because these conditions are important precursors to implant failure.

REFERENCES

1. Mombelli A, Muller N, Cionca N. The epidemiology of peri-implantitis. Clin Oral Implants Res 2012;23(Suppl 6):67–76.
2. Peri-implant mucositis and peri-implantitis: a current understanding of their diagnoses and clinical implications. J Periodontol 2013;84(4):436–43.
3. Al-Ahmad A, Wiedmann-Al-Ahmad M, Fackler A, et al. In vivo study of the initial bacterial adhesion on different implant materials. Arch Oral Biol 2013;58(9): 1139–47.
4. Schmidlin PR, Muller P, Attin T, et al. Polyspecies biofilm formation on implant surfaces with different surface characteristics. J Appl Oral Sci 2013;21(1):48–55.
5. Greenstein G, Cavallaro J Jr, Tarnow D. Dental implants in the periodontal patient. Dent Clin North Am 2010;54(1):113–28.
6. Kumar PS, Mason MR, Brooker MR, et al. Pyrosequencing reveals unique microbial signatures associated with healthy and failing dental implants. J Clin Periodontol 2012;39(5):425–33.
7. Cortelli SC, Cortelli JR, Romeiro RL, et al. Frequency of periodontal pathogens in equivalent peri-implant and periodontal clinical statuses. Arch Oral Biol 2013; 58(1):67–74.
8. Koyanagi T, Sakamoto M, Takeuchi Y, et al. Comprehensive microbiological findings in peri-implantitis and periodontitis. J Clin Periodontol 2013;40(3):218–26.
9. Dabdoub SM, Tsigarida AA, Kumar PS. Patient-specific analysis of periodontal and peri-implant microbiomes. J Dent Res 2013;92(12 Suppl):168S–75S.
10. Kocar M, Seme K, Hren NI. Characterization of the normal bacterial flora in peri-implant sulci of partially and completely edentulous patients. Int J Oral Maxillofac Implants 2010;25(4):690–8.

11. Aloufi F, Bissada N, Ficara A, et al. Clinical assessment of peri-implant tissues in patients with varying severity of chronic periodontitis. Clin Implant Dent Relat Res 2009;11(1):37–40.
12. Cho-Yan Lee J, Mattheos N, Nixon KC, et al. Residual periodontal pockets are a risk indicator for peri-implantitis in patients treated for periodontitis. Clin Oral Implants Res 2012;23(3):325–33.
13. Lagervall M, Jansson LE. Treatment outcome in patients with peri-implantitis in a periodontal clinic: a retrospective study. J Periodontol 2013;84(10): 1365–73.
14. Pjetursson BE, Helbling C, Weber HP, et al. Peri-implantitis susceptibility as it relates to periodontal therapy and supportive care. Clin Oral Implants Res 2012;23(7):888–94.
15. Lefever D, Van Assche N, Temmerman A, et al. Aetiology, microbiology and therapy of periapical lesions around oral implants: a retrospective analysis. J Clin Periodontol 2013;40(3):296–302.
16. Chen H, Liu N, Xu X, et al. Smoking, radiotherapy, diabetes and osteoporosis as risk factors for dental implant failure: a meta-analysis. PLoS One 2013;8(8): e71955.
17. Clementini M, Rossetti PH, Penarrocha D, et al. Systemic risk factors for peri-implant bone loss: a systematic review and meta-analysis. Int J Oral Maxillofac Surg 2014;43(3):323–34.
18. Bergstrom J, Preber H. Tobacco use as a risk factor. J Periodontol 1994; 65(5 Suppl):545–50.
19. Johnson GK, Hill M. Cigarette smoking and the periodontal patient. J Periodontol 2004;75(2):196–209.
20. Burt B. Position paper: epidemiology of periodontal diseases. J Periodontol 2005;76(8):1406–19.
21. Karbach J, Callaway A, Kwon YD, et al. Comparison of five parameters as risk factors for peri-mucositis. Int J Oral Maxillofac Implants 2009;24(3):491–6.
22. D'Haese J, De Bruyn H. Effect of smoking habits on accuracy of implant placement using mucosally supported stereolithographic surgical guides. Clin Implant Dent Relat Res 2013;15(3):402–11.
23. Stoker G, van Waas R, Wismeijer D. Long-term outcomes of three types of implant-supported mandibular over dentures in smokers. Clin Oral Implants Res 2012;23(8):925–9.
24. Wahlström M, Sagulin GB, Jansson LE. Clinical follow-up of unilateral, fixed dental prosthesis on maxillary implants. Clin Oral Implants Res 2010;21(11): 1294–300.
25. Vervaeke S, Collaert B, Vandeweghe S, et al. The effect of smoking on survival and bone loss of implants with a fluoride-modified surface: a 2-year retrospective analysis of 1106 implants placed in daily practice. Clin Oral Implants Res 2012;23(6):758–66.
26. Haas R, Haimbock W, Mailath G, et al. The relationship of smoking on peri-implant tissue: a retrospective study. J Prosthet Dent 1996;76(6):592–6.
27. Kourtis SG, Sotiriadou S, Voliotis S, et al. Private practice results of dental implants. Part I: survival and evaluation of risk factors–part II: surgical and prosthetic complications. Implant Dent 2004;13(4):373–85.
28. Sayardoust S, Grondahl K, Johansson E, et al. Implant survival and marginal bone loss at turned and oxidized implants in periodontitis-susceptible smokers and never-smokers: a retrospective, clinical, radiographic case-control study. J Periodontol 2013;84(12):1775–82.

29. Aalam AA, Nowzari H. Clinical evaluation of dental implants with surfaces roughened by anodic oxidation, dual acid-etched implants, and machined implants. Int J Oral Maxillofac Implants 2005;20(5):793–8.

30. Balshe AA, Eckert SE, Koka S, et al. The effects of smoking on the survival of smooth- and rough-surface dental implants. Int J Oral Maxillofac Implants 2008;23(6):1117–22.

31. Strietzel FP, Reichart PA, Kale A, et al. Smoking interferes with the prognosis of dental implant treatment: a systematic review and meta-analysis. J Clin Periodontol 2007;34(6):523–44.

32. Chung DM, Oh TJ, Lee J, et al. Factors affecting late implant bone loss: a retrospective analysis. Int J Oral Maxillofac Implants 2007;22(1):117–26.

33. d'Avila S, dos Reis LD, Piattelli A, et al. Impact of smoking on human bone apposition at different dental implant surfaces: a histologic study in type IV bone. J Oral Implantol 2010;36(2):85–90.

34. Levin L, Hertzberg R, Har-Nes S, et al. Long-term marginal bone loss around single dental implants affected by current and past smoking habits. Implant Dent 2008;17(4):422–9.

35. Leonhardt A, Dahlen G, Renvert S. Five-year clinical, microbiological, and radiological outcome following treatment of peri-implantitis in man. J Periodontol 2003;74(10):1415–22.

36. Bayat E, Bauss O. Effect of smoking on the failure rates of orthodontic miniscrews. J Orofac Orthop 2010;71(2):117–24.

37. Jansson H, Hamberg K, De Bruyn H, et al. Clinical consequences of IL-1 genotype on early implant failures in patients under periodontal maintenance. Clin Implant Dent Relat Res 2005;7(1):51–9.

38. Gruica B, Wang HY, Lang NP, et al. Impact of IL-1 genotype and smoking status on the prognosis of osseointegrated implants. Clin Oral Implants Res 2004; 15(4):393–400.

39. Lindquist LW, Carlsson GE, Jemt T. Association between marginal bone loss around osseointegrated mandibular implants and smoking habits: a 10-year follow-up study. J Dent Res 1997;76(10):1667–74.

40. Takamiya AS, Goiato MC, Filho HG. Effect of smoking on the survival of dental implants. Biomedical papers of the Medical Faculty of the University Palacky, Olomouc, Czechoslovakia 2013. [Epub ahead of print].

41. Heinikainen M, Vehkalahti M, Murtomaa H. Influence of patient characteristics on Finnish dentists' decision-making in implant therapy. Implant Dent 2002; 11(3):301–7.

42. Yilmazel Ucar E, Araz O, Yilmaz N, et al. Effectiveness of pharmacologic therapies on smoking cessation success: three years results of a smoking cessation clinic. Multidiscip Respir Med 2014;9(1):9.

43. Yasin SM, Retneswari M, Moy FM, et al. Predictors of sustained six months quitting success: efforts of smoking cessation in low intensity smoke-free workplaces. Ann Acad Med Singapore 2013;42(8):401–7.

44. Chapple IL, Genco R, Working Group 2 of Joint EFPAAP Workshop. Diabetes and periodontal diseases: consensus report of the Joint EFP/AAP Workshop on periodontitis and systemic diseases. J Clin Periodontol 2013;40(Suppl 14):S106–12.

45. Taylor JJ, Preshaw PM, Lalla E. A review of the evidence for pathogenic mechanisms that may link periodontitis and diabetes. J Clin Periodontol 2013; 40(Suppl 14):S113–34.

46. Chapple IL, Genco R, Working Group 2 of the Joint EFPAAP Workshop. Diabetes and periodontal diseases: consensus report of the Joint EFP/AAP

Workshop on periodontitis and systemic diseases. J Periodontol 2013; 84(4 Suppl):S106–12.

47. Preshaw PM, Bissett SM. Periodontitis: oral complication of diabetes. Endocrinol Metab Clin North Am 2013;42(4):849–67.

48. Tervonen T, Oliver RC. Long-term control of diabetes mellitus and periodontitis. J Clin Periodontol 1993;20(6):431–5.

49. Mattson JS, Cerutis DR. Diabetes mellitus: a review of the literature and dental implications. Compend Contin Educ Dent 2001;22(9):757–60, 762, 764 passim; [quiz: 773].

50. Marchand F, Raskin A, Dionnes-Hornes A, et al. Dental implants and diabetes: conditions for success. Diabetes Metab 2012;38(1):14–9.

51. Bornstein MM, Cionca N, Mombelli A. Systemic conditions and treatments as risks for implant therapy. Int J Oral Maxillofac Implants 2009;24(Suppl):12–27.

52. Schlegel KA, Prechtl C, Most T, et al. Osseointegration of SLActive implants in diabetic pigs. Clin Oral Implants Res 2013;24(2):128–34.

53. Quintero DG, Winger JN, Khashaba R, et al. Advanced glycation endproducts and rat dental implant osseointegration. J Oral Implantol 2010;36(2):97–103.

54. de Morais JA, Trindade-Suedam IK, Pepato MT, et al. Effect of diabetes mellitus and insulin therapy on bone density around osseointegrated dental implants: a digital subtraction radiography study in rats. Clin Oral Implants Res 2009;20(8): 796–801.

55. Gomez-Moreno G, Aguilar-Salvatierra A, Rubio Roldan J, et al. Peri-implant evaluation in type 2 diabetes mellitus patients: a 3-year study. Clin Oral Implants Res 2014. [Epub ahead of print].

56. Oates TW, Huynh-Ba G, Vargas A, et al. A critical review of diabetes, glycemic control, and dental implant therapy. Clin Oral Implants Res 2013;24(2): 117–27.

57. Colombo JS, Balani D, Sloan AJ, et al. Delayed osteoblast differentiation and altered inflammatory response around implants placed in incisor sockets of type 2 diabetic rats. Clin Oral Implants Res 2011;22(6):578–86.

58. Venza I, Visalli M, Cucinotta M, et al. Proinflammatory gene expression at chronic periodontitis and peri-implantitis sites in patients with or without type 2 diabetes. J Periodontol 2010;81(1):99–108.

59. Nibali L, Tatarakis N, Needleman I, et al. Clinical review: association between metabolic syndrome and periodontitis: a systematic review and meta-analysis. J Clin Endocrinol Metab 2013;98(3):913–20.

60. Chaffee BW, Weston SJ. Association between chronic periodontal disease and obesity: a systematic review and meta-analysis. J Periodontol 2010;81(12): 1708–24.

61. Bullon P, Morillo JM, Ramirez-Tortosa MC, et al. Metabolic syndrome and periodontitis: is oxidative stress a common link? J Dent Res 2009;88(6):503–18.

62. Montebugnoli L, Venturi M, Cervellati F, et al. Peri-implant response and microflora in organ transplant patients 1 year after prosthetic loading: a prospective controlled study. Clin Implant Dent Relat Res 2014. [Epub ahead of print].

63. Montebugnoli L, Venturi M, Cervellati F. Bone response to submerged implants in organ transplant patients: a prospective controlled study. Int J Oral Maxillofac Implants 2012;27(6):1494–500.

64. Gu L, Yu YC. Clinical outcome of dental implants placed in liver transplant recipients after 3 years: a case series. Transplant Proc 2011;43(7):2678–82.

65. Tsolaki IN, Madianos PN, Vrotsos JA. Outcomes of dental implants in osteoporotic patients. A literature review. J Prosthodont 2009;18(4):309–23.

66. Gaetti-Jardim EC, Santiago-Junior JF, Goiato MC, et al. Dental implants in patients with osteoporosis: a clinical reality? J Craniofac Surg 2011;22(3):1111–3.

67. Holahan CM, Koka S, Kennel KA, et al. Effect of osteoporotic status on the survival of titanium dental implants. Int J Oral Maxillofac Implants 2008;23(5):905–10.

68. Fu JH, Bashutski JD, Al-Hezaimi K, et al. Statins, glucocorticoids, and nonsteroidal anti-inflammatory drugs: their influence on implant healing. Implant Dent 2012;21(5):362–7.

69. Giro G, Coelho PG, Pereira RM, et al. The effect of oestrogen and alendronate therapies on postmenopausal bone loss around osseointegrated titanium implants. Clin Oral Implants Res 2011;22(3):259–64.

70. Gomez-Moreno G, Cutando A, Arana C, et al. The effects of growth hormone on the initial bone formation around implants. Int J Oral Maxillofac Implants 2009; 24(6):1068–73.

71. Tresguerres IF, Blanco L, Clemente C, et al. Effects of local administration of growth hormone in peri-implant bone: an experimental study with implants in rabbit tibiae. Int J Oral Maxillofac Implants 2003;18(6):807–11.

72. Tresguerres IF, Clemente C, Donado M, et al. Local administration of growth hormone enhances periimplant bone reaction in an osteoporotic rabbit model. Clin Oral Implants Res 2002;13(6):631–6.

73. Stenport VF, Olsson B, Morberg P, et al. Systemically administered human growth hormone improves initial implant stability: an experimental study in the rabbit. Clin Implant Dent Relat Res 2001;3(3):135–41.

74. Moy PK, Medina D, Shetty V, et al. Dental implant failure rates and associated risk factors. Int J Oral Maxillofac Implants 2005;20(4):569–77.

75. Attard NJ, Zarb GA. A study of dental implants in medically treated hypothyroid patients. Clin Implant Dent Relat Res 2002;4(4):220–31.

76. Sakakura CE, Marcantonio E Jr, Wenzel A, et al. Influence of cyclosporin A on quality of bone around integrated dental implants: a radiographic study in rabbits. Clin Oral Implants Res 2007;18(1):34–9.

77. Ruggiero SL. Bisphosphonate-related osteonecrosis of the jaws. Compend Contin Educ Dent 2008;29(2):96–8, 100–2, 104–5.

78. Mavrokokki T, Cheng A, Stein B, et al. Nature and frequency of bisphosphonate-associated osteonecrosis of the jaws in Australia. J Oral Maxillofac Surg 2007; 65(3):415–23.

79. Shabestari GO, Shayesteh YS, Khojasteh A, et al. Implant placement in patients with oral bisphosphonate therapy: a case series. Clin Implant Dent Relat Res 2010;12(3):175–80.

80. Zahid TM, Wang BY, Cohen RE. Influence of bisphosphonates on alveolar bone loss around osseointegrated implants. J Oral Implantol 2011;37(3):335–46.

81. Abtahi J, Agholme F, Sandberg O, et al. Effect of local vs. systemic bisphosphonate delivery on dental implant fixation in a model of osteonecrosis of the jaw. J Dent Res 2013;92(3):279–83.

82. Shibutani T, Inuduka A, Horiki I, et al. Bisphosphonate inhibits alveolar bone resorption in experimentally-induced peri-implantitis in dogs. Clin Oral Implants Res 2001;12(2):109–14.

83. Kumar MN, Honne T. Survival of dental implants in bisphosphonate users versus non-users: a systematic review. Eur J Prosthodont Restor Dent 2012;20(4): 159–62.

84. Lazarovici TS, Yahalom R, Taicher S, et al. Bisphosphonate-related osteonecrosis of the jaw associated with dental implants. J Oral Maxillofac Surg 2010;68(4): 790–6.

85. Chambrone L, Mandia J Jr, Shibli JA, et al. Dental implants installed in irradiated jaws: a systematic review. J Dent Res 2013;92(12 Suppl):119S–30S.
86. Mancha de la Plata M, Gias LN, Diez PM, et al. Osseointegrated implant rehabilitation of irradiated oral cancer patients. J Oral Maxillofac Surg 2012;70(5): 1052–63.
87. Nooh N. Dental implant survival in irradiated oral cancer patients: a systematic review of the literature. Int J Oral Maxillofac Implants 2013;28(5):1233–42.
88. Granstrom G. Osseointegration in irradiated cancer patients: an analysis with respect to implant failures. J Oral Maxillofac Surg 2005;63(5):579–85.
89. Buddula A, Assad DA, Salinas TJ, et al. Survival of dental implants in irradiated head and neck cancer patients: a retrospective analysis. Clin Implant Dent Relat Res 2012;14(5):716–22.
90. Jacobi-Gresser E, Huesker K, Schutt S. Genetic and immunological markers predict titanium implant failure: a retrospective study. Int J Oral Maxillofac Surg 2013;42(4):537–43.
91. Vaz P, Gallas MM, Braga AC, et al. IL1 gene polymorphisms and unsuccessful dental implants. Clin Oral Implants Res 2012;23(12):1404–13.
92. Huynh-Ba G, Lang NP, Tonetti MS, et al. Association of the composite IL-1 genotype with peri-implantitis: a systematic review. Clin Oral Implants Res 2008; 19(11):1154–62.
93. Casado PL, Villas-Boas R, de Mello W, et al. Peri-implant disease and chronic periodontitis: is interleukin-6 gene promoter polymorphism the common risk factor in a Brazilian population? Int J Oral Maxillofac Implants 2013;28(1):35–43.
94. Pigossi SC, Alvim-Pereira F, Montes CC, et al. Genetic association study between Interleukin 10 gene and dental implant loss. Arch Oral Biol 2012;57(9): 1256–63.
95. Khadivi V, Anderson J, Zarb GA. Cardiovascular disease and treatment outcomes with osseointegration surgery. J Prosthet Dent 1999;81(5):533–6.

Use of Cone-Beam Computed Tomography in Early Detection of Implant Failure

Juan F. Yepes, DDS, MD, MPH, MS, DrPH, FDS RCSEd[a],*,
Mohanad Al-Sabbagh, DDS, MS[b]

KEYWORDS

- Cone-beam computed tomography (CBCT) • Postimplant assessment
- Implant failure assessment

KEY POINTS

- Cone-beam computed tomography (CBCT) has become a helpful tool in assessing the stability of the dental implant site.
- Little is known about the ability of CBCT to evaluate peri-implant bone wall morphology or about its performance compared with conventional radiographic modalities, such as peri-apical radiography.
- For patients with postoperative complications, diagnostic imaging, including CBCT, may be indicated as a supplement to the clinical examination, although in most cases conventional radiographs will provide the necessary information.
- More studies are needed to determine the actual role of CBCT in detecting early implant failure.

INTRODUCTION

Radiological examination is crucial in planning and assessing dental implants. In 1998, cone-beam computed tomography (CBCT) was introduced to dentistry. Depending on the specific machine, CBCT enables clinicians to obtain 3-dimensional (3D) images with a low dose of radiation.[1] Standard 2-dimensional images do not provide detailed discrimination of the areas suitable for dental implants or of the areas close to an implant. CBCT is widely used in implant dentistry for several indications, including pre-implant assessment of anatomy, implant placement, visualization of important anatomic structures, assessment of bone mineral density, and, recently, early

[a] Department of Pediatric Dentistry, James Whitcomb Riley Hospital for Children, Indiana University School of Dentistry, Indianapolis, IN 46202, USA; [b] Division of Periodontology, Department of Oral Health Practice, College of Dentistry, University of Kentucky, Lexington, KY 40536, USA
* Corresponding author.
E-mail address: jfyepes@iupui.edu

Dent Clin N Am 59 (2015) 41–56
http://dx.doi.org/10.1016/j.cden.2014.09.003
0011-8532/15/$ – see front matter

assessment of implant failure. CBCT is helpful in assessing the stability of the implant site. However, little is known about the utility and validity of CBCT in evaluating peri-implant bone wall morphology, particularly after bone augmentation procedures performed to improve the implant site.

One potential limitation of CBCT in evaluating implant placement is the presence of metal in the area to be scanned; in these cases, CBCT images are susceptible to artifact, some of which are caused by a phenomenon called *beam hardening*. When an x-ray beam travels through an object, more low-energy photons are absorbed than high-energy photons; this difference produces beam-hardening artifacts that limit the image quality.[2] Although certain techniques can be used to decrease the number of these artifacts, such as changing the exposure conditions, decreasing the field of view, or changing the patient's position, the use of CBCT for early detection of implant failure is still limited.[3,4] This article presents a summary of current knowledge about the use of CBCT in implant dentistry, evaluates the potential use of CBCT in detecting early implant failures, compares the performance of CBCT with that of other traditional imaging techniques, and examines the limitations of CBCT.

INDICATIONS FOR CONE-BEAM COMPUTED TOMOGRAPHY IN IMPLANT DENTISTRY

Selection of the potential implant site is crucial to the success or failure of the implant. The potential implant site must be evaluated to determine the quantity and quality of available bone, the angulation of the alveolar process, the relationship of the site to anatomic structures, and the possible problems in the area.[5] Radiologic techniques can provide information crucial to an assessment of all of these factors. CBCT allows cross-sectional evaluation of the dental arch for a determination of the width, height, and quality of bone at the potential implant site. CBCT technology provides the clinician with the ability to fully assess the potential implant site using a relatively low radiation dose (compared with traditional computed tomography [CT]), and at a reasonable cost to the patient. Considering the quality of the images, the low radiation dose, and the favorable cost, CBCT is currently one of the most recommended imaging modalities for assessing potential implant sites. The use of 3D information in diagnosis and treatment planning has been enhanced by the availability of CBCT. **Box 1** shows the main indications of CBCT in implant dentistry.

Use in Measuring Bone Mineral Density

The most frequently reported indications for the use of CBCT in implant planning are to measure the alveolar ridge and map the bone morphology of potential implant sites (**Figs. 1–3**). CBCT images have been found to provide information for the clinician beyond linear measurements, such as measurement of bone mineral density.[6] Several

---

Box 1
Main indications of CBCT in implant dentistry

- Evaluation of the quality, height, and width of available bone
- Three-dimensional assessment of alveolar ridge topography
- Identification of vital anatomic structures
- Identification of potential problems
- Fabrication of CBCT-derived surgical guides
- Patient education

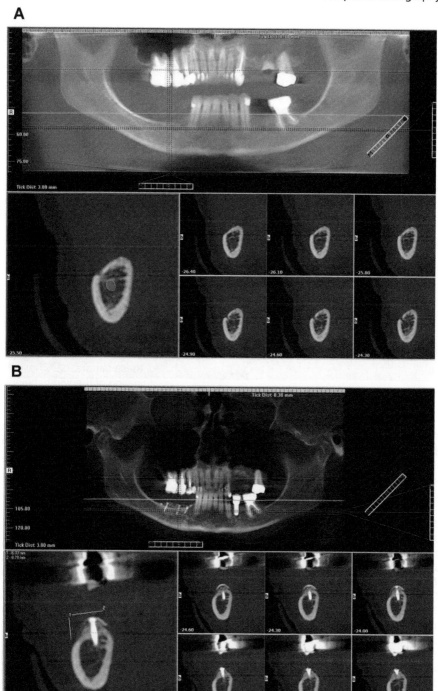

Fig. 1. (*A*) Red dot indicates the location of inferior alveolar canal. Limited bone height is available for implant placement. (*B*) Guided bone regeneration was performed to increase alveolar bone height for implant placement. (*C*) Gain of approximately 5 mm in alveolar ridge bone height after guided bone regeneration procedure.

C

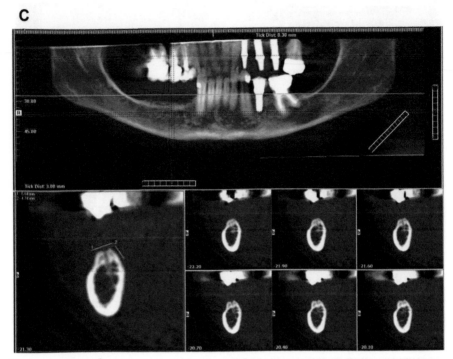

Fig. 1. (*continued*)

studies have found that the gray values of CBCT images are positively correlated with the known density of reference materials, including bone.[7,8] In an vitro study using a water phantom, Nomura and colleagues[9] found a high correlation between the voxel values of CBCT and CT. However, Hua and colleagues[10] reported that the voxel values of CBCT seemed inappropriate for evaluating bone mineral density.

When the same CBCT scanner is used, the gray value of scanned bone can be directly converted to the corresponding bone mineral density value using a calibration curve.[6] However, imaging errors during processing should be addressed when CBCT images obtained under different conditions are used to determine bone mineral density. Using human jaws, Parsa and colleagues[11] compared micro-CT and multislice CT (MSCT) in evaluating the accuracy of CBCT for determining trabecular bone density. Their results showed a strong correlation between CBCT and MSCT, suggesting that CBCT can be used to assess bone mineral density at the implant site. Monje and colleagues[12] analyzed the relationship between bone density as determined by CBCT, and morphologic parameters of bone as determined by micro-CT. Their results supported the use of CBCT for assessing bone mineral density. However, additional studies are necessary to provide clinicians with better tools for assessing bone mineral density with CBCT.

Limitations

CBCT has some of the same limitations inherent to all imaging modalities. The most important limitations for implant planning are the lack of accurate representation of soft tissue structures, such as the gingiva, and the various artifacts produced primarily by metal restorations; such artifacts may interfere with the diagnostic process by

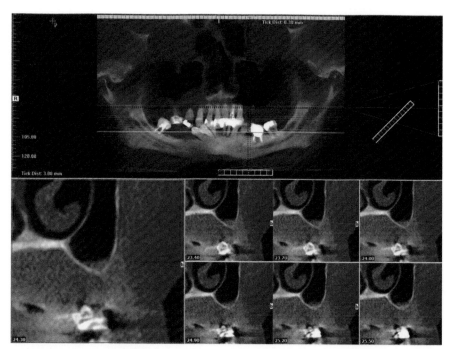

Fig. 2. CBCT showing limited alveolar bone height in the maxillary left region.

masking underlying structures. Furthermore, the cost of CBCT is higher than that of other traditional modalities. The advent of CBCT has also introduced the issue of liability in interpreting the image. CBCT is increasingly being performed by dentists who do not have training in interpreting the image beyond what they see frequently or are familiar with. The dentists assume liability in reading and interpreting all of the anatomy of the entire CBCT image (**Box 2**).

Associated Radiation Dose

Radiation dose is a crucial factor associated with the use of CBCT or any other imaging modality in implant planning. The ALARA principle (As Low As Reasonably Achievable) must always be applied to the decision process of image selection. Although the concept of using one imaging modality (CBCT) in lieu of obtaining multiple images (eg, periapical, panoramic) is attractive, some authors have expressed concerns about the cost to the patient in terms of radiation dose.[13]

Potential radiation risk is an important topic in the dental literature. A potential relationship exists between exposing the thyroid gland to ionizing radiation and adverse outcomes, such as low-birth-weight infants.[14] In 2007, the International Commission on Radiological Protection reviewed and reassessed tissue-weighting factors in an effort to calculate more accurately the dosage delivered to various organs.[15] The effective radiation dose to various oral and maxillofacial organs varies according to several parameters, including the field of view and the type of CBCT scanner used.[13] For example, the effective dose delivered to the thyroid gland during large field of view examinations is reported to range from 447 to 2045 µGy, depending on the type of scanner used.

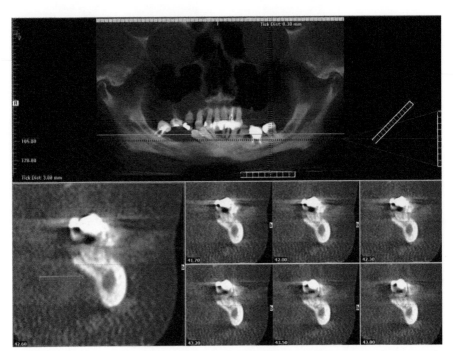

Fig. 3. Morphology of alveolar ridge in the left mandibular posterior region. Red arrow indicates the undercut and the risk of invasion of the submandibular fossa during implant placement.

Use in Detecting Implant Failure

Monitoring the condition of bone and tissue condition around dental implants is essential not only during follow-up under functional loading but also during the assessment of strategies for regenerating peri-implant bone (**Figs. 4** and **5**). Periapical radiolucencies with a strict projection protocol can assess mesial and distal peri-implant bone levels almost as accurately as histologic studies, assuming that the project level of peri-implant bone is located in the sectioning plane of the implant or is of uniform height around the implant.[16] However, in the case of buccal or lingual bone defects, CBCT has the same limitations as periapical radiographs (**Figs. 6–8**). CBCT allows 3D visualization of the bone around the implant but with the inherent limitation of the presence of artifacts caused by a titanium surface.

Among the 5 criteria for implant success proposed by Albrektsson and colleagues[17–19] in 1986, is the absence of any radiographic evidence of peri-implant

---

Box 2
Limitations of CBCT

- Radiation exposure higher than that associated with traditional radiographs (intraoral or panoramic)
- Limited soft tissue visualization
- Artifacts created by metal objects
- Cost and liability

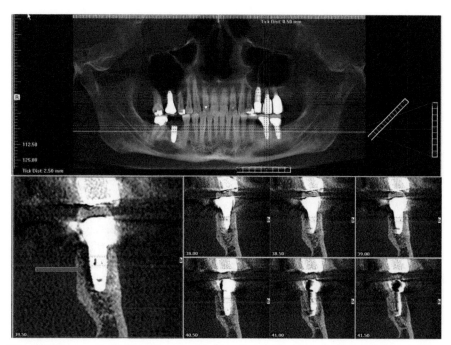

Fig. 4. Red arrow indicates reduced bone density on the lingual aspect of bone-implant interface.

radiolucency. This criterion is still regarded as essential, and radiographs are frequently used in combination with clinical examination to evaluate the success of dental implants.[20] Although one study has reported a correspondence between clinical symptoms and radiographic findings,[21] some limitations are associated with the use of radiographs to detect implant failure. Furthermore, the probability of diagnosing early implant failure with radiographs is low when the prevalence of unstable implants is low.

Marginal bone loss is a crucial outcome variable in evaluating the success of implant therapy. It has been suggested that the data regarding bone loss that are obtained during the first year of function should be distinguished from those obtained during the subsequent period of service.[22] Furthermore, according to Albrektsson's criteria,[17] marginal bone loss should not exceed 1.5 mm during the first year of function and should be less than 0.2 mm per year thereafter. In 1999, a consensus report from the European Workshop on Periodontology modified Albrektsson's criteria to indicate that no more than 2 mm of bone loss should occur during the first 5 years after installation of the prosthesis.[23] In 2010, Fransson and colleagues[22] reported that, for 182 subjects, the average bone loss after the first year of function, as determined by intraoral periapical radiographs, was 1.68 mm and that 32% of the implants exhibited bone loss of more than 2.0 mm. The crucial question is whether CBCT will detect these bone defects earlier than conventional radiographs and whether these early bone defects will have an effect on the overall success and prognosis of the implants. In 2006, a cross-sectional study by Roos-Jansaker and colleagues[24] assessed the severity of peri-implantitis–associated bone loss and found that the relative proportion of implants with peri-implantitis and bone loss of more than 2 mm was

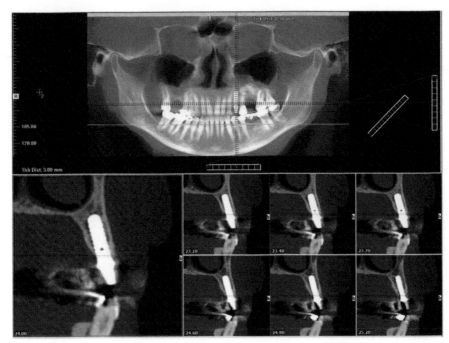

Fig. 5. Cross-sectional image showing healthy bone-implant interface and intact buccal bone.

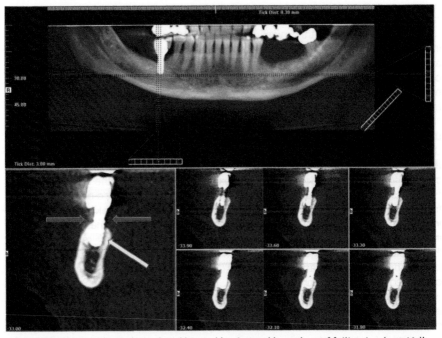

Fig. 6. Red arrows indicate buccal and lingual horizontal bone loss of failing implant. Yellow arrow indicates reduced bone density on the lingual aspect of bone-implant interface.

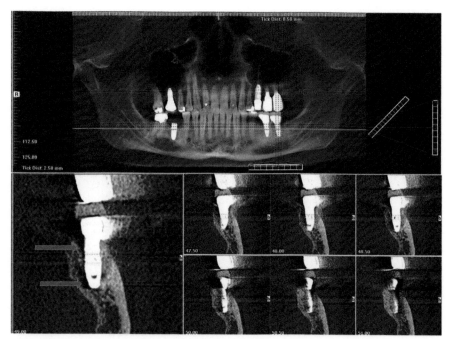

Fig. 7. Red arrows indicate bony defect on lingual aspect of failing implant.

31%. The radiographic techniques used for bone-level assessment demonstrated a lack of accuracy for bone defects smaller than 2.0 mm.

According to the general principles of radiographic imaging, difficulties are evident in diagnosing a thin connective tissue layer lining the surface of an implant. The quality and density of bone vary, as does the contrast between implant radiopacity and adjacent bone radiolucency. CBCT offers the advantage that osseous structures can be represented in 3 planes, true to scale, and without overlay or distortion. Dental practitioners have made wide use of the 3D information obtained by CBCT in the areas of diagnosis and treatment planning; however, few studies have evaluated the role of imaging in detecting early implant failure.

The success of an implant depends on the ability of the titanium implant surfaces to establish contact with the surrounding bone tissues at the cellular level, without the interference of a fibrous tissue layer.[18] A substantial number of research studies have helped clinicians understand the healing mechanisms at the bone-implant interface. The gaps between the biomaterial and the host tissue may be of fundamental importance in predicting the outcome of implant treatment.[25] Radiologic follow-up of dental implants is a standard of care in clinical practice. Predictable success rates for endosseous dental implants can be achieved through a careful combination of clinical and radiologic evaluations. In the past 10 years, several studies[26–30] have confirmed the 3D geometric accuracy of CBCT.

The postoperative use of CBCT must be restricted to specific situations (eg, when implant retrieval is anticipated or a patient presents with implant mobility or altered sensation). Postoperative cross-sectional imaging is used to evaluate implant success based on 2 fundamental areas: integration and postoperative complications (**Box 3, Figs. 9–11**).

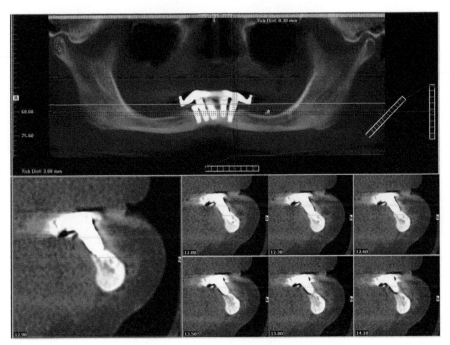

Fig. 8. Complete disintegration of bone around failed implant.

Accuracy in Evaluating Implants After Placement

Few studies have evaluated the accuracy of CBCT in detecting early bone defects after implant placement. In a study using dogs, Fienitz and colleagues[1] assessed the accuracy of CBCT in determining buccal-wall configuration and regeneration of peri-implant bone defects after alveolar bone augmentation. Radiologic evaluation with CBCT was compared with histomorphometric measures at the site of the implant. The authors found that CBCT is not accurate in evaluating of bone defects smaller than 0.5 mm. In a clinical study, Vera and colleagues[31] evaluated whether CBCT could be used to measure buccal alveolar bone changes 1 year after implant placement.

Box 3
Areas of postoperative assessment using cross-sectional imaging

- Integration
  - Marginal peri-implant bone height
  - Bone-implant interface
  - Postaugmentation assessment of bone
- Postoperative complications
  - Altered sensation
  - Infection or postoperative integration failure
  - Implant mobility
  - Rhinosinusitis

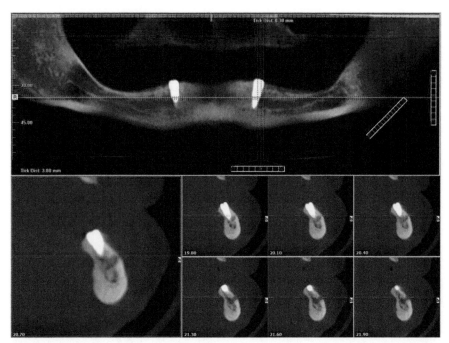

Fig. 9. Cross-sectional images showing possible nerve injury of the inferior alveolar by dental implant.

They found that CBCT can visualize buccal bone changes if the implant is appropriately displaced from the buccal wall of the socket.

COMPARISON WITH OTHER IMAGING MODALITIES

Recently, research publications have focused on the performance of CBCT with that of other imaging modalities. The main purpose of these studies has been to compare the performance of CBCT with that of traditional radiographic methods, such as periapical and panoramic radiographs, and to determine whether the use of CBCT to evaluate implant placement can be justified despite its disadvantages (radiation exposure and cost).

In an experimental study, Sirin and colleagues[32] evaluated the diagnostic potential and practical advantages of CBCT in detecting bone defects around dental implants. They created crestal bone defects around implants and compared images obtained with conventional periapical radiography, panoramic radiography, and CBCT. They found that periapical radiographs allowed a faster and more confident assessment of peri-implant radiolucencies than either of the other modalities. CBCT was found to have a comparable ability to detect peri-implant radiolucencies but was associated with slower decision making and lower image quality than traditional imaging modalities. Panoramic films were accurate if the diameter of the bone defect was at least 1.5 mm larger than that of the implant. In an in vitro study using bovine ribs, Dave and colleagues[33] compared the diagnostic accuracy of conventional periapical radiographs and CBCT in detecting peri-implant bone defects. They found that digital periapical images (using a long cone) were better than CBCT images in diagnosing peri-implant bone defects when the bone defect was smaller than 0.35 mm.

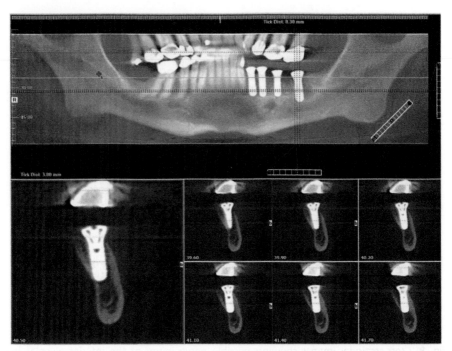

Fig. 10. Assessment after implant placement in the mandibular second molar site. Cross-sectional image showing no violation to the submandibular fossa or to the inferior alveolar canal.

However, when the bone defect was larger than 0.675 mm, no significant difference was seen in diagnostic accuracy between the imaging methods. Using pig mandibles, Mengel and colleagues[34] compared the accuracy and quality of the representation of peri-implant defects using intraoral periapical radiographs, panoramic radiographs, CT images, and CBCT images. The authors concluded that, overall, CT and CBCT images showed only slight deviations in the extent of the peri-implant defects, whereas intraoral periapical images detected only mesiodistal defects.

The authors concluded, based on the few available publications, that traditional image modalities, such as periapical radiographs, bitewing radiographs, and panoramic radiographs, perform at least as well as CBCT when the goal is evaluation of implant placement. Additional studies are needed to help clinicians decide on the most accurate image modality for detecting early implant failure.

ARTIFACTS AND ASSESSMENT OF IMPLANT PLACEMENT

The placement of dental implants involves the insertion of metallic bodies into the jaw bone. The artifacts produced by the implants can cause significant interference when images are reviewed to assess implant placement and performance. Noise artifacts and beam-hardening artifacts caused by the titanium surface are the most prominent artifacts induced by high-density objects in the beam (**Fig. 12**).[35] For many high-density dental filling materials, such as amalgam or gold, the complete absorption of the beam leads to extinction artifacts rather than to beam-hardening artifacts.[36] Dental implants, however, are commonly made of titanium, a light metal with the

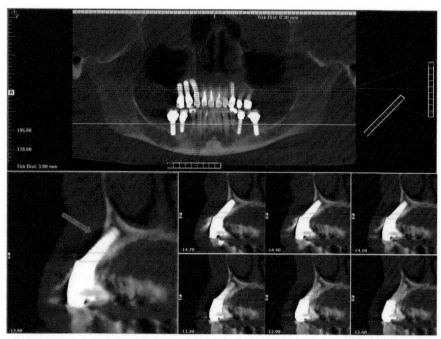

Fig. 11. Red arrow indicates loss of bony plate and presence of bony defect on the facial aspect of failing implant.

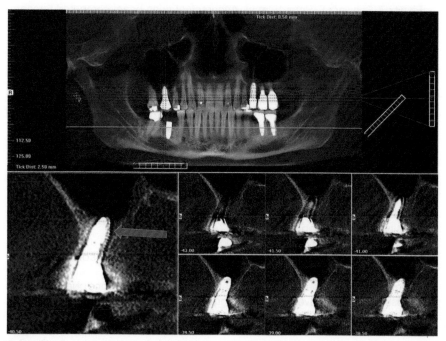

Fig. 12. Red arrow indicates radiolucency around implant caused by beam hardening artifact.

atomic number of 22. Titanium produces artifacts that interfere with the assessment of implant placement and performance.

Schulze and colleagues[2] used a hard-plaster phantom containing 2 titanium implants to review the mathematical background of beam-hardening artifacts in CBCT reconstruction. They found that massive beam-hardening artifacts were associated with the typical diameter of implants and the typical energies used by CBCT machines. Decreasing the number of beam-hardening artifacts associated with CBCT will require more sophisticated mathematical modeling of the process used to acquire the actual physical image. Research aimed at reducing the number of artifacts caused by titanium implants in CBCT images is currently underway.

SUMMARY

Radiologic examination is a crucial factor in the planning, assessment, and follow-up of dental implants. In 1998, CBCT was introduced to dentistry, and this modality has become a helpful tool in assessing implant stability. However, little is known about the ability of CBCT in the evaluation of peri-implant bone-wall morphology or about its performance compared with conventional radiographic procedures, such as periapical radiography. For patients with postoperative complications, diagnostic imaging, including CBCT, may be indicated as a supplement to the clinical examination, although in most cases conventional radiographs will provide the necessary information. More studies are necessary to determine the actual role of CBCT in detecting early implant failure.

REFERENCES

1. Fienitz T, Schwarz F, Ritter L, et al. Accuracy of cone beam computed tomography in assessing peri-implant bone defect regeneration: a histologically controlled study in dogs. Clin Oral Implants Res 2012;23(7):882–7.
2. Schulze RK, Berndt D, d'Hoedt B. On cone-beam computed tomography artifacts induced by titanium implants. Clin Oral Implants Res 2010;21(1):100–7.
3. Wang G, Vannier MW, Cheng PC. Iterative X-ray cone-beam tomography for metal artifact reduction and local region reconstruction. Microsc Microanal 1999;5(1):58–65.
4. Zhang Y, Zhang L, Zhux R, et al. Reducing metal artifacts in cone-beam CT images by preprocessing projection data. Int J Radiat Oncol Biol Phys 2007;67(3):924–32.
5. Frederiksen NL. Diagnostic imaging in dental implantology. Oral Surg Oral Med Oral Pathol Oral Radiol Endod 1995;80(5):540–54.
6. Kim DG. Can dental cone beam computed tomography assess bone mineral density? J Bone Metab 2014;21(2):117–26.
7. Reeves TE, Mah P, McDavid WD. Deriving Hounsfield units using grey levels in cone beam CT: a clinical application. Dentomaxillofac Radiol 2012;41(6):500–8.
8. Taylor TT, Gans S, Jones E, et al. Comparison of micro-CT and cone beam CT-based assessments for relative difference of grey level distribution in a human mandible. Dentomaxillofac Radiol 2013;42(3):25117764.
9. Nomura Y, Watanabe H, Honda E, et al. Reliability of voxel values from cone-beam computed tomography for dental use in evaluating bone mineral density. Clin Oral Implants Res 2010;21(5):558–62.

10. Hua Y, Nackaerts O, Duyck J, et al. Bone quality assessment based on cone beam computed tomography imaging. Clin Oral Implants Res 2009;20(8):767–71.
11. Parsa A, Ibrahim N, Hassan B, et al. Bone quality evaluation at dental implant site using multislice CT, micro-CT, and cone beam CT. Clin Oral Implants Res 2013. [Epub ahead of print].
12. Monje A, Monje F, Gonzalez-Garcia R, et al. Comparison between microcomputed tomography and cone-beam computed tomography radiologic bone to assess atrophic posterior maxilla density and microarchitecture. Clin Oral Implants Res 2014;25(6):723–8.
13. Ludlow JB, Ivanovic M. Comparative dosimetry of dental CBCT devices and 64-slice CT for oral and maxillofacial radiology. Oral Surg Oral Med Oral Pathol Oral Radiol Endod 2008;106(1):106–14.
14. Hujoel PP, Bollen A, Noonan C, et al. Antepartum dental radiography and infant low birth weight. JAMA 2004;291(16):1987–93.
15. Gonzalez AJ, Mason G, Clarke R, et al. Scope of radiological protection control measures. Ann ICRP 2007;37(5):1–105.
16. Hermann JS, Schoolfield JD, Nummikoski PV, et al. Crestal bone changes around titanium implants: a methodologic study comparing linear radiographic with histometric measurements. Int J Oral Maxillofac Implants 2001;16(4):475–85.
17. Albrektsson T, Zarb G, Worthington P, et al. The long-term efficacy of currently used dental implants: a review and proposed criteria of success. Int J Oral Maxillofac Implants 1986;1(1):11–25.
18. Albrektsson T, Jansson T, Lekholm U. Osseointegrated dental implants. Dent Clin North Am 1986;30(1):151–74.
19. Carlsson L, Rostlund T, Albrektsson B, et al. Osseointegration of titanium implants. Acta Orthop Scand 1986;57(4):285–9.
20. Buser D, Weber HP, Bragger U, et al. Tissue integration of one-stage ITI implants: 3-year results of a longitudinal study with Hollow-Cylinder and Hollow-Screw implants. Int J Oral Maxillofac Implants 1991;6(4):405–12.
21. Hansson HA, Albrektsson T, Branemark PI. Structural aspects of the interface between tissue and titanium implants. J Prosthet Dent 1983;50(1):108–13.
22. Fransson C, Tomasi C, Pikner SS, et al. Severity and pattern of peri-implantitis-associated bone loss. J Clin Periodontol 2010;37(5):442–8.
23. Wennstrom J, Palmer R. Consensus report of session 3: clinical trials. In: Lang N, Karring T, Lindhe J, editors. Proceedings of the 3rd European Workshop on Periodontology. Quintessence; 1999. p. 1–40.
24. Roos-Jansaker AM, Renvert H, Lindahl C, et al. Nine- to fourteen-year follow-up of implant treatment. Part II: presence of peri-implant lesions. J Clin Periodontol 2006;33(4):290–5.
25. Colnot C, Romero DM, Huang S, et al. Molecular analysis of healing at a bone-implant interface. J Dent Res 2007;86(9):862–7.
26. Kobayashi K, Shirmoda S, Nakagawa Y, et al. Accuracy in measurement of distance using limited cone-beam computerized tomography. Int J Oral Maxillofac Implants 2004;19(2):228–31.
27. Lascala CA, Panella J, Marques MM. Analysis of the accuracy of linear measurements obtained by cone beam computed tomography (CBCT-NewTom). Dentomaxillofac Radiol 2004;33(5):291–4.
28. Marmulla R, Wortche R, Muhling J, et al. Geometric accuracy of the NewTom 9000 Cone Beam CT. Dentomaxillofac Radiol 2005;34(1):28–31.
29. Pinsky HM, Dyda S, Pinsky RW, et al. Accuracy of three-dimensional measurements using cone-beam CT. Dentomaxillofac Radiol 2006;35(6):410–6.

30. Ludlow JB, Laster WS, See M, et al. Accuracy of measurements of mandibular anatomy in cone beam computed tomography images. Oral Surg Oral Med Oral Pathol Oral Radiol Endod 2007;103(4):534–42.
31. Vera C, De kok IJ, Chen W, et al. Evaluation of post-implant buccal bone resorption using cone beam computed tomography: a clinical pilot study. Int J Oral Maxillofac Implants 2012;27(5):1249–57.
32. Sirin Y, Horasan S, Yaman D, et al. Detection of crestal radiolucencies around dental implants: an in vitro experimental study. J Oral Maxillofac Surg 2012; 70(7):1540–50.
33. Dave M, Davies J, Wilson R, et al. A comparison of cone beam computed tomography and conventional periapical radiography at detecting peri-implant bone defects. Clin Oral Implants Res 2013;24(6):671–8.
34. Mengel R, Kruse B, Flores-de-Jacoby L. Digital volume tomography in the diagnosis of peri-implant defects: an in vitro study on native pig mandibles. J Periodontol 2006;77(7):1234–41.
35. Kalender WA, Hebel R, Ebersberger J. Reduction of CT artifacts caused by metallic implants. Radiology 1987;164(2):576–7.
36. Haramati N, Staron RB, Mazel-Sperling K, et al. CT scans through metal scanning technique versus hardware composition. Comput Med Imaging Graph 1994; 18(6):429–34.

Surgical Complications After Implant Placement

Igor Batista Camargo, DDS, MSc[a,b,c,d], Joseph E. Van Sickels, DDS[d,*]

KEYWORDS

- Bleeding • Infection • Dental injury • Mandibular fracture
- Displacement of the implant • Anatomic concerns • Prevention • Management

KEY POINTS

- Many of the issues that arise at surgery can be traced to the preoperative evaluation of the patient and assessment of the underlying anatomy.
- Prevention of all surgical complications is impossible; however, many can be minimized with proper planning.
- Failure to recognize variations in the regional anatomy of the maxilla and mandible can be the cause of major bleeding during implant placement.
- Consultation with restorative colleagues, computed tomography when the anatomy is in question, and a thorough review of the patient's medical history will help.

INTRODUCTION

Any number of complications can occur during or after the placement of dental implants. Most are immediately apparent; however, some can occur much later. Most complications can be traced to treatment planning and execution and are therefore preventable. Christman and colleagues[1] recommended the use of a safety checklist before the placement of implants; this checklist includes a review of the patient's medical and dental history, a diagnostic workup, a determination of the periodontal stability of adjacent teeth, and effective communication with restorative partners. We agree that a thorough review of all of the patient's records before the procedure will help to prevent some of the common complications seen during implant placement. This article reviews some of the more common and a few of the more severe surgical

This work was not supported by any external funds.

The authors have nothing to disclose.

Sponsored by CAPES/CNPq Scholarship and Brazilian Army (I.B. Camargo).

[a] Department of Oral and Maxillofacial Surgery, College of Dentistry of Pernambuco, University of Pernambuco, 1650 General Newton Cavalcalte Avenue, Recife, Pernambuco, Brazil 54753-020; [b] Brazilian Army, Brazil; [c] Military Hospital Area of Recife, 95 General Salgado Road, Office 103 Recife, Pernambuco, Brazil 51130-320; [d] Department of Oral and Maxillofacial Surgery, University of Kentucky, College of Dentistry, D-508, 800 Rose Street, Lexington, KY 40536-0297, USA

* Corresponding author.

E-mail address: vansick@email.uky.edu

http://dx.doi.org/10.1016/j.cden.2014.08.003
dental.theclinics.com

complications associated with the placement of implants. Additionally, we discuss short-term surgical complications, those seen either at the time of placement or during the weeks or months thereafter, with an emphasis on their management and prevention. In a few cases, the discussion also includes longer term complications related to the surgical procedure. When the material overlaps with that presented in other articles in this issue, the reader is referred to those works.

COMMON AND UNCOMMON COMPLICATIONS WITH IMPLANT PLACEMENT
Bleeding

Minor bleeding is inherent during the placement of dental implants, as with any surgical procedure. However, major bleeding is uncommon and can be life threatening. The causes of major bleeding may be related to systemic issues or regional anatomy. A wide variety of systemic issues can increase bleeding in a given patient. They may be broadly divided into those related to medications and those related to an underlying bleeding coagulopathy. Although a complete discussion of the management of every type of congenital or developmental bleeding disorder is beyond the scope of this discussion, it is worth noting that many patients with coagulopathies can undergo routine dentoalveolar surgery either in an office or in a hospital environment. Perhaps the most common potential bleeding issue seen in an office setting occurs with patients who are taking warfarin. These patients can undergo implant dentistry according to the protocols developed for dentoalveolar surgery. Most guidelines suggest that patients with an International Normalized Ratio of less than 3.5 can have a simple single extraction without any adjustment in anticoagulation. For patients taking warfarin, the overall frequency of persistent bleeding (2%) is low when all dental procedures are considered.[2] However, when extractions are combined with placement of an implant, the incidence of persistent bleeding increases to 4.8%.[2] This suggests that patients taking warfarin are at a higher risk of postoperative bleeding after simultaneous extraction and implant placement are combined if coagulation levels are not adjusted before the procedure. When such adjustments are not possible, the extraction and implant placement can be performed as a staged procedure.

It is important to understand that many patients who require anticoagulation but do not have prosthetic heart valves may be taking a newer class of anticoagulant drugs. The mechanism of action of these newer medications is different from that of warfarin: they directly inhibit either thrombin (dabigatran) or factor Xa (apixaban and rivaroxaban). The half-life of the drugs currently on the market ranges from 9 to 28 hours. The number of patients using these medications is increasing, and bleeding in association with dentoalveolar surgery is a distinct possibility. A systematic literature review concluded that the evidence and the recommendations of published guidelines all point to the same conclusion: Oral antithrombotic medication, including dual antiplatelet therapy, should not be interrupted for simple dental procedures.[3] Currently, there are no established protocols for managing patients taking these drugs who are undergoing dentoalveolar surgery, and the reversal of these newer medications is difficult.[4,5] For these reasons, we suggest a consultation with the patient's physician so that perioperative anticoagulation scenarios can be discussed.

Anatomic concerns
Failure to recognize variations in the regional anatomy of the maxilla and mandible can be the cause of major bleeding during implant placement. In some cases, the bleeding may have life-threatening consequences. The primary focus of the rest of this section is to review the specific anatomy of the maxilla and mandible and its relationship to cases of bleeding during and after surgery.

Maxilla

Bleeding with the placement of maxillary implants is rare. Moderate or severe maxillary bleeding may result from injury to intraosseous vessels lying within the walls of the maxilla. The vessels can be seen on computed tomography (CT), but not on plain radiographic films (**Fig. 1**). Anterior or posterior nasal bleeding, which may be profuse, and rapid swelling of the gingiva are common signs associated with an injury to one of these vessels. Aggressive surgery is necessary when the bleeding cannot be controlled by local means. Cauterization of the bleeding site using a nasal endoscope is the most common operative technique, but if an endoscope is not available, a Caldwell-Luc procedure can be used to identify and coagulate the injured vessel.[6] Careful evaluation of a CT of the maxilla in the areas of interest can prevent this type of maxillary bleeding during implant placement or sinus lifts.

Mandible

Multiple publications have reported bleeding, in some cases life-threatening hemorrhage, after the placement of implants in the anterior mandible.[7–9] Dubois and colleagues[10] reviewed 18 reported cases of life-threatening hemorrhage after implant surgery, most of which occurred when implants were placed in the region between the canines. Eight patients required intubation and 7 needed tracheostomies to ensure patency of the airway. Three of the 18 cases were managed by observation.[10]

The cause of bleeding during implant placement in the anterior mandible is perforation of the lingual cortex, resulting in injury to the terminal branches of the sublingual or submental artery.[9,11] The risk of perforation is high when the lingual fossa is very deep and is even higher when no flap is elevated during the procedure. One study involving 100 participants found that in 80% the depth of the submandibular fossa was more than 2 mm.[7]

Several techniques are available for assessing potential implant sites in both the anterior and posterior regions of the mandible, including both clinical assessment and radiographic evaluation of the intended site. The results of palpation of the ridge are variable; however, during the procedure, dissection of the lingual aspect of the mandible can determine its curvature and help to prevent perforation. Examining a

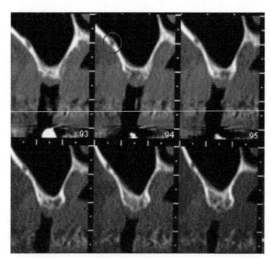

Fig. 1. Cone beam computerized tomography of a patient who had a large hematoma after a sinus lift. Red circle indicates vessel in the bony of the maxillary sinus.

facial CT with attention to the lingual aspect of the mandible also alerts the surgeon to possible risks of perforation in this region.

Management of bleeding once perforation has occurred requires both control of the hemorrhage and protection of the airway. In the early stages, when hemorrhage is seen in the floor of the mouth, basic measures should be taken, including immediate bimanual compression at the suspected perforation site and control of the patient's blood pressure if it is elevated. The injection of local anesthesia with a vasoconstrictor through the perforation may be helpful. If there is any doubt about control of bleeding, the airway should be secured in the dental office or the patient should be transported to the nearest hospital by emergency medical services so that the airway can be secured without delay. Once the airway has been secured, then isolation of the vessel(s) that has been injured can be identified. It is mandatory that the surgeon be alert for delayed hematomas on the floor of the mouth when patients complain of a protruding tongue, hemorrhage, or respiratory distress. If hemorrhage is severe, it is almost impossible to visualize the anatomy in the affected area. Retraction of the artery after laceration makes ligation difficult or impossible. If operative intervention is necessary for controlling the hemorrhage, an extraoral approach for ligation procedures is preferred. The facial and submental arteries can easily be accessed and should be ligated first.[8] Surgical intervention for ligation of vessels is usually not necessary, but the patient may need to be intubated for several days for protection of the airway. Antibiotics should be used to prevent infection when hematomas are extensive, especially if intraoral communication is present. Administration of steroids for reducing swelling should also be considered.[8]

Although published reports show that severe bleeding with hematoma formation is a very rare complication, the consequences of such a complication for the patient can be tremendous when the lingual cortex is perforated. We suggest that, if there is any question regarding the mandibular anatomy, a CT should be included in the planning stages for implant placement in the anterior region of the mandible.[9,10]

Infection

Postoperative infections can occur after implant placement with or without grafting of the site. A variety of local and systemic factors may play a role in the development of such infection. Our review of the literature suggests an inconsistency in the definition of postoperative infection. In this section, we define postoperative infection as the presence of purulent drainage (either spontaneously or by incision) or fistula in the operative region, together with pain or tenderness, localized swelling, redness, or fever (>38°C). Early infection is defined as infection occurring within 1 week postoperatively, and late infection, as infection occurring from 1 week postoperatively to the time of abutment connection (3–8 months postoperatively).[12]

It is believed that bacterial contamination during implant insertion can cause early failure of the dental implant. Contamination of the implant surface by bacterial biofilms during operative procedures can lead to an inflammatory process in the hard and soft tissues, thus decreasing the implant success rate. Infections around biomaterials are very difficult to treat and nearly all infected implants may fail at some time after placement.

Although massive infection after the placement of dental implants is possible, most early infections occur when grafts are used, and most of these occur with a sinus lift. We refer the reader to the article by Drs Fugazzotto and Kenney elsewhere in this issue for additional details regarding the management and prevention of infections associated with sinus lifts.

Prophylactic antibiotics

Prophylactic antibiotics may prevent postoperative infections and thus decrease implant failure. The benefit of antibiotic prophylaxis for healthy patients undergoing routine placement of dental implants is controversial. For an otherwise healthy patient, intraoperative tissue manipulation and clinical technique seem to be the most important factors in determining whether the implant site becomes infected after surgery.[12,13]

Some studies have found that the use of prophylactic antibiotics of little or no benefit, whereas others have found the opposite.[14] Those opposed to the routine use of antibiotics note that such drugs are associated with risks, including diarrhea, anaphylaxis, and antibiotic resistance with the development of resistant strains.[15–17] Even those published reports that advocates the use of antibiotics do not discuss a standard regimen or protocol for their use during implant placement.[12,14] A number of regimens have been suggested including preoperative single or multiple doses, postoperative single or multiple doses for several days, or a preoperative dose followed by a postoperative dose.[14] Conceptually, when antibiotic prophylaxis is indicated an appropriate-spectrum antibiotic should be administered preoperatively as a single dose. The drug must be present at an adequate concentration in the blood stream before the incision is made, and its use should be discontinued postoperatively. A recent report illustrated this point by comparing 2 antibiotic protocols (a single dose before surgery and a 3-day course of antibiotic). The outcome assessed was the reduction of early failure of dental implant. A several-day course of antibiotics after implant placement was not shown to have an advantage over a single preoperative dose. Although the authors suggested the need for a larger sample size, they concluded that a single dose of antibiotics before implant placement is sufficient to prevent infection and implant failure.[14]

Another study compared 4 antibiotic protocols: A single dose of amoxicillin administered preoperatively, 3 days postoperatively, 5 days postoperatively, 7 days postoperatively, and a placebo. The outcome assessed was the success of osseointegration of the dental implant in an animal model. The results of the study suggested that prolonged use of antibiotics may have a negative effect on bone formation around implants. The authors recommended a single preoperative dose of amoxicillin because it has minimal adverse effects on the host and on osseointegration.[18]

Late infection

Actinomycosis has been implicated in a number of cases of implant failures. *Actinomyces odontolyticus* was present in 84% of *Actinomyces*-positive failed implants.[19] Oral actinomycosis is uncommon, but it can cause infection and in some instances massive bone destruction. A published report described an implant that failed 1.5 years after placement and 3 years after tooth extraction. Radiographs revealed a large radiolucency on the mesial aspect of the implant, which was placed in the lower second bicuspid region. The implant was surgically removed, and the lesion thoroughly debrided. A course of antibiotics was prescribed. Histologic examination noted sulfur granules, which were confirmed to be actinomycotic colonies. The authors reported no recurrence of the infection 1 year after the procedure.[20]

Fungal infection

Fungal infections after implant surgery are also rare. However, the incidence of fungal infection of the paranasal sinuses is increasing.[21] More than 10% of all patients with chronic sinusitis have an aspergilloma, the most common type of chronic noninvasive fungal sinusitis.[22] An unusual case of *Aspergillus* infection associated with dental implants and sinus bone grafting has been reported.[23]

Successful treatment of patients with noninvasive fungal sinusitis requires surgical curettage with removal of the mycotic masses. Both a Caldwell-Luc procedure and endoscopic techniques have been used for this purpose.[22] In general, fungal infections do not tend to recur after successful removal of mycotic masses. Systemic antifungal therapy may be required if the patient continues to exhibit symptoms after surgical treatment. Invasive and fulminant fungal sinusitis is the rarest form of fungal sinusitis and occurs primarily in immunosuppressed patients. Because fulminant fungal sinusitis may be fatal, an invasive infection requires not only aggressive surgical debridement of abnormal bone and soft tissue, but also prolonged antifungal chemotherapy.

Nerve Injury

Injuries to the inferior alveolar nerve and, less frequently, the lingual nerve have been reported and are of concern when posterior mandibular implants are placed. Management of these injuries is predicated on the degree of nerve injury. Prevention can be simplified to careful preoperative planning. The readers are referred to the article by Drs Al-Sabbagh, Okeson, Khalaf and Bertolli elsewhere in this issue for more details about the management and prevention of these injuries.

Malpositioning of Implants

Malpositioning of implants can occur during implant surgery and may be the result of a number of factors, such as the quantity or quality of residual available bone, dental inclinations adjacent to the surgical implant site, and lack of previous prosthodontic planning. Managing an implant that is poorly positioned may require a modified prosthetic attachment or surgical removal. The choice of treatment depends on the degree to which the poorly positioned implant will compromise the restorative plan. The reader is referred to the articles by Drs Kim, Sadid-Zadeh and Kutkut elsewhere in this issue.

Injury to Adjacent Teeth

When partially edentulous patients are treated, there is a risk of direct or indirect (thermal) injury to the roots of the adjacent teeth (**Fig. 2**).[24] Depending on the severity of the injury, the tooth may be sensitive to cold and tender to percussion, and may cause mild discomfort when the patient is eating,[25] although the injured tooth may respond normally to vitality tests. Treatment may involve extraction or endodontic treatment.[26] When an implant is in direct contact with an adjacent tooth, immediate removal of the implant may avoid major complications to the tooth. In some instances, implant removal may be accomplished with counterclockwise movement. In other instances, an internal device (Implant Retrieval Tool, Nobel Biocare, Kloten, Switzerland) can be used to unscrew the implant (**Fig. 3**).

Several published reports have described the histologic response of the periodontium, cementum, and pulp after intentional root injury created with titanium

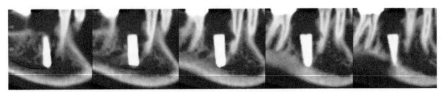

Fig. 2. Cone beam images obtained 3 months after placement of an implant in a lower first molar site. The second bicuspid was sensitive to percussion.

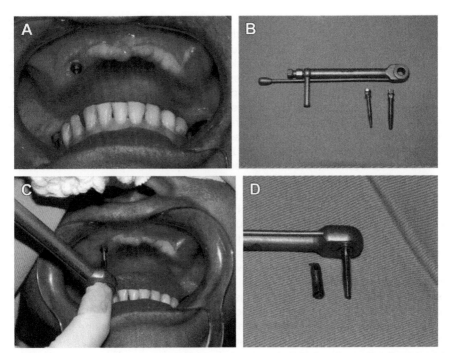

Fig. 3. (*A*) Malpositioned osseointegrated implant associated with peri-implantitis. (*B*) Generic retriever devices of 2 diameters with clockwise threads on the body. This device should be used with a torque wrench. (*C*) Generic retriever inside the implant platform. Counterclockwise force is used. (*D*) Osseointegrated implant after removal. (*Courtesy of David M. Oliveira, DDS, MSc, PhD, Recife, Pernambuco, Brazil.*)

orthodontic screws.[27] Unlike implant surgery, this protocol required insertion of the screws without the use of drills. However, the injuries were similar to those occur when implants are placed. The authors concluded that permanent damage to the pulp and supporting tissues does not routinely occur when miniscrews abrade or even enter the root surface.[28] Immediate removal of the mini-implant leads to cementum repair, but leaving the mini-implant in place leads to either a delay in repair or no repair. Placing mini-implants less than 1 mm from the surface of the root causes root–surface resorption.[29] Another study found that, when titanium screws penetrated cementum or dentin, no pulpal necrosis or inflammation was observed after 12 weeks. Cementum regenerated at every injury site, but ankylosis was possible when root fragmentation was present. Woven bone was seen at the screw–bone interface, even when root contact suggested osteointegration.[24] Increased resistance is an indicator of possible root contact during implant placement.[30]

Although these studies are interesting, prevention of injury to adjacent teeth starts with the preoperative assessment and planning of the procedure and the assessment of the amount of space available for implant placement. Surgical guides are helpful if they are well designed.

Fracture of the Mandible

Rehabilitation of a severely resorbed mandible (greatest height <7 mm) with implants is a surgical and prosthetic challenge because of the minimal amount of residual bone.[31] Fractures can occur in less dense or poorly mineralized bone when stress or strain develops as implants are placed. Excess tightening of a screw-type implant can result in microfractures in the surrounding bone caused by the strain generated by placing the implant in unhealthy bone. Additionally, unfavorable biomechanics can also increase the risk of a mandibular fracture.[32] Although the exact mechanism by which such fractures occur is not known, the most likely cause is the concentration of stress at the implant site. Before osseointegration occurs, the implant site acts as a region of tensile stress concentration and ultimately an area of weakness. Consequently, this area of weakness is more prone than others to applied functional forces. Repeated submaximal functional forces may lead to a spontaneous fracture with no associated macrotrauma. With these factors in mind, several extra precautions should be taken when implants are placed in thin or weak mandibles.[33]

Before the use of implant restorations become routine, various surgical techniques were used to augment the severely atrophic mandible, prevent fractures, and facilitate prosthetic usage. These procedures included onlay grafts, sandwich osteotomy, visor osteotomy, and grafts to the border of the lower mandible. Although most of these techniques are no longer used, some can increase the stability and longevity of implants placed in atrophic mandibles. Newer strategies include short implants, autogenous bone grafts or implants, and distraction osteogenesis for augmenting mandibles 10 mm or less in height. The use of short implants is an attractive treatment option because it requires a simple surgical procedure with limited morbidity. The disadvantages of placing short implants in an atrophic mandible include long vertical lever arms and, often, the need for a tissue-borne prosthesis. Both of these mechanical issues are problematic for the patient with an atrophic mandible in which the inferior alveolar nerve is often very superficial.

Treatment

Several published reports describe fracture of the mandible after placement of implants.[33,34] The incidence of fracture is approximately 0.2%, but when it occurs it can lead to osteomyelitis, paresthesia, malunion, nonunion, and prolonged functional and nutritional disturbances.[35] Our experience is that fractures most frequently occur on 1 side or the other of the most distal implant. When a fracture is well aligned, an effective treatment is to discontinue the use dentures and keep the patient on a soft diet. Although this treatment may be successful, our experience is that these fractures frequently require open reduction with the application of a large bone plate placed through an extraoral approach (**Fig. 4**).[36] When a fracture occurs between implants, an alternative treatment is to use a wire-reinforced acrylic splint over the implants to the abutments on either side spanning and connecting each side of the mandibular fracture (external intraoral splint).[33]

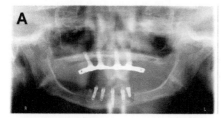 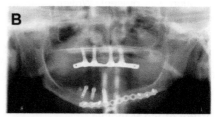

Fig. 4. (A) This patient presented to our clinic with a mobile implant and mandible on the left side. The implant had been recently placed at another office. The mobile implant was removed, and the patient chose conservative therapy for the fractured mandible. (B) Ultimate treatment of the fractured mandible with the loss of another implant.

A final option is an intraoral open reduction and internal fixation using a locking reconstruction plate. Although this type of reconstruction is more challenging to place, it is associated with a lower risk of injury to the marginal mandibular branch of the facial nerve, and it also avoids a facial scar.[35] We believe that larger plates with low profiles are necessary with both the extraoral and intraoral approaches because of diminished bone stock and the loss of internal buttressing.[37]

Prevention

A number of alternative techniques can be used to prevent a fracture in patients with atrophic mandibles.[38–40] In 2009 and again in 2012, Lopes and co-workers[38,39] described novel approaches to the prevention of fracture of the mandible with a 2-mm locking reconstruction bone plate. The plate was placed to reinforce the atrophic mandible before the placement of implants (**Fig. 5**). Korpi and associates[40] described the use of a reconstruction plate combined with the "tent pole technique" (implants stabilized in the basilar bone, leaving exposed threads above the bone covered with autogenous bone graft). These authors achieved good results by

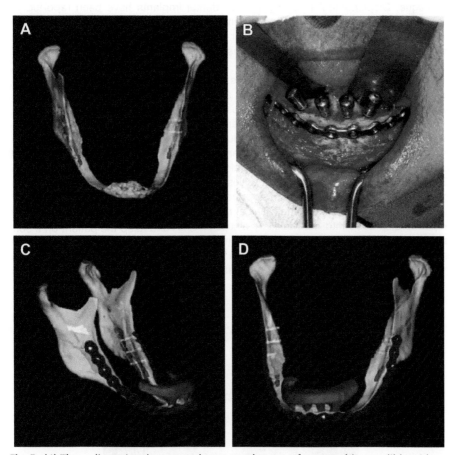

Fig. 5. (*A*) Three-dimensional computed tomography scan of an atrophic mandible without a reconstruction plate. (*B*) Implants placed in the interforaminal region. (*C*, *D*) Postoperative computed tomography. (*Courtesy of* André Vajgel Fernandes, DDS, MSc, Recife, Pernambuco, Brazil.)

treating patients with atrophic mandible fractures with either simultaneous or delayed implant placement.

Displacement or Infringement on Adjacent Spaces

Numerous cases of displacement or migration of implants into adjacent spaces have been published, generally as case reports.

Maxilla

Displacement of an implant can occur intraoperatively or shortly thereafter because of surgical technique or anatomic variances. In contrast, migration involves the relatively long-term movement of an implant. In either case, the quantity and quality of bone is usually poor. Mechanisms that have been proposed to explain implant migration into the sinus include changes in sinus and nasal pressure, autoimmune reactions to the implant, and poor distribution of occlusal forces. Intraoperative and early displacement of dental implants has been attributed to low bone density, thin cortical bone, anatomic variances, previous infection, osteopenia or osteoporosis, and poor surgical technique. Displacement and migration of dental implants have been reported to occur in the maxillary sinus, sphenoid sinus, and ethmoid sinus.[41] They have also been reported to perforate the nasal floor and, in 1 case, the anterior cranial fossa. In general, these types of complications result from planning errors or surgical inexperience.

When implants migrate into the sinuses, there may or may not be signs or symptoms of infection, but there will likely be an oral–antral communication. If infection occurs, it may involve the adjacent sinuses. We recommend the removal of displaced implants (**Fig. 6**). Implants that are displaced into the maxillary sinus can be removed by a Caudwell-Luc procedure (**Fig. 7**) or by a transnasal approach with functional endoscopic sinus surgery. An intraoral approach (Caldwell-Luc) can also be used to close an oral–antral communications. The disadvantage of a Caldwell-Luc procedure is that it gives the infection adequate access to an obstructed maxillary sinus ostium and may result in concomitant sinusitis of other paranasal sinuses. A multicenter clinical report compared 3 methods of managing implants displaced into the maxillary sinus. They concluded that functional endoscopic sinus surgery in combination with an intraoral approach can be used to safely treat complications associated with the displacement or migration of grafting materials or oral implants into the paranasal sinuses.[42] An alternative approach is

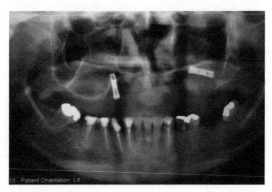

Fig. 6. Implant displaced in the maxillary sinus. (*Courtesy of* André Vajgel Fernandes, DDS, MSc, Recife, Pernambuco, Brazil.)

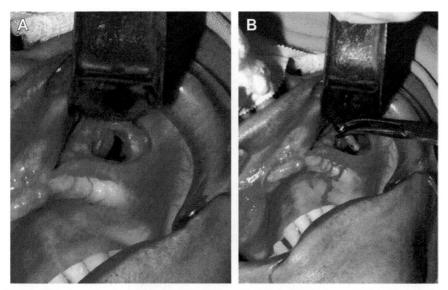

Fig. 7. (*A*) Intraoral access with lateral windows in the maxillary sinus. (*B*) Removal of the displaced implant using a hemostatic clamp. (*Courtesy of* André Vajgel Fernandes, DDS, MSc, Recife, Pernambuco, Brazil.)

the use of intraoral videolaparoscopic trocars for removing implants form the maxillary sinus.[43] This technique is called the double barrier approach because it uses 2 trocars. One trocar is rotated parallel to the sagittal plane to penetrate the anterior wall of the maxillary sinus. This trocar is removed from the sheath, and diagnostic endoscopy of the sinus is performed using a 45° endoscope. A second trocar is inserted through the anterior wall in close proximity to the first. Under visual control, a biopsy forceps is introduced through the second sheath. The implant is grasped under endoscopic control and extracted by removing the forceps and the cannula of the trocar.

Mandible
Although displacement of implants into the maxillary sinus is well known, there are fewer reports of displacement of a dental implant into the medullary space of the mandible. Focal osteoporotic bone marrow defects of the jaws and other asymptomatic radiolucent lesions occur predominantly in the molar region of middle-aged women and may be associated with a higher risk of implant displacement.[44] In a case report, Bayram and Alaaddinoglu[45] described the elevation of a mucoperiosteal flap on an edentulous ridge of the posterior mandible; they observed type IV bone quality during the osteotomy. As they inserted an implant with a diameter of 4.2 mm, bleeding suddenly started. After controlling the hemorrhage, they noted that the implant was not where they had placed it. A bone osteotomy was performed at the lateral corpus of the mandible. After a rectangular cortical bone window had been removed, the implant was exposed and removed. The inner aspect of the corpus was devoid of cancellous bone; the authors noted only yellow soft tissue filling the space. The osteotomy window was replaced and fixed with a microplate and screws. We experienced a similar case in a private practice with one of our colleagues (courtesy Dr André Vajgel) with an internal hexagonal platform implant. We chose to fill the defect with demineralized bone graft (**Fig. 8**).

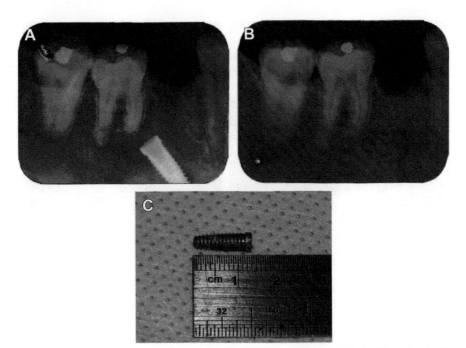

Fig. 8. (*A*) Implant displaced in the mandibular medulla. (*B*) Defect filled with grafted with inorganic bovine bone (Bioss) after creation removal of a window using a 702 bur at low speed. (*C*) Hexagonal intern 3I implant (4.1 × 13 mm). (*Courtesy of* André Vajgel Fernandes, DDS, MSc, Recife, Pernambuco, Brazil.)

Other anatomic regions

One case report described the displacement of a dental implant into the anterior cranial fossa (the region of the cribriform plate) and its endoscopic removal. A dural repair was necessary for treating a subsequent leak of cerebral spinal fluid. The authors did not describe the placement of this implant.[46] A retrospective analysis of 244 cases of complications after the placement of zygomatic implants found 2 cases of subcutaneous malar emphysema caused by dislocation of the tip of the implant burs in the zygomatic–facial region. The subcutaneous emphysema resolved spontaneously by resorption of the air.[47]

Salivary gland injury

The sublingual salivary gland can be injured when an implant is placed in the posterior mandible.[48] The proximity of the sublingual gland to the lingual cortex of the mandible, which lies directly below the mylohyoid muscle, makes it susceptible to injury if a penetration occurs in this area. This traumatic insult could induce the formation of a ranula. Preoperative planning, good surgical technique, and experience in dental implant placement will help avoid these types of complications. Additional imaging studies and CT are helpful in planning anatomically challenging procedures.

Miscellaneous Surgical Complications: Swallowing and Aspiration of Implants or Surgical Devices

Any dentoalveolar procedure may result in aspiration or ingestion of instruments or parts of crowns. Common signs and symptoms of aspiration of an implant or a surgical part may include coughing, choking, wheezing, and hoarseness.[49] These are serious medical emergencies. We suggest that the patient be given supplemental oxygen and that emergency medical services be called to transport the patient to the nearest emergency department. Standard basic life support techniques should be used, including the Heimlich maneuver.

Ingestion of foreign bodies can also occur, although it may not be as dramatic as aspiration. Current protocols suggest that the patient be transferred to a local emergency department for chest and abdominal radiography. Depending on the shape of the instrument or part, it may need to be removed rather than allowed to pass.

The key to managing aspiration and ingestion of foreign bodies is prevention. Although no technique can completely eliminate this complication, the cornerstone of preventive procedures in the office is placement of a gauze screen posterior to the surgical site so that access to the oropharynx is blocked. The entire oral cavity should be clearly visualized with an adequate light source and high-vacuum suction. A finger sweep should be used to dislodge implant pieces before they pass behind the gauze pack. In patients with strong gag reflexes who cannot tolerate this safety precaution, chair positioning is very important during extraction or implant procedures. These patients should be seated more upright. All small devices, such as implant instruments, should be fastened to a long length of dental floss hanging from the mouth for quick retrieval in case of displacement. All instruments should be properly applied and maintained to minimize instrument fracture and loss in the oral cavity.[50]

SUMMARY

Prevention of all surgical complications is impossible; however, many can be minimized with proper planning. Consultation with restorative colleagues, CT when the anatomy is in question, and a thorough review of the patient's medical history will help. When complications do occur, the surgeon and the office staff should be prepared to deal with them expeditiously.

ACKNOWLEDGMENTS

The authors thank CAPES/CNPq (Conselho Nacional de Desenvolvimento Científico e Tecnológico) and the Brazilian Army (Departamento Geral do Pessoal – Diretoria de Saúde - Exército Brasileiro).

REFERENCES

1. Christman A, Schrader S, John V, et al. Designing a safety checklist for dental implant placement: a Delphi Study. J Am Dent Assoc 2014;145:131–40.
2. Hong C, Napenas JJ, Brennan M, et al. Risk of postoperative bleeding after dental procedures in patients on warfarin: a retrospective study. Oral Surg Oral Med Oral Pathol Oral Radiol 2012;114:464–8.
3. van Diermen DE, van der Waal I, Hoogstraten J. Management recommendations for invasive dental treatment in patients using oral antithrombotic medication, including novel oral anticoagulants. Oral Surg Oral Med Oral Pathol Oral Radiol 2013;116:709–16.
4. UK Chandler Medical. Critical bleeding reversal protocol. Available at: https://docs.google.com/viewer?url=http://www.hosp.uky.edu/pharmacy/formulary/criteria/Critical%20Bleeding%20Reversal%20Protocol.pdf. Accessed April 2014.

5. UC Davis Health System. Anticoagulation services recommendations for anticoagulation management before & after dental procedures. Available at: http://www.ucdmc.ucdavis.edu/anticoag/pdf/AnticoagDentalProcedure.pdf. Accessed May 2014.

6. Hong YH, Mun SK. A case of massive maxillary sinus bleeding after dental implant. Int J Oral Maxillofac Surg 2011;40:758–60.

7. Parnia F, Fard EM, Marboub F, et al. Tomographic volume evaluation of submandibular fossa in patients requiring dental implants. Oral Surg Oral Med Oral Pathol Oral Radiol Endod 2010;109:32–6.

8. Niamtu J 3rd. Near-fatal airway obstruction after routine implant placement. Oral Surg Oral Med Oral Pathol Oral Radiol Endod 2001;92:597–600.

9. Woo BM, Al-Bustani S, Ueeck BA. Floor of mouth haemorrhage and life-threatening airway obstruction during immediate implant placement in the anterior mandible. Int J Oral Maxillofac Surg 2006;35:961–4.

10. Dubois L, de Lange J, Baas E, et al. Excessive bleeding in the floor of the mouth after endosseus implant placement: a report of two cases. Int J Oral Maxillofac Surg 2010;39:412–5.

11. Tarakji B, Nassani MZ. Factors associated with hematoma of the floor of the mouth after placement of dental implants. Saudi Dent J 2012;24:11–5.

12. Gynther GW, Köndell PA, Lars-Erik Moberg LE, et al. Dental implant installation without antibiotic prophylaxis. Oral Surg Oral Med Oral Pathol Oral Radiol Endod 1998;85:509–11.

13. Pye AD, Lockhart DE, Dawson MP, et al. A review of dental implants and infection. J Hosp Infect 2009;72:104–10.

14. El-Kholey KE. Efficacy of two antibiotic regimens in the reduction of early dental implant failure: a pilot study. Int J Oral Maxillofac Surg 2014;43(4):487–90.

15. Zix J, Schaller B, Iizuka T, et al. The role of postoperative prophylactic antibiotics in the treatment of facial fractures: a randomised, double-blind, placebo-controlled pilot clinical study. Part 1: orbital fractures in 62 patients. Br J Oral Maxillofac Surg 2013;51:332.

16. Granowitz EV, Brown RB. Antibiotic adverse reactions and drug interactions. Crit Care Clin 2008;24:421.

17. Pallasch TJ. Antibiotic resistance. Dent Clin North Am 2003;47:623.

18. Giro G, In J, Witek L, et al. Amoxicillin administrations and its influence on bone repair around osseointegrated implants. J Oral Maxillofac Surg 2014;72:305.e1–5.

19. Sarkonen N, Könönen E, Eerola E, et al. Characterization of Actinomyces species isolated from failed dental implant fixtures. Anaerobe 2005;11:231–7.

20. Sun CX, Henkin JM, Ririe C, et al. Implant Failure Associated With Actinomycosis in a Medically Compromised Patient. J Oral Implantol 2013;39(2):206–9.

21. Krennmair G, Lenglinger F. Maxillary sinus aspergillosis: diagnosis and differentiation of the pathogenesis based on computed tomography densitometry of sinus concretions. J Oral Maxillofac Surg 1995;53:657–63.

22. Loidolt D, Mangge H, Wilders-Truschnig M, et al. In vivo and in vitro suppression of lymphocyte function in Aspergillus sinusitis. Arch Otorhinolaryngol 1989;246:321–3.

23. Sohn DS, Lee JK, Shin HI, et al. Fungal infection as a complication of sinus bone grafting and implants: a case report. Oral Surg Oral Med Oral Pathol Oral Radiol Endod 2009;107:375–80.

24. Dao V, Renjen R, Prasad HS, et al. Cementum, pulp, periodontal ligament, and bone response after direct injury with orthodontic anchorage screws: a histomorphologic study in an animal model. J Oral Maxillofac Surg 2009;67:2440–5.

25. Margelos JT, Verdelis KG. Irreversible pulpal damage of teeth adjacent to recently placed osseointegrated implants. J Endod 1995;21(9):479–82.
26. Sussman HI. Tooth devitalization via implant placement: a case report. Periodontal Clin Investig 1998;20:22–4.
27. Alves M Jr, Baratieri C, Araújo MT, et al. Root damage associated with intermaxillary screws: a systematic review. Int J Oral Maxillofac Surg 2012;41:1445–50.
28. Renjen R, Maganzini AL, Rohrer MD, et al. Root and pulp response after intentional injury from miniscrew placement. Am J Orthod Dentofacial Orthop 2009; 136:708–14.
29. Kim H, Kim TW. Histologic evaluation of root-surface healing after root contact or approximation during placement of mini-implants. Am J Orthod Dentofacial Orthop 2011;139:752–60.
30. Brisceno CE, Rossouw PE, Carrillo R, et al. Healing of the roots and surrounding structures after intentional damage with miniscrew implants. Am J Orthod Dentofacial Orthop 2009;135:292–301.
31. Bell RB, Blakey GH, White RP, et al. Staged reconstruction of the severely atrophic mandible. J Oral Maxillofac Surg 2002;60:1135.
32. Stellingsma C, Vissink A, Meijer HJ, et al. Implantology and the severely resorbed edentulous mandible. Crit Rev Oral Biol Med 2004;15:240.
33. Manson ME, Triplett RG, Van Sickels JE, et al. Mandibular fractures through endosseous cylinder implants: report of cases and review. J Oral Maxillofac Surg 1990;49:311–7.
34. Raghoebar GM, Stellingsma K, Batenburg RH, et al. Etiology and management of mandibular fractures associated with endosteal implants in the atrophic mandible. Oral Surg Oral Med Oral Pathol Oral Radiol Endod 2000;89:553–9.
35. Almasri M, El-Hakim M. Fracture of the anterior segment of the atrophic mandible related to dental implants. Int J Oral Maxillofac Surg 2012;41:646–9.
36. Oh WS, Roumanas ED, Beumer J 3rd. Mandibular fracture in conjunction with bicortical penetration, using wide-diameter endosseous dental implants. J Prosthodont 2010;19(8):625–9.
37. Vajgel A, Camargo IB, Willmersdorf RB, et al. Comparative finite element analysis of the biomechanical stability of 2.0 fixation plates in atrophic mandibular fractures. J Oral Maxillofac Surg 2013;71:335–42.
38. Lopes N, Oliveira DM, Vajgel A, et al. A new approach for reconstruction of a severely atrophic mandible. J Oral Maxillofac Surg 2009;67:2455–9.
39. Lopes N, Vajgel A, Oliveira DM, et al. Use of rhBMP-2 to reconstruct a severely atrophic mandible: a modified approach. Int J Oral Maxillofac Surg 2012;41:1566–70.
40. Korpi JT, Kainulainen VT, Sándor GK, et al. Tent-pole approach to treat severely atrophic fractured mandibles using immediate or delayed protocols: preliminary case series. J Oral Maxillofac Surg 2013;71:83–9.
41. Dimitriou C, Karavelis A, Triardis K. Foreign body in the sphenoid sinus. J Craniomaxillofac Surg 1992;20:228–9.
42. Chiapasco M, Felisati G, Maccari A, et al. The management of complications following displacement of oral implants in the paranasal sinuses: a multicenter clinical report and proposed treatment protocols. Int J Oral Maxillofac Surg 2009;38:1273–8.
43. Albu S. The 'double-barrel' approach to the removal of dental implants from the maxillary sinus. Int J Oral Maxillofac Surg 2013;42:1529–32.
44. Carvalho A, Barros MM, Garcia FB, et al. Displacement of dental implant into the focal osteoporotic bone marrow defect [abstracts]. Oral Surg Oral Med Oral Pathol Oral Radiol Endod 2014;117:e154.

45. Bayram B, Alaaddinoglu E. Implant-box mandible: dislocation of an implant into the mandible. J Oral Maxillofac Surg 2011;69:498–501.
46. Cascone P, Ungari C, Filiaci F, et al. A dental implant in the anterior cranial fossae. Int J Oral Maxillofac Surg 2010;39:92–3.
47. Fernandez H, Gomez-Delgado A, Trujillo-Saldarriaga S, et al. Zygomatic: implants for the management of the severely atrophied maxilla: a retrospective analysis of 244 implants. J Oral Maxillofac Surg 2014;72:887–91.
48. Loney WW Jr, Termini S, Sisto J. Ranula formation and dental implant surgery. J Oral Maxillofac Surg 2006;64:1204–8.
49. Bergermann M, Donald PJ, aWengen DE. Screwdriver aspiration. A complication of dental implant placement. Int J Oral Maxillofac Surg 1992;21:339–41.
50. Fields RT Jr, Schow SR. Aspiration and ingestion of foreign bodies in oral and maxillofacial surgery: a review of the literature and report of five cases. J Oral Maxillofac Surg 1998;56:1091–8.

Immediate Implant Placement

Surgical Techniques for Prevention and Management of Complications

Mohanad Al-Sabbagh, DDS, MS[a],*, Ahmad Kutkut, DDS, MS[b]

KEYWORDS

- Immediate implant placement • Complications of immediate placement
- Techniques for immediate placement • Prevention of complications

KEY POINTS

- Clinical studies have reported successful outcome of immediate placement of dental implants in fresh extraction sockets.
- Although immediate implant placement has advantages over delayed implant placement, like any other procedure, it is associated with risks and complications.
- Case selection and evaluation of patient-related and implant-related factors are keys to the success of immediate implant placement.
- A thorough discussion between practitioner and the patient is indispensable to discern patient's desires.

INTRODUCTION
Healing of Extraction Socket

Wound healing in an extraction socket is characterized by resorption of alveolar bone, which may result in restorative complications.[1,2] Healing of extraction sites when no socket preservation techniques are used results in the resorption of an average of 1 to 2 mm of vertical alveolar bone height and an average of 4 to 5 mm of horizontal alveolar bone width. Most of this bone loss occurs during the first year after extraction, and two thirds of this bone loss occurs within the first 3 months after extraction. Therefore, preservation of alveolar bone immediately after tooth extraction has an important impact on the functional and esthetic outcomes of subsequent prosthetic treatment.[2] The purpose of preserving the extraction socket is to maintain the architecture of the

[a] Division of Periodontology, Department of Oral Health Practice, College of Dentistry, University of Kentucky, 800 Rose Street, Lexington, KY 40536, USA; [b] Division of Restorative Dentistry, Department of Oral Health Practice, College of Dentistry, University of Kentucky, 800 Rose Street, Lexington, KY 40536, USA
* Corresponding author.
E-mail address: malsa2@email.uky.edu

Dent Clin N Am 59 (2015) 73–95
http://dx.doi.org/10.1016/j.cden.2014.09.004
0011-8532/15/$ – see front matter © 2015 Elsevier Inc. All rights reserved.

alveolar bone, prevent soft tissue collapse, and minimize or eliminate the need for future bone augmentation procedures.

Histologically, 4 important changes may occur during the 5 stages of normal healing of the extraction site: External dimensional changes at the extraction socket, internal dimensional changes within the extraction socket, dimensional changes in a damaged extraction socket, and dimensional changes in the mucosa. The first stage of healing is characterized by the formation of a blood clot as a coagulum of red and white blood cells. The second stage is characterized by the formation of granulation tissue, which replaces the clot over 4 to 5 days. The third stage is characterized by the formation of connective tissue, which replaces granulation tissue over 14 to 16 days. The fourth stage is characterized by the appearance of osteoid calcification, which begins at the base and the periphery of the socket (early osteoid calcification is present within 7–10 days, and trabecular bone fills the socket by 6 weeks). The fifth stage is characterized by complete epithelial closure of the socket after 24 to 35 days (bone filling occurs between 5 and 10 weeks, and complete filling occurs by 16 weeks). Maximum osteoblastic activity occurs within 4 to 6 weeks.[3,4]

External dimensional changes at the extraction socket consist of horizontal or buccolingual ridge reduction of approximately 5 to 7 mm (almost 50% of the initial ridge width); this reduction occurs over a period of 6 to 12 months, although most of the changes occur during the first 3 months. Reduction in the apicocoronal or vertical height of 2.0 to 4.5 mm accompanies the horizontal change. Internal dimensional changes within extraction sockets, consisting of a reduction of 3 to 4 mm in the vertical height of the socket, or approximately 50% of the initial socket height, have been reported after 6 months of healing. Most of this bone loss occurs during the first 3 months after tooth extraction. Dimensional changes in damaged extraction sockets most likely consist of fibrous tissue that may occupy a portion of the socket, thereby preventing normal healing and osseous regeneration.[5]

Elevating the flap after extraction may compromise the blood supply of the thin buccal plate, which has little or no cancellous bone, resulting in partial or complete resorption of the buccal plate. At the surgically treated tooth site (full-thickness flap elevation) in dogs, the mean amount of bone loss is 1.0 mm buccal and 0.1 mm lingual. Surface bone resorption has a more pronounced effect on the delicate buccal bone than on the lingual bone.[6]

Fate of Buccal Bone

Buccal bone generally is thinner than lingual and palatal bone (**Fig. 1**). The crest of the buccal bone is composed solely of bundle bone. Buccal dehiscence and fenestration

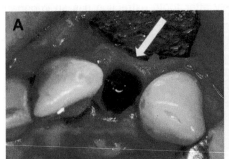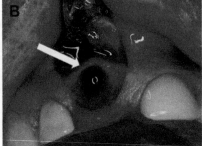

Fig. 1. (*A*) Thick buccal bone (*arrow*) of an extraction socket. (*B*) Thin buccal bone (*arrow*) of an extraction socket.

of the buccal plate of socket are frequently present. There are 3 main sources of blood supply to the alveolar bone around teeth: The periodontal ligament blood vessels, the periosteal blood vessels, and the alveolar bone blood vessels. After tooth removal, 20% of the blood supply from periodontal ligament blood vessels is discontinued. If a flap is elevated on the buccal side, the periosteal blood supply will be discontinued for 4 to 6 days, until new anastomoses occur. The thin cortical bone buccal plate has no endosteal blood vessels; therefore, complete resorption of the buccal plate may occur if no socket preservation technique is used.[7] Bone grafting is frequently used to prevent collapse and to minimize resorption of the thin buccal plate.[8] However, no comparative clinical studies have evaluated the fate and stability of the buccal bone over time with or without bone regeneration.

Immediate Implant Placement

Immediate implant placement is defined as the placement of an implant into the extraction socket at the time of tooth extraction. Immediate loading is defined as the placement of full occlusal or incisal loading on a dental implant restoration. Immediate provisionalization is a clinical protocol for the placement of an interim prosthesis, either with occlusal contact with the opposing dentition (ie, immediate occlusal loading) or without such occlusal contact (ie, immediate nonocclusal loading) at the same clinical visit during which the implant is placed. Delayed loading refers to applying force on an implant at some point after initial placement; a prosthesis is attached or secured after a conventional healing period (for the maxilla, 3–4 months; for the mandible, 2–3 months). Early loading refers applying force on an implant after initial placement; a prosthesis is attached to the implant(s) before the end of the conventional healing period.

There is variation in the descriptive terminology used in the dental literature to describe the timing of implant placement. In 2004, Hammerle and colleagues[9] published a consensus report containing a new classification system for the timing of implant placement. This classification is based on the structural changes that occur after extraction on and knowledge derived from clinical observations (**Table 1**).

OUTCOME AND ADVANTAGES OF IMMEDIATE IMPLANT PLACEMENT

Several retrospective, prospective, and randomized, controlled clinical studies have evaluated the clinical outcome of immediate placement of an implant in an extraction socket. Generally, clinical studies reported similar short-term and long-term survival rates (1–7 years) for immediate and delayed implant placement.[10–16] As reported by

Table 1
Timing of implant placement

Classification	Terminology	Time After Extraction	Clinical Findings
Type 1	Immediate implant placement	Immediately	Fresh extraction socket
Type 2	Early implant placement	4–6 wk	Healed soft tissue
Type 3	Delayed implant placement	3–4 mo	Healed soft tissue and substantial bone healing
Type 4	Late implant placement	>4 mo	Completely healed bone

Adapted from Hammerle CH, Chen ST, Wilson TG Jr. Consensus statements and recommended clinical procedures regarding the placement of implants in extraction sockets. Int J Oral Maxillofac Implants 2004;19(Suppl):26–8.

Lang and associates,[17] the survival rate of immediate implants is 97.3% to 99%. The effect of apical pathology on the survival of an implant immediately placed in an extraction socket is debatable. Some studies have found that the survival rates for implants placed immediately into infected sockets[18] and those for implants placed in noninfected socket or healed ridges are similar.[19,20]

Traditional guidelines have stressed the need for complete healing of the alveolar bone before an implant is placed into a fresh extraction socket, a process that usually requires several months.[21,22] This lengthy undisturbed healing period extends the time of oral functional disability and substantial resorption of the alveolar ridge may occur. Shanaman[23] and Denissen and co-workers[24] reported that the dimensions of the alveolar ridge can be maintained after immediate implant placement, whereas Werbitt and Goldberg[25] reported that soft tissue preservation is optimal after immediate implant placement. Immediate implant placement may reduce the number of operative interventions required and the treatment time.[26] The ideal orientation of the implant may be achieved.[27] Preserving the architecture of the hard and soft tissues at the extraction site may provide optimal restorative esthetics (**Table 2**).[23,28]

GUIDELINES FOR IMMEDIATE IMPLANT PLACEMENT

Several indications suggest that immediate placement may be an appropriate procedure with good oral hygiene; the presence of a single failing tooth with good adjacent dentition; the presence of adequate and harmonious gingival architecture with the surrounding dentition; adequate bone volume to accommodate an implant, with minimum dimensions of 3.5 × 10 mm and without the need for bone grafting; no dental trauma affecting the alveolar bone; osseous-level dental decay without purulence; and endodontic failure without periapical infection, a residual nonrestorable root, or root fracture (**Fig. 2**).[29] On the other hand, the following are contraindications for immediate placement: Active infection, lack of bone beyond the apex, a close relationship to anatomic vital structures (ie, mandibular canal, maxillary sinus, nasal cavity), dental history of bruxism, parafunctional habits, lack of stable posterior occlusion, perforation or loss of the labial bony plate after tooth removal, and inability to achieve primary stability (**Fig. 3**).[29] The most predictable method of successful immediate implant placement are maintenance of the soft tissue architecture with conservative tissue manipulation (ie, leaving the periosteum intact) to preserve the blood supply, maintenance of the buccal plate, and firm implant stability with a minimum torque value of 30 Ncm and an implant stability quotient of at least 60 (**Box 1**).

Micromovement

Micromovement caused by load peaks higher than friction hold is crucial. Micromovement of the implant can grind and slowly smooth the bone surface, thereby reducing

Table 2 Advantages and disadvantages of immediate implant placement	
Advantages	**Disadvantages**
One surgical procedure	Surgically demanding; complex procedure
Less treatment time	Risk of marginal mucosal recession
Preservation of bone at extraction site	Adjunct connective tissue graft
Reduction in cost	Adjunct bone graft or guided bone regeneration

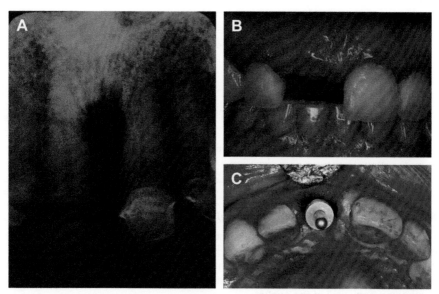

Fig. 2. Maxillary right incisor is nonrestorable. Site is suitable for immediate implant placement. (*A*) Adequate bone past the root apex for primary stability and no evidence of radiographic infection. (*B*) Thick gingival biotype with good adjacent dentition. (*C*) Intact thick buccal plate of the extraction socket.

the interlock between bone and titanium and ultimately resulting in a loss of primary stability. It is critical that there are no occlusal implant overloads during the early healing stage. Primary stability is important during the first days after implant installation. The first weeks are a crucial period because primary stability can decrease to critical levels before secondary stability develops. Any micromotion of more than 150 μm causes fibrous encapsulation of the implant. Therefore, patients should be compliant and should avoid high masticatory forces by eating only soft foods for at least for 6 weeks postoperatively.[30,31]

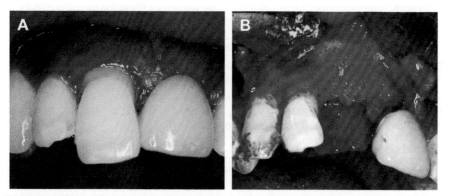

Fig. 3. Maxillary right central incisor has periodontal abscess. Site is not suitable for immediate implant placement. (*A*) Clinical sign of active infection (pus). (*B*) Significant loss of the extraction socket walls.

> **Box 1**
> **Criteria for immediate implant placement**
>
> - Low-risk patient
> - Low esthetic expectations
> - Adequate quality and quantity of soft tissue
> - Adequate quality and quantity of socket bone
> - Absence of diffuse infection
> - Healthy condition of adjacent teeth and supporting structures
> - Primary stability

Horizontal Bone Defect (Jumping Distance)

A horizontal bone defect is defined as the longest distance in a perpendicular direction from the implant surface to the socket wall.[32] In 2003, Botticelli and associates[33] introduced the term *jumping distance* at implant sites with a horizontal defect dimension; the jumping distance is the horizontal distance between the implant surface and the surrounding bony wall of the socket.

The need for bone grafting and the use of a barrier after immediate implant placement depend on the thickness of the labial plate and the size of the gap between the implant and the adjacent alveolar bone. Although a thick labial plate is generally resistant to resorption and grafting is unnecessary, bone grafting is frequently used to prevent collapse and minimize resorption of the thin labial plate, regardless of the gap size. Bone grafting aids in osteoconduction of osteogenic cells by preserving space and promoting the formation of new bone (the scaffold effect).[8] Human and animal studies have shown that, in implant sites with an horizontal defect dimension of 2 mm or less, spontaneous bone regeneration and osseointegration with adequate bone-to-implant contact can occur; however, if the horizontal defect dimension is larger than 2 mm, the use of a barrier membrane with or without membrane-supporting bone grafting material is warranted for achieving adequate bone-to-implant contact and proper osseointegration.[32,34,35] Botticelli and colleagues[36] reported that no bone grafting is needed even if the jumping distance is greater than 2 mm. In a case report study, Tarnow and colleagues[37] concluded that no bone graft, membrane, or primary closure is necessary for filling the jumping distance, provided that the buccal plate is intact after extraction (**Fig. 4**).

Submerged or Transmucosal Implant Placement

The submerged placement protocol was introduced by Brånemark and colleagues.[38] With this approach, the implant is sealed from the outer environment by the mucosa, and this sealing may decrease the chances of implant contamination.[39] However, several publications of clinical trials using the transmucosal approach for immediate implant placement reported successful outcome.[11,12,40]

Tapered or Parallel Side Implant Design

Tapered design implants were used in several clinical studies, and were reported with high success and survival rates in the immediate implant protocol. Because tapered implants are narrow apically and wide coronally, they have the advantage of filling the gap between the implant body and the socket wall at the crest level. It also improves the implant's primary stability, avoiding buccal wall engagement in the anterior

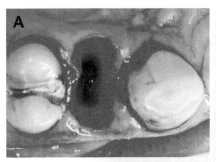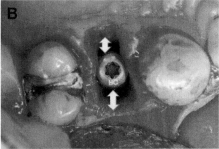

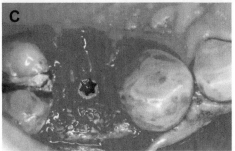

Fig. 4. Horizontal defect dimension (jumping distance). (*A*) Fresh extraction socket with intact walls. (*B*) Longest distance in a perpendicular direction from the implant surface to the socket wall (*arrows*). (*C*) The jumping distance was grafted with bone particulate.

region, and reducing the need for jumping distance augmentation.[41–43] McAllister and associates[41] reported safe and effective application after using variable thread tapered implants. Although the difference was not significant, Sanz and colleagues[43] reported less vertical and horizontal space using tapered implants than of cylindrical implants after immediate implant placements. However, Lang and colleagues[40] found in a clinical trial that both cylindrical and tapered implants have shown similar short-term outcomes with regard to wound healing and primary stability. Bone augmentation at the time of implant placement was required for both designs in transmucosal placement approach.

Rough Surface

Increased surface roughness of an implant can help to improve primary stability.[44] In a clinical study involving 1925 immediate implants placed from 1988 to 2004, Wagenberg and Froum[45] reported a higher success rate for immediate implants with rough surface than for immediate implants with machined surfaces.

Implant Design

The effect of the design of the implant collar or neck placed immediately after the tooth extraction on the peri-implant soft and hard tissues has been explored in several experimental studies.[46–48] They reported that implants with roughened and micro-threaded neck would cause less resorption of the crestal bone than implants with roughened and not microthreaded neck. These studies are in agreement with 1 clinical study involving delayed implant placement, which showed less marginal bone resorption around roughened and microthreaded neck than of machined neck.[49] The use of tapered platform-switched internal connection implants at the implant shoulder is recommended for immediate implant placement, because these implants can allow rapid rehabilitation with no adverse impact on implant survival.

GUIDELINES FOR PROVISIONALIZATION AND LOADING

The outcome of conventional implant loading is predictable in all clinical situations. It is highly recommended in instances of poor primary implant stability, substantial bone augmentation, small-diameter implants, and compromised host conditions.

Achieving primary stability is the key factor in the success of dental implants. Insertion torque is among the methods used for clinical assessment of primary stability. Insertion torque is the amount of torque required to place the dental implant into the prepared osteotomy. With the introduction of newer dental implant systems, various manufacturers have recommended different insertion torques: Low insertion torque, moderate insertion torque, and high insertion torque (32–70 Ncm).[50–52] Ottoni and colleagues[51] compared immediate-loading implants (test group) that were restored within 24 hours with a provisional crown and conventional-loading implants (control group) after healing. A minimal insertion torque of 20 Ncm was standard for attaining primary stability. The insertion torque was associated with the risk of implant failure for the test group but not for the control group, in which 9 implants failed when the insertion torque was 20 Ncm. The authors concluded that an initial insertion torque of greater than 32 Ncm is necessary for immediate loading of a dental implant with provisional restoration. Furthermore, adding 9.8 Ncm to the insertion torque decreases the risk of implant failure by 20%.[51] Atieh and colleagues[52] investigated the influence of insertion torque (32, 50, or 70 Ncm) and stress distribution on wide-diameter, tapered oral implants placed immediately in extraction sockets of mandibular molars. The authors found that the use of moderate insertion torque (32–50 Ncm) may reduce the risk of implant failure in an extraction socket. Furthermore, they found that the highest insertion torque of 70 Ncm introduced substantial stress and should be avoided during immediate placement of an implant into a fresh extraction socket. The use of higher insertion torque is linked to the introduction of stresses to the bone. These stresses can directly affect the stability of the dental implant or hinder the process of osseointegration by inducing micromovements, which can lead to failure. Cannizzaro and colleagues[50] used the split-mouth design to investigate the effect of medium insertion torque (25–35 Ncm) and high insertion torque (>80 Ncm) on single implants with immediate loading placed without flaps into 50 patients.[50] The patients were observed for 6 months after initial loading. Osseointegration failed for 7 implants placed with medium insertion torque (between 25 and 35 Ncm). On the other hand, none of the implants placed with insertion torque higher than 35 Ncm failed. The authors concluded that single implants with immediate loading should be placed with a higher insertion torque so that early implant failure can be prevented.

Marginal bone loss around immediately loaded implants is comparable with that associated with conventionally loaded implants. Ericsson and colleagues[53] reported crestal bone loss of 0.14 mm for immediate implant loading and 0.07 mm for conventional implant loading. Recent systematic reviews reported that immediate loading is associated with significantly less bone loss than conventional loading.[54,55]

Early implant failure can be minimized by avoiding lower insertion torque, especially for an implant associated with immediate or early loading. Immediate and early loading require high insertion torque (30–35 Ncm), an implant stability quotient of at least 60, and minimal implant length (≥10 mm), as well as the absence of contraindications such as parafunctional activities, large bone defects, and the need for sinus floor elevation.

SURGICAL TECHNIQUES

Implant placement in a fresh extraction socket was first introduced by Schulte and associates.[56] Since then, the immediate replacement of a missing tooth has been considered a time-effective approach.[26,57] The buccal plate is usually more vulnerable to resorption after extraction.[2] Using an atraumatic extraction technique that results in minimal trauma to hard and soft tissues is a key factor in immediate or delayed implant placement.[58] Generally, surgical elevation of a mucoperiosteal flap and tooth sectioning are used when the clinician believes that excessive force would be necessary to remove the tooth, when a substantial amount of the crown is missing or covered by tissue, or when access to the root of a tooth is difficult, such as when a fragile crown is present.[59] Flapless and flap techniques for immediate implant placement have favorable hard tissue and soft tissue outcomes.[60] Flapless implants are feasible and have been shown to reduce postoperative discomfort for correctly selected patients.[61,62]

The concept of atraumatic extraction includes managing the soft and hard tissues around the tooth. Atraumatic extraction may include placing an intrasulcular incision 360° around the tooth to cut the connective tissue fibers above the bone and to detach the connective tissue fibers from the cementum.[58] The interproximal contact surfaces should be trimmed to facilitate the application of the periotome and the elevator and to clear the path of tooth removal.[58] The periotome is usually pushed into to the periodontal ligament space with light mallet tapping along the crestal third of the interproximal bone. This process should take 10 to 30 seconds, after which a forceps is used with controlled force to luxate the tooth before extraction (**Fig. 5**).[58] For

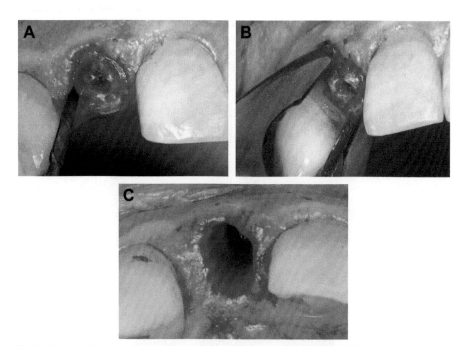

Fig. 5. Atraumatic extraction with integrity of alveolus maintained. (*A*) Periotome is pushed into the periodontal ligament along the crestal third of the interproximal bone to luxate the maxillary right lateral tooth. (*B*) Titan forceps is used to atraumatically extract the tooth. (*C*) The tooth was extracted with the preservation of soft and bone tissues of the extraction socket.

multirooted teeth, root sectioning and separation are advisable (**Fig. 6**).[63] A drilling depth of 4 to 6 mm is required for sectioning the upper first and second molars, whereas a drilling depth of 3 to 4 mm is required for the lower first and second molars. A long fine bur is recommended for sectioning the roots.[64] All granulation tissue should be removed from the extraction socket.

The osteotomy for an immediate placement of anterior implant could be initiated more palatally (**Fig. 7**), whereas for premolars and molars the osteotomy could be initiated toward the center of the socket. A Lindemann bur (Komet Dental, Lemgo, Germany) or a small (number 2) round bur is recommended for creating the initial hole in the extraction socket before the implant twist drills are used.

For the posterior region, the crown of the molar should be cut off horizontally. The roots should be carefully separated, and the inter-radicular bone within the socket should be maintained for use in osteotomy preparation. The Piezo procedure may be used to assist in removal of the ankylosed roots. A round bur should be positioned off center toward the lingual side of the inter-radicular septum. This positioning allows for preparation of the implant placement site in a centrally located position but away from the buccal bone plate. To compensate for natural bone resorption after tooth extraction, the implant site must allow the implant to be seated 1 to 2 mm below the margin of the intact buccal bony wall. If the residual jumping distance is more than 2 mm wide, a bone graft should be used.[65–68]

Special attention should be paid to the restoratively driven 3-dimensional positioning of the implants.[69] Immediate implant placement should always follow the rule of restorative-driven 3-dimensional placement not only to provide functional replacement of missing teeth, but also to satisfy the esthetic needs of the patient particularly in the esthetic zone. More guidance on the proper 3-dimensional placement of dental implants is provided by an article published in 2006 (**Fig. 8**).[70]

For adequate primary stability, immediate implants should be placed few millimeters beyond the socket[39] or 3 to 5 mm past the apex.[63] The diameter of the implant

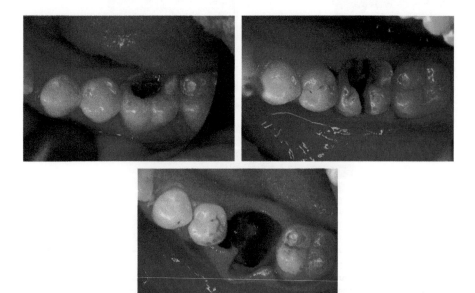

Fig. 6. Root sectioning in the buccal lingual direction of mandibular molar.

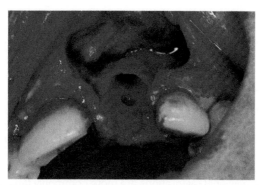

Fig. 7. The initial hole for the preparation of implant osteotomy should be placed on the conjunction of the middle and apical thirds of the lingual wall of the extraction socket of maxillary anterior teeth.

should exceed the root diameter, and primary stability must be obtained with a pristine apical and lateral socket wall.[63]

If the clinician believes that the existing socket precludes the attainment of primary stability for an appropriately sized implant in an ideal restorative position, immediate implant placement should be avoided, and guided bone regeneration and delayed implant placement can be undertaken. The implant should not touch the buccal plate of the socket wall in the maxillary anterior teeth, because such touching could cause resorption of buccal plate and esthetic risk.[71–73] The implant must be placed at least 1 mm subcrestally, especially if the buccal or lingual plates are thin,[63] or 2 to 3 mm below the gingival margin.[74] The extraction and the placement of the implant should be flapless, when possible,[62] or can use a sulcular incision, 1 tooth mesial and 1 tooth distal to the implant site, which could help to expose the buccal bone.[61]

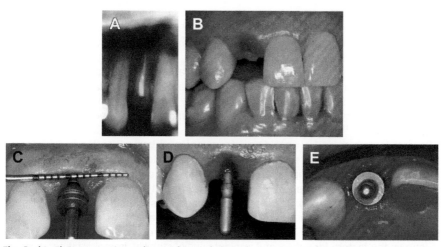

Fig. 8. (*A, B*) Preoperative radiographic and clinical assessment of maxillary right lateral for immediate implant placement. (*C*) Intraoperative assessment of apicocoronal placement of immediate implant. (*D*) Intraoperative assessment of mesiodistal placement of immediate implant. (*E*) Intraoperative assessment of buccolingual placement of immediate implant.

After immediate implant placement, the jumping distance or the horizontal gap between the implant and the buccal surface should be filled with bone fill if the gap is larger than 2 mm.[35,75] All types of bone fill are effective for closing the horizontal gap (**Tables 3** and **4**).[5]

Provisional Options

The key elements in preserving ridge contour are protection and maintenance of the bone graft during the healing phase of treatment, which can extend for several months. A contoured healing abutment or provisional restoration provides these elements to the bone graft. The alternative to using a contoured healing abutment is the fabrication of a screw-retained provisional restoration.

Screw-retained provisional restorations are more commonly fabricated of autopolymerizing acrylic resin in infra-occlusion than are cement-retained restorations. Excess cement may compromise peri-implant tissues if it is not completely removed. The provisional restorations should have subgingival contours that conform to support the soft tissue emergence profile and help to protect the blood clot as well as any graft particles that may be placed.

In cases that do not involve immediate provisional restoration, a straight healing abutment or a stock contoured healing abutment should be placed. A fixed partial denture is more suitable than a removable partial denture in preventing any pressure or movement at the surgical site. Moreover, the pontic can be modified to avoid contact with the healing abutment.

Immediate provisional restoration can control displacement of the available soft tissue around a single implant to create the desired soft tissue contour. Provisional restorations allow evaluation of esthetic parameters before treatment is completed and provide comfort and psychological advantages for the patient. The cervical contour of the temporary restoration will guide the scallop of the gingival margin and the height of the interdental papillae.[77,78]

Loading of Single or Multiple Implants

Published studies have shown that the success rate for immediately loaded implants is similar to that for delayed loaded implants.[79,80] Patients who are partially or fully edentulous may be predictably restored with a fixed prosthesis immediately upon implant placement if certain criteria are met.

Immediate loading of implants has biologic advantages: It increases bone density around the implant, increases bone remodeling around the implant, and provides bone-to-implant contact similar that achieved by delayed loading of implants, as demonstrated histologically. Immediately loaded implants exhibited bone-to-implant contact of 92.9%.[81,82]

Several factors must be considered for successful immediate loading. Creating cross-arch stabilization by splinting multiple implants together, placing implants in bone of higher density, using tapered implants to provide a wedging effect, placing long wide-diameter implants with a minimum height of 10 mm and a minimum width of 4 mm, and using a rough surface implant increases the surface area for better osseointegration.[83] A major disadvantage of immediate loading of implants is that no second-stage procedure is performed, so there is no chance to modify soft tissue. As long as the factors for successful implants (initial stability, immobilization, and patient compliance) are met and the principle of no movement greater than 150 μm is fulfilled, even in bone with poor quality, and even in periodontally involved cases, success can be achieved with immediate loading.

Table 3
Surgical exploration for immediate implant placement

Consideration	Details
Difficulty of extraction	a. Atraumatic (careful luxation, possible use of a periosteotome for anterior teeth, consider flapless procedure) b. Difficult
Anatomy of the socket	a. Buccal cortical wall thickness b. Buccal wall integrity: Fenestration or dehiscence The most important aspects of an extraction site in determining its suitability for immediate implantation are: The number of remaining walls The preexisting amount of attachment loss The position and condition of the arch This is one of the most important parts of decision making because it determines the need for more advanced procedures, such as GBR or CTG
Availability of bone past the apex of the root	a. Ample $\geq$4 mm: Suitable for immediate implant placement b. Limited: Primary stability may not be achieved in certain sites
Primary stability	a. Absence of axial or lateral mobility with physical resistance to rotation b. Place depth gauge and compare depth with proposed length and width of implant c. If inadequate primary stability, immediate implant placement is not recommended
Implant positioning	Restoration-driven implant positioning should be achieved in 3 dimensions for optimal esthetic treatment outcome a. Buccolingual b. Mesiodistal c. Apicocoronal d. Angulation
HDD	a. HDD < 2 mm: Augmentation not required, defect will heal spontaneously b. HDD > 2 mm: Will not heal predictably; augmentation required
Adjunct therapy	a. Intact thick buccal bone with thick gingival biotype: Immediate implant placement, consider flapless procedure b. Intact thick buccal bone, thin scalloped biotype: Immediate implant placement, consider CTG c. Intact thin buccal bone and thick scalloped biotype: Immediate implant placement with flapless procedure and grafting of facial jumping distance d. Intact thin buccal bone and thin scalloped biotype: Possible immediate implant placement in low-risk patients with flapless procedure and grafting of facial jumping distance in addition to staged CTG c. Small defect in buccal bone, but implant can be placed with stability: Possible immediate implant placement with GBR with or without staged CTG d. Major defect in buccal bone, implant will not be placed in optimal position: Consider delayed implant placement

Abbreviations: CTG, connective tissue graft; GBR, guided bone regeneration; HDD, horizontal defect dimension.

Table 4
Recommendations for osteotomy preparation for immediate implant placement

Teeth	Initial Osteotomy Preparation	Attainment of Primary Stability
Maxillary anterior teeth	Initial hole should be placed on the conjunction of the middle and apical thirds of the lingual wall of the extraction socket. Engagement of buccal wall of the extraction socket with implant body should be avoided.	Apical: Provide the prime stability by engaging 3–4 mm of native bone past the apex of the socket. Horizontal: Provide additional stability by engaging the palatal wall of the socket with the implant body.
Maxillary premolar teeth	Attempt to place the initial hole in the middle but slightly toward the lingual of the socket. If a furcation septum exists, slightly remove the inter-radicular bone crest until enough septal bone width is attained. If initial drilling through the septum is unsuccessful, the initial hole can be placed in the apical side of the palatal socket and more toward the center. No engagement of the buccal bone by the body of the implant.	Apical: Provide additional stability by engaging 3–4 mm of native bone past the apex of socket, if available. Horizontal: Provide the prime stability by engaging the mesial and distal, and sometime the palatal, wall of the socket with the implant body.
Maxillary molar teeth	Immediate placement is generally is not recommended; however, if roots are divergent, osteotomy preparation can be initiated by drilling into the center of the inter-radicular bone. If a narrow septum exists, slightly remove the inter-radicular bone crest until enough septal bone width is attained. It is not recommend using the palatal root as a site of immediate implant placement because restorative-driven 3-dimensional placement of the implant may not be achieved. The implant neck may engage the mesial, distal, and palatal plate of the extraction socket.	Apical: Provide the prime stability by engaging 3–4 mm of native bone past the apex of socket. Horizontal: May provide primary stability in case of neumatized maxillary sinus by engaging the palatal, mesial, and distal wall of the socket with the wide implant body.
Mandibular anterior teeth	Initial osteotomy preparation should be straight through the middle of the socket.	Apical: Provide the prime stability by engaging 3–4 mm of native bone past the apex of the socket. Horizontal: No engagement of buccal, lingual, mesial, or distal walls of the socket by the narrow implant body is recommended.
Mandibular premolar teeth	Initial osteotomy preparation should be straight through the middle of the socket.	Apical: Provide additional stability by engaging 3–4 mm of native bone past the apex of socket, if available. Horizontal: Provide the prime stability by engaging the lingual, mesial, and distal walls of the socket with the implant body.

(continued on next page)

Teeth	Initial Osteotomy Preparation	Attainment of Primary Stability
Table 4 (*continued*)		
Mandibular molars	If roots are divergent, osteotomy preparation can be initiated by drilling into the center of the inter-radicular bone. If a narrow furcation septum exists, slightly remove the inert-radicular bone crest until enough septal bone width is attained. If unsuccessful, the initial hole can be placed in the apical of mesial or distal root of the socket and more toward the center, opposing the lingual maxillary cusp. It is not recommend using the mesial or distal root as a site of immediate implant placement because restorative-driven 3-dimensional placement of the implant may not be achieved.	Apical: Provide additional stability by the engagement of 3–4 mm of native bone pass the apex of socket, if available. Horizontal: Provide the prime stability by the engagement of the buccal, lingual, mesial and distal wall of socket by the wide implant body.

Data from Refs.[63,69,76]

PREVENTION OF COMPLICATIONS ASSOCIATED WITH IMMEDIATE IMPLANT PLACEMENT

Although immediate implant placement is associated with high success rates and survival rates, complications can occur. The most common complications are poor 3-dimensional implant positioning, inadequate band of keratinized tissue, gingival recession, unacceptable esthetics, and implant failure because of surgical trauma, contamination of the surgical field, premature loading, implant design, anatomic limitations such as quality and quantity of bone, systemic factors, and unknown factors. Implant failure can be classified as early when osseointegration is not achieved or as late when achieved osseointegration is lost after function begins. Early implant failure is caused by inability to regenerate intimate bone-to-implant contact, resulting in impaired wound healing after implant placement. Clinical indications of early implant failure are bone loss, implant mobility, pain or other symptoms during function, and biological infection.[84,85]

Fenestration or Dehiscence

The complications of fenestration and dehiscence have been reported to occur after immediate implant placement.[39] The most commons area for fenestration during the immediate implant placement are the maxillary anterior and premolar sockets. The socket apex can be more facially oriented and is frequently misleading during the initiation of the osteotomy preparation. A round bur positioned off center toward the palatal side and along the alveolar ridge angulation reduces the chance of fenestration of facial plate of the alveolar ridge. When these complications occur, spontaneous bone regeneration may be possible; however, in some cases, delayed implant placement is advisable.[86,87] For managing fenestration or dehiscence, a resorbable or nonresorbable membrane can be used with or without bone particulate from various sources.[5,88] However, bone augmentation techniques may lead to suboptimal bone-to-implant contact and soft tissue esthetics, especially when achieving primary closure of the surgical site is difficult (**Fig. 9**).[89,90]

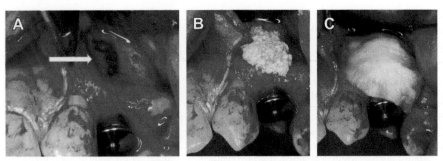

Fig. 9. Fenestration of the buccal plate during immediate placement of implant in a fresh extraction socket of maxillary premolar. (*A*) Penetration of apex of the implant through the buccal bony plate (*arrow*). (*B*) Primary stability is achieved and bone graft particles were placed. (*C*) Collagen membrane was placed on the bone particulates.

Bone Quality and Quantity

Implant failure rates are higher when the quality and quantity of bone at the implant site are insufficient. Attaining primary stability is a prerequisite for successful osseointegration, and accomplishing primary stability requires adequate bone quantity and density. An osteotome can be used to condense spongy trabecular bone, such as that found in the posterior maxillary region. Packing of bone graft particulate and the simultaneous use of an osteotome may transform very spongy bone into more dense bone (**Fig. 10**).

Gingival Biotype and Width of Keratinized Gingiva

The dental literature is inconclusive with regard to the effect of the presence or absence of adequate keratinized gingiva around dental implants on the success or

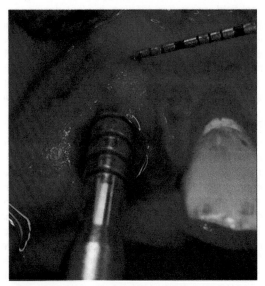

Fig. 10. The use of osteotome with packing of bone graft material into an extraction socket to expand the extraction socket and condense the spongy trabecular bone to increase the primary stability.

failure of an implant. Recession can be avoided and the long-term stability of the mucosal tissue around the implant can be ensured by the use of adjunct soft tissue grafting. Authors of current article recommend following the adjunct soft tissue therapy guidelines described in **Table 3**.

Surgical Trauma

Bone is viable and is sensitive to temperature. Overheating the bone during preparation of the implant osteotomy site can lead to necrosis of the bone tissue surrounding the dental implant. Less surgical trauma is expected when clinicians are skillful and experienced, and the clinician's skill is an important factor in the successful outcome of dental implants.

Overheating the bone should be avoided by using copious irrigation and periodic replacement of twist drills to ensure sharpness. The implant manufacturer's guidelines for drilling speed should be followed, and low hand pressure is warranted during high-speed drilling in dense bone.

Infection

Strict antiseptic protocol should be followed during surgical implant placement. Premedication with broad-spectrum antibiotics is recommended. Thorough debridement of contained infection in the extraction socket and excavation of all of the soft and granulation tissues are necessary. In cases of active diffuse infection, delayed implant placement is recommended.

Violation of Anatomic Structure

The availability of 3 to 5 mm of bone past the apex of the root is often necessary for primary stability and is helpful for avoiding the violation of surrounding anatomic structures. The implementation of a vertical sinus lift with an osteotome and the placement of a wide-neck implant decrease the likelihood of introducing an immediate implant into the maxillary sinus cavity. Obtaining cross-sectional radiographic images for locating the maxillary sinus, the nasal cavity, the inferior alveolar canal, and the lingual undercut (submandibular fossa) is helpful for avoiding the violation of these anatomic structure because it ensures at least 2 mm of clearance between the implant apex and the surrounding structures.

Implant Stability

Primary stability and success of implants are more likely when implants are supported by cortical bone. Bicortical anchorage is associated with some complications, but it results in good primary stability and better distribution of loading forces than moncortical anchorage.

Malpositioning of Implant

Restoration-driven implant position must be correct in 3 dimensions for optimal functional and esthetic outcomes. Correction of integrated malpositioned implants is difficult and limited to prosthetic correction; otherwise, removal of the implant is warranted. Buccolingual, mesiodistal, and apicocoronal angulation of an implant immediately placed into an extraction socket is reviewed in an article published in 2006.[70]

Unesthetic Outcome

Certain esthetic complications are associated with immediate implant placement. For example, tissue alterations leading to recession of the facial mucosa and papillae are common after immediate placement. Indicators of risk of recession after immediate placement include a thin tissue biotype, a facial malpositioning of the implant, and a thin or damaged facial bone wall. A history of chronic periodontitis is an indicator of risk of lack of survival of postextraction implants.[91,92]

In studies with observation period of 3 years or longer, approximately 20% of patients who underwent immediate implant placement and delayed restoration experienced suboptimal aesthetic outcomes because of buccal soft tissue recession[17]

For optimal esthetic outcome and limiting of buccal mucosal recession, Tarnow and colleagues[37] recommend placing a bone graft and contoured healing abutment or provisional restoration at the time of flapless implant placement in a postextraction socket. For long-term stability of the mucosal tissue around the implant, the authors of current article recommend following the guidelines of the use of an adjunct soft and bone tissue grafting (see **Table 3**).

SUMMARY

Several clinical studies have reported successful outcome of immediate placement of dental implants in fresh extraction sockets. Although immediate implant placement has several advantages over delayed implant placement, it, like any other procedure, is associated with risks and complications. Treatment protocols and guidelines should be followed to prevent complications. Case selection and evaluation of patient-related and implant-related factors are keys to the success of immediate implant placement. A thorough discussion between practitioner and patient is indispensable to discern patient's desires. Practitioners need to consider these desires when planning immediate, early, or delayed implant placement.

REFERENCES

1. Mecall RA, Rosenfeld AL. Influence of residual ridge resorption patterns on implant fixture placement and tooth position. 1. Int J Periodontics Restorative Dent 1991;11(1):8–23.
2. Schropp L, Wenzel A, Kostopoulos L, et al. Bone healing and soft tissue contour changes following single-tooth extraction: a clinical and radiographic 12-month prospective study. Int J Periodontics Restorative Dent 2003;23(4):313–23.
3. Amler MH. The time sequence of tissue regeneration in human extraction wounds. Oral Surg Oral Med Oral Pathol 1969;27(3):309–18.
4. Cardaropoli G, Araujo M, Lindhe J. Dynamics of bone tissue formation in tooth extraction sites. An experimental study in dogs. J Clin Periodontol 2003;30(9): 809–18.
5. Chen ST, Wilson TG Jr, Hammerle CH. Immediate or early placement of implants following tooth extraction: review of biologic basis, clinical procedures, and outcomes. Int J Oral Maxillofac Implants 2004;19(Suppl):12–25.
6. Araujo MG, Sukekava F, Wennstrom JL, et al. Ridge alterations following implant placement in fresh extraction sockets: an experimental study in the dog. J Clin Periodontol 2005;32(6):645–52.
7. Lindhe J, Lang NP, Karring T. Clinical periodontology and implant dentistry 2008. 5th edition. New York: Wiley-Blackwell; 2008.
8. Kan JY, Rungcharassaeng K. Immediate placement and provisionalization of maxillary anterior single implants: a surgical and prosthodontic rationale. Pract Periodontics Aesthet Dent 2000;12(9):817–24 [quiz: 826].

9. Hammerle CH, Chen ST, Wilson TG Jr. Consensus statements and recommended clinical procedures regarding the placement of implants in extraction sockets. Int J Oral Maxillofac Implants 2004;19(Suppl):26–8.

10. Gelb DA. Immediate implant surgery: three-year retrospective evaluation of 50 consecutive cases. Int J Oral Maxillofac Implants 1993;8(4):388–99.

11. Lang NP, Bragger U, Hammerle CH, et al. Immediate transmucosal implants using the principle of guided tissue regeneration. I. Rationale, clinical procedures and 30-month results. Clin Oral Implants Res 1994;5(3):154–63.

12. Bragger U, Hammerle CH, Lang NP. Immediate transmucosal implants using the principle of guided tissue regeneration (II). A cross-sectional study comparing the clinical outcome 1 year after immediate to standard implant placement. Clin Oral Implants Res 1996;7(3):268–76.

13. Rosenquist B, Grenthe B. Immediate placement of implants into extraction sockets: implant survival. Int J Oral Maxillofac Implants 1996;11(2):205–9.

14. Schwartz-Arad D, Grossman Y, Chaushu G. The clinical effectiveness of implants placed immediately into fresh extraction sites of molar teeth. J Periodontol 2000; 71(5):839–44.

15. Gomez-Roman G, Kruppenbacher M, Weber H, et al. Immediate postextraction implant placement with root-analog stepped implants: surgical procedure and statistical outcome after 6 years. Int J Oral Maxillofac Implants 2001;16(4): 503–13.

16. Goldstein M, Boyan BD, Schwartz Z. The palatal advanced flap: a pedicle flap for primary coverage of immediately placed implants. Clin Oral Implants Res 2002; 13(6):644–50.

17. Lang NP, Pun L, Lau KY, et al. A systematic review on survival and success rates of implants placed immediately into fresh extraction sockets after at least 1 year. Clin Oral Implants Res 2012;23(Suppl 5):39–66.

18. Waasdorp JA, Evian CI, Mandracchia M. Immediate placement of implants into infected sites: a systematic review of the literature. J Periodontol 2010;81(6): 801–8.

19. Crespi R, Cappare P, Gherlone E. Fresh-socket implants in periapical infected sites in humans. J Periodontol 2010;81(3):378–83.

20. Crespi R, Cappare P, Gherlone E. Immediate loading of dental implants placed in periodontally infected and non-infected sites: a 4-year follow-up clinical study. J Periodontol 2010;81(8):1140–6.

21. Adell R, Lekholm U, Rockler B, et al. A 15-year study of osseointegrated implants in the treatment of the edentulous jaw. Int J Oral Surg 1981;10(6):387–416.

22. Albrektsson T, Zarb G, Worthington P, et al. The long-term efficacy of currently used dental implants: a review and proposed criteria of success. Int J Oral Maxillofac Implants 1986;1(1):11–25.

23. Shanaman RH. The use of guided tissue regeneration to facilitate ideal prosthetic placement of implants. Int J Periodontics Restorative Dent 1992;12(4): 256–65.

24. Denissen HW, Kalk W, Veldhuis HA, et al. Anatomic consideration for preventive implantation. Int J Oral Maxillofac Implants 1993;8(2):191–6.

25. Werbitt MJ, Goldberg PV. The immediate implant: bone preservation and bone regeneration. Int J Periodontics Restorative Dent 1992;12(3):206–17.

26. Lazzara RJ. Immediate implant placement into extraction sites: surgical and restorative advantages. Int J Periodontics Restorative Dent 1989;9(5):332–43.

27. Schultz AJ. Guided tissue regeneration (GTR) of nonsubmerged implants in immediate extraction sites. Pract Periodontics Aesthet Dent 1993;5(2):59–65 [quiz: 66].

28. Kalk W, Denissen HW, Kayser AF. Preventive goals in oral implantology. Int Dent J 1993;43(5):483–91.
29. Schwartz-Arad D, Chaushu G. Placement of implants into fresh extraction sites: 4 to 7 years retrospective evaluation of 95 immediate implants. J Periodontol 1997; 68(11):1110–6.
30. Wohrle PS. Single-tooth replacement in the aesthetic zone with immediate provisionalization: fourteen consecutive case reports. Pract Periodontics Aesthet Dent 1998;10(9):1107–14 [quiz: 1116].
31. Gapski R, Wang HL, Mascarenhas P, et al. Critical review of immediate implant loading. Clin Oral Implants Res 2003;14(5):515–27.
32. Wilson TG Jr, Schenk R, Buser D, et al. Implants placed in immediate extraction sites: a report of histologic and histometric analyses of human biopsies. Int J Oral Maxillofac Implants 1998;13(3):333–41.
33. Botticelli D, Berglundh T, Buser D, et al. The jumping distance revisited: an experimental study in the dog. Clin Oral Implants Res 2003;14(1):35–42.
34. Wilson TG Jr. Guided tissue regeneration around dental implants in immediate and recent extraction sites: initial observations. Int J Periodontics Restorative Dent 1992;12(3):185–93.
35. Paolantonio M, Dolci M, Scarano A, et al. Immediate implantation in fresh extraction sockets. A controlled clinical and histological study in man. J Periodontol 2001; 72(11):1560–71.
36. Botticelli D, Berglundh T, Lindhe J. Hard-tissue alterations following immediate implant placement in extraction sites. J Clin Periodontol 2004;31(10):820–8.
37. Tarnow DP, Chu SJ, Salama MA, et al. Flapless postextraction socket implant placement in the esthetic zone: part 1. The effect of bone grafting and/or provisional restoration on facialpalatal ridge dimensional change-a retrospective cohort study. Int J Periodontics Restorative Dent 2014;34(3):323–31.
38. Brånemark PI, Adell R, Breine U, et al. Intra-osseous anchorage of dental prostheses. I. Experimental studies. Scand J Plast Reconstr Surg 1969; 3(2):81–100.
39. Schropp L, Isidor F. Timing of implant placement relative to tooth extraction. J Oral Rehabil 2008;35(Suppl 1):33–43.
40. Lang NP, Tonetti MS, Suvan JE, et al. Immediate implant placement with transmucosal healing in areas of aesthetic priority. A multicentre randomized-controlled clinical trial I. Surgical outcomes. Clin Oral Implants Res 2007; 18(2):188–96.
41. McAllister BS, Cherry JE, Kolinski ML, et al. Two-year evaluation of a variable-thread tapered implant in extraction sites with immediate temporization: a multicenter clinical trial. Int J Oral Maxillofac Implants 2012;27(3):611–8.
42. Kolinski ML, Cherry JE, McAllister BS, et al. Evaluation of a variable-thread tapered implant in extraction sites with immediate temporization: a 3-year multicenter clinical study. J Periodontol 2014;85(3):386–94.
43. Sanz M, Cecchinato D, Ferrus J, et al. A prospective, randomized-controlled clinical trial to evaluate bone preservation using implants with different geometry placed into extraction sockets in the maxilla. Clin Oral Implants Res 2010; 21(1):13–21.
44. Simon Z, Watson PA. Biomimetic dental implants–new ways to enhance osseointegration. J Can Dent Assoc 2002;68(5):286–8.
45. Wagenberg B, Froum SJ. A retrospective study of 1925 consecutively placed immediate implants from 1988 to 2004. Int J Oral Maxillofac Implants 2006;21(1): 71–80.

46. Calvo-Guirado JL, Lopez-Lopez PJ, Mate Sanchez de Val JE, et al. Influence of collar design on peri-implant tissue healing around immediate implants: a pilot study in Foxhound dogs. Clin Oral Implants Res 2014. [Epub ahead of print].

47. Calvo-Guirado JL, Boquete-Castro A, Negri B, et al. Crestal bone reactions to immediate implants placed at different levels in relation to crestal bone. A pilot study in Foxhound dogs. Clin Oral Implants Res 2014;25(3):344–51.

48. Negri B, Calvo-Guirado JL, Pardo-Zamora G, et al. Peri-implant bone reactions to immediate implants placed at different levels in relation to crestal bone. Part I: a pilot study in dogs. Clin Oral Implants Res 2012;23(2):228–35.

49. Nickenig HJ, Wichmann M, Schlegel KA, et al. Radiographic evaluation of marginal bone levels adjacent to parallel-screw cylinder machined-neck implants and rough-surfaced microthreaded implants using digitized panoramic radiographs. Clin Oral Implants Res 2009;20(6):550–4.

50. Cannizzaro G, Leone M, Ferri V, et al. Immediate loading of single implants inserted flapless with medium or high insertion torque: a 6-month follow-up of a split-mouth randomised controlled trial. Eur J Oral Implantol 2012;5(4):333–42.

51. Ottoni JM, Oliveira ZF, Mansini R, et al. Correlation between placement torque and survival of single-tooth implants. Int J Oral Maxillofac Implants 2005;20(5):769–76.

52. Atieh MA, Alsabeeha NH, Payne AG, et al. Insertion torque of immediate wide-diameter implants: a finite element analysis. Quintessence Int 2012;43(9):e115–26.

53. Ericsson I, Nilson H, Lindh T, et al. Immediate functional loading of Branemark single tooth implants. An 18 months' clinical pilot follow-up study. Clin Oral Implants Res 2000;11(1):26–33.

54. Sanz-Sanchez I, Sanz-Martin I, Figuero E, et al. Clinical efficacy of immediate implant loading protocols compared to conventional loading depending on the type of the restoration: a systematic review. Clin Oral Implants Res 2014. [Epub ahead of print].

55. Kinaia BM, Shah M, Neely AL, et al. Crestal bone level changes around immediately placed implants: a systematic review and meta-analyses with at least 12 months follow up after functional loading. J Periodontol 2014. [Epub ahead of print].

56. Schulte W, Kleineikenscheidt H, Lindner K, et al. The Tubingen immediate implant in clinical studies. Dtsch Zahnarztl Z 1978;33(5):348–59 [in German].

57. Parel SM, Triplett RG. Immediate fixture placement: a treatment planning alternative. Int J Oral Maxillofac Implants 1990;5(4):337–45.

58. Misch CE, Suzuki JB. Tooth extraction, socket grafting, and barrier membrane bone regeneration. In: Misch CE, editor. Contemporary implant dentistry. 3rd edition. St Louis (MO): Mosby; 2008. p. 870–6.

59. Hupp JR, Ellis E, Tucker MR, editors. Contemporary oral and maxillofacial surgery. 5th edition. St Louis (MO): Mosby; 2008.

60. Esposito M, Grusovin MG, Pdyzos IP, et al. Interventions for replacing missing teeth: different times for loading dental implants. Cochrane Database Syst Rev 2009;(1):CD003878.

61. Capelli M, Testori T, Galli F, et al. Implant-buccal plate distance as diagnostic parameter: a prospective cohort study on implant placement in fresh extraction sockets. J Periodontol 2013;84(12):1768–74.

62. Guarnieri R, Ceccherini A, Grande M. Single-tooth replacement in the anterior maxilla by means of immediate implantation and early loading: clinical and aesthetic results at 5 years. Clin Implant Dent Relat Res 2013. [Epub ahead of print].

63. Greenstein G, Cavallaro J. Immediate dental implant placement: technique, part I. Dent Today 2014;33(1):98, 100–4; [quiz: 105].

64. Greenstein G, Caton J, Polson A. Trisection of maxillary molars: a clinical technique. Compend Contin Educ Dent 1984;5(8):624–6, 631–2.

65. Annual award for clinical research in periodontology. Int J Periodontics Restorative Dent 2003;23(2):111.

66. Wilson TG Jr, Roccuzzo M, Ucer C, et al. Immediate placement of tapered effect (TE) implants: 5-year results of a prospective, multicenter study. Int J Oral Maxillofac Implants 2013;28(1):261–9.

67. Vandeweghe S, Hattingh A, Wennerberg A, et al. Surgical protocol and short-term clinical outcome of immediate placement in molar extraction sockets using a wide body implant. J Oral Maxillofac Res 2011;2(3):e1.

68. Froum SJ. Immediate placement of implants into extraction sockets: rationale, outcomes, technique. Alpha Omegan 2005;98(2):20–35.

69. Buser D, Martin W, Belser UC. Optimizing esthetics for implant restorations in the anterior maxilla: anatomic and surgical considerations. Int J Oral Maxillofac Implants 2004;19(Suppl):43–61.

70. Al-Sabbagh M. Implants in the esthetic zone. Dent Clin North Am 2006;50(3):391–407, vi.

71. Caneva M, Salata LA, de Souza SS, et al. Hard tissue formation adjacent to implants of various size and configuration immediately placed into extraction sockets: an experimental study in dogs. Clin Oral Implants Res 2010;21(9):885–90.

72. Caneva M, Botticelli D, Salata LA, et al. Collagen membranes at immediate implants: a histomorphometric study in dogs. Clin Oral Implants Res 2010;21(9):891–7.

73. Vela X, Mendez V, Rodriguez X, et al. Crestal bone changes on platform-switched implants and adjacent teeth when the tooth-implant distance is less than 1.5 mm. Int J Periodontics Restorative Dent 2012;32(2):149–55.

74. Sorni-Broker M, Penarrocha-Diago M. Factors that influence the position of the peri-implant soft tissues: a review. Med Oral Patol Oral Cir Bucal 2009;14(9):e475–9.

75. Covani U, Cornelini R, Barone A. Bucco-lingual bone remodeling around implants placed into immediate extraction sockets: a case series. J Periodontol 2003;74(2):268–73.

76. Cavallaro J, Greenstein G. Immediate dental implant placement: technique, part 2. Dent Today 2014;33(2):94, 96–8; [quiz: 99].

77. Mitrani R, Phillips K, Kois JC. An implant-supported, screw-retained, provisional fixed partial denture for pontic site enhancement. Pract Proced Aesthet Dent 2005;17(10):673–8 [quiz: 680].

78. Bichacho N, Landsberg CJ. A modified surgical/prosthetic approach for an optimal single implant-supported crown. Part II. The cervical contouring concept. Pract Periodontics Aesthet Dent 1994;6(4):35–41 [quiz: 41].

79. Glauser R, Ruhstaller P, Windisch S, et al. Immediate occlusal loading of Branemark TiUnite implants placed predominantly in soft bone: 1-year results of a prospective clinical study. Clin Implant Dent Relat Res 2003;5(Suppl 1):47–56.

80. Rocci A, Martignoni M, Gottlow J. Immediate loading of Branemark system TiUnite and machined-surface implants in the posterior mandible: a randomized open-ended clinical trial. Clin Implant Dent Relat Res 2003;5(Suppl 1):57–63.

81. Romanos GE, Toh CG, Siar CH, et al. Histologic and histomorphometric evaluation of peri-implant bone subjected to immediate loading: an experimental study with Macaca fascicularis. Int J Oral Maxillofac Implants 2002;17(1):44–51.

82. Rocci A, Martignoni M, Burgos PM, et al. Histology of retrieved immediately and early loaded oxidized implants: light microscopic observations after 5 to 9 months of loading in the posterior mandible. Clin Implant Dent Relat Res 2003; 5(Suppl 1):88–98.

83. Tarnow DP, Emtiaz S, Classi A. Immediate loading of threaded implants at stage 1 surgery in edentulous arches: ten consecutive case reports with 1- to 5-year data. Int J Oral Maxillofac Implants 1997;12(3):319–24.

84. Badell CL, Palaiologou A, Vastardis SA. Early dental implant failure after immediate placement. J West Soc Periodont Periodontal Abstr 2009;57(3):67–77.

85. Schwartz-Arad D, Laviv A, Levin L. Survival of immediately provisionalized dental implants placed immediately into fresh extraction sockets. J Periodontol 2007; 78(2):219–23.

86. Schropp L, Kostopoulos L, Wenzel A. Bone healing following immediate versus delayed placement of titanium implants into extraction sockets: a prospective clinical study. Int J Oral Maxillofac Implants 2003;18(2):189–99.

87. Dahlin C, Andersson L, Linde A. Bone augmentation at fenestrated implants by an osteopromotive membrane technique. A controlled clinical study. Clin Oral Implants Res 1991;2(4):159–65.

88. Schwartz-Arad D, Chaushu G. The ways and wherefores of immediate placement of implants into fresh extraction sites: a literature review. J Periodontol 1997; 68(10):915–23.

89. Gher ME, Quintero G, Assad D, et al. Bone grafting and guided bone regeneration for immediate dental implants in humans. J Periodontol 1994;65(9):881–91.

90. Augthun M, Yildirim M, Spiekermann H, et al. Healing of bone defects in combination with immediate implants using the membrane technique. Int J Oral Maxillofac Implants 1995;10(4):421–8.

91. Chen ST, Buser D. Clinical and esthetic outcomes of implants placed in postextraction sites. Int J Oral Maxillofac Implants 2009;24(Suppl):186–217.

92. Martin W, Lewis E, Nicol A. Local risk factors for implant therapy. Int J Oral Maxillofac Implants 2009;24(Suppl):28–38.

Complications When Augmenting the Posterior Maxilla

Paul Fugazzotto, DDS[a],*, Philip R. Melnick, DMD[b],
Mohanad Al-Sabbagh, DDS, MS[c]

KEYWORDS

- Sinus lift • Complications of sinus lift • Lateral window • Osteotome
- Bone augmentation

KEY POINTS

- Sinus augmentation is considered a successful procedure to provide adequate vertical bone augmentation in the maxillary posterior atrophic alveolar ridge for the placement of dental implant.
- Complications of maxillary sinus augmentation may occur during or after the surgical procedure.
- The most frequent intraoperative complication of maxillary sinus lift is perforation of the sinus membrane.
- The most common postoperative complication is sinus infection.

INTRODUCTION
Definition of Problem

A discussion of augmentation of the posterior maxilla is inadequate in view of therapeutic capabilities. Increasing the vertical dimension of bone alone should no longer be considered a successful treatment outcome. Rather, the clinician must look toward reconstruction of the posterior maxilla in a three-dimensional manner. Such reconstruction must have specific goals, which are attainable and address the multilevel concerns of both the clinician and the patient regarding comfort, function, aesthetics, and long-term predictability.

Sinus augmentation was once considered successful if adequate bone was present posttherapeutically for placement of at least a 10-mm-long implant. No consideration

[a] Private Practice, 25 High Street, Milton, MA 02186, USA; [b] Private Practice, 4281 Katella Avenue, Suite 112, Los Alamitos, CA 90720, USA; [c] Division of Periodontology, Department of Oral Health Practice, College of Dentistry, University of Kentucky, 800 Rose Street, Lexington, KY 40536, USA
* Corresponding author.
E-mail address: progressiveperio@aol.com

Dent Clin N Am 59 (2015) 97–130
http://dx.doi.org/10.1016/j.cden.2014.09.005
0011-8532/15/$ – see front matter © 2015 Elsevier Inc. All rights reserved.

was given to the buccopalatal positioning of the implant, nor its diameter. The definitions of success often used after sinus augmentation, and subsequent implant placement and restoration, are flawed at best.

The surgical rehabilitation of the atrophic maxillary has been established as a predictable treatment.[1–7] Several recent reviews have shown implant survival rates using lateral window[2,5,7] and transcrestal techniques[8,9] for sinus elevation surgery to be more than 95%. Jensen,[7] in a review of 85 studies, reported survival rates for the rough-surfaced implants of 88.6% to 100%. These rates were found to be comparable with nongrafted sites.

The concept of implant success versus implant survival is still debated. Initially, all implants that attained osseointegration and fulfilled the criteria of Albrektsson and colleagues[10] regarding immobility, lack of suppuration, or tissue inflammation, and so forth were considered successful. As has long been evident through a historical analysis of the development of knowledge, concepts once believed revolutionary become foundational building blocks on which to evolve a more nuanced understanding and outlook. Although the Albrektsson criteria were an invaluable starting point, such criteria do not assess the stability of bone on the buccal or palatal/lingual aspects of an implant.

Any discussion of implant success must include an implant assessment, which combines the Albrektsson and colleagues' criteria with buccal and lingual/palatal bone assessment to ensure peri-implant marginal bone stability. Once these measurements are taken, the clinician can truly claim a successful implant therapeutic outcome. Such considerations are not purely semantic. To appropriately assess therapeutic efficacy in the long-term, criteria must be used that separate true success from mere survival. Unless the clinician is to assume the role of an actuarial, success is the only true goal.

As already mentioned, reconstruction of the posterior maxilla should always be viewed in a three-dimensional manner. Adequate bone must be present after regenerative efforts to place an implant in the ideal, prosthetically driven position. However, such a regenerative outcome is not in itself adequate. Although the concept of prosthetically driven implant placement is popular and well intentioned, it does not take into account the diameter of the tooth being replaced, or the fact that functional and parafunctional forces have their greatest effect on the peri-implant crestal bone. The greater the implant diameter, the greater the potential surface area of the osseointegrative bond at the crest of bone, to help better dissipate these forces. Therefore, buccopalatal/lingual regenerative efforts should be aimed at rebuilding adequate bone for prosthetically driven placement of an implant of the ideal diameter for the tooth being replaced (**Fig. 1**). Of course, when such placement results in a thin patina of bone on the buccal or palatal/lingual aspect of the implant, treatment should not be deemed successful. The likelihood of this thin patina of bone resorbing under function over time is high. Such resorption results in significant compromise of the osseous support of the implant. Buccopalatal/lingual regeneration should be considered successful if the following criteria are met.

An implant of ideal dimensions for the tooth being replaced may be placed in a prosthetically driven position, and show a minimum of 2 mm of bone buccally and palatally/lingually at the osseous crest. Such a treatment result helps ensure long-term stability of the bony support of the implant under function. Another and most important criterion for success is a maximization of treatment outcomes in conjunction with a minimization of therapeutic insult to the patient. The most conservative treatment approach possible must always be used, assuming that the final treatment

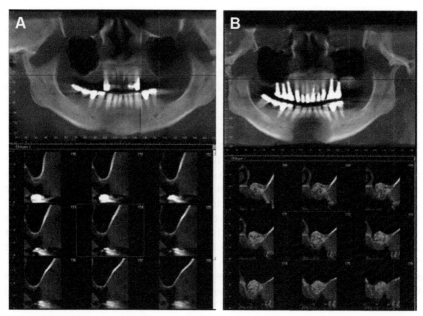

Fig. 1. (*A, B*) Before and after CT scans of an augmented sinus. Implants are placed in the maxillary left posterior sextants.

outcome is not compromised. A treatment approach that is easier or faster is of no use if the final treatment outcome is not equal in all respects to the therapeutic result after a more complex approach.

Treatment Options

When reconstructing the posterior maxilla, regenerative options include the following:

a. Lateral wall Caldwell-Luc sinus augmentation
b. Lateral wall Caldwell-Luc sinus augmentation in conjunction with buccal or palatal ridge augmentation
c. Trephine and osteotome use in anticipation of implant placement at a second stage
d. Trephine and osteotome use with simultaneous implant placement
e. Trephine and osteotome use followed by a second procedure of trephine and osteotome use, with simultaneous implant placement

Although complications may arise with any of these procedures, it is imperative to understand that an appropriate consideration of complications goes beyond surgical or postsurgical problems. Complications may occur before active therapy, during the surgical procedure, immediately after the surgical procedure, before implant loading, after implant loading, and after months or years of implant loading.

Pretreatment Evaluation

Complete medical, dental, social, and habit histories are required. The avoidance of complications must include addressing both absolute and relative contraindications.[11–13] Absolute contraindications include systemic conditions such as radiation therapy, poorly controlled diabetes, hypertension, immune compromise, neoplasm, and associated polypharmacies. However, it is valuable to know that well-controlled type 2 diabetics have shown implant survival rates comparable with nondiabetics. Tawil and colleagues[13] treated 45 well-controlled and fairly well-controlled (hemoglobin A_{1c} <7% vs 7%–9%) diabetic patients (143 implants) and 45 nondiabetic controls (142 implants) with classic protocol sinus elevation and bone grafting. Followed for 1 to 12 years the overall implant survival for the diabetic patients was 97.2% versus 98.8% for the nondiabetic control group.

Other significant risk factors for complications include active periodontitis, active sinusitis, large cysts, and history of chronic sinus disease.[14–17] Active periodontics has been shown to reduce the survival rates for dental implants and, prospectively, even if successfully treated, as a risk for peri-implantitis.[18] Acute or chronic sinusitis must be resolved before sinus elevation. Brook[19] suggested that 10% to 13% of maxillary sinusitis is attributable to odontogenic infection. Conventional dental and medical treatment should be undertaken to eliminate these factors.

Smoking is a relative risk factor and has been linked to reduced implant survival outcomes. In an 8-year follow-up study of 13,147 implants placed in 4316 patients, Busenlechner and colleagues,[20] found a 3-fold failure rate in the smokers compared with nonsmokers. In a recent systematic review, Pjetursson and colleagues[5] found that there was almost twice the rate of implant failures in smokers compared with nonsmokers.

Assuming a noncontributory medical history, a thorough clinical examination must be carried out to assess both the patient's regenerative needs and the feasibility of performing the proposed regenerative therapy. An accurate assessment of the condition of the soft tissues, not only of the site to be regenerated but throughout the mouth, must occur. A full occlusal examination must also be carried out.

At the least, digital clinical photographs must be taken, including photographs in various lateral and protrusive positions. A formatted computed tomography (CT) scan is usually necessary in addition to properly angled individual digital radiographs, to assess the presence or absence of various diseases and the morphology of the site to be treated. Face bow mounted models are a key component in facilitating an accurate diagnosis and helping to formulate a comprehensive treatment plan. In addition, face bow mounted models allow for fabrication of regenerative and implant placement stents, to help guide the clinician in assessing regenerative needs, and thus rebuilding the necessary hard and soft tissues.

Failure to perform a thorough examination and accomplish a comprehensive diagnosis often lead to either use of a less than ideal surgical approach, selection of an inappropriate restorative modality, postoperative complications, or implant loss after restoration and varying lengths of time in function. In addition, failure to identify either the etiologic factors, or cofounding factors that must be managed to ensure long-term maximization of treatment outcomes, compromises patient care. For example, an undiagnosed parafunctional habit often leads to loss of bony support around implants under function and a poorer prognosis.

All treatment plans must be grounded in biological principles and therapeutic possibilities. Such treatment plans must strive to attain the most optimal treatment outcomes possible with the available technologies and techniques. To do so, the treating clinician(s) must constantly visualize ideal treatment outcomes and strive to attain them. For example, the determination of whether or not buccal or palatal ridge augmentation therapy is necessary should be based on neither specific clinician's limitations nor manufacturer's claims. Rather, an implant of the ideal diameter for the tooth being replaced must be able to be inserted in a restoratively driven position and show 2 mm of bone buccally and palatally, at the alveolar crests.

SINUS ANATOMY

Any discussion of treatment of complications related to sinus elevation procedures must include sinus anatomy. The maxillary sinus is a pyramidal cavity, volume of 12 to 15 mL, contained within the maxillary bone. It is bounded superiorly by the orbital floor, inferiorly by the alveolar process, medially by the lateral nasal wall, and laterally by the zygomatic process and buccal alveolus.[8,21] The sinus is lined with a thin layer of mucoperiosteum, the Schneiderian membrane, of variable thickness, with an average of approximately 1.0 mm.[21,22] The sinus drains medially and superiorly into the nasal cavity via the ostium. The maxillary artery and nerve provide blood supply and innervation. The posterior superior branch of the maxillary artery may pass through the area of the posterior lateral window preparation, with average distance from the artery to the alveolar crest 16.9 mm. However, this distance has been found to be as little as 11.25 ± 2.99 mm (standard deviation) mean vertical distance from the lowest point of the bony canal to the alveolar crest.[23]

COMPLICATIONS AFTER VARIOUS TREATMENT APPROACHES

Complications may be divided into intraoperative and postoperative events, and they may be interrelated (**Table 1**).[8]

Moreno Vasquez and colleagues,[21] in a retrospective study, reported on the complication rate of 200 consecutive sinus lift procedures in 127 patients. The complications included Schneiderian membrane perforation, 25.7% (with no postoperative complications), 14.7% had wound infections, abscesses, drainage, dehiscence, maxillary sinusitis, graft exposure; and loss of graft (2 cases). Nolan and colleagues[23] reported on 359 sinus augmentation procedures in 208 patients. The incidence of sinus perforation was 41%. Of the 6.7% of the sinus grafts that failed, 70.8% had perforated sinus membranes. Lee and colleagues[33] reported a complication rate of almost 28% in a retrospective analysis of 97 sinus elevations. Although the sinus lift surgery is a reliable procedure, it is not without risk.

Complications do not automatically imply failure. The most common complications of sinus floor elevation and their effect on the final outcome of therapy have been extensively discussed.[34–36]

LATERAL WALL CALDWELL-LUC SINUS AUGMENTATION
Conceptual Complication

It is important to adequately visualize the shape of the sinus to be augmented. Failure to do so may result in an attempt to prepare a sinus window in the alveolar ridge.

Treatment

When this problem occurs, the solution is to reassess the area with appropriate imaging and adjust the position of the osteotomy window accordingly.

Technical Complications

The most frequent technical complication is perforation of the sinus membrane. Various investigators reported incidence of sinus membrane perforation during sinus augmentation therapy to range between 19.5% and 41% (**Table 2**). Numerous factors have been described as risk providers related to membrane perforation, including the presence of septa,[44] the width of the sinus, the angle of the sinus walls, residual height,[39,45] and membrane thickness. This complication may happen during window preparation, initial reflection, final reflection, or graft placement. The chances of

Table 1
Clinical reports on sinus augmentation complications

Article	Aim	Materials	Criteria	Results	Conclusion
Maxillary sinus functions and complications with lateral window and osteotome sinus floor elevation procedures, followed by dental implants placement: a retrospective study in 60 patients[24]	Evaluate maxillary sinus functions and complications by using lateral window and osteotome sinus floor elevation then implants placement	60 patients sinus floor elevation using lateral window with residual subsinus alveolar bone height (RSABH) of 3 mm and osteotome with RSABH of >4 mm No bone grafting with osteotome procedures followed by implants (ITI implants) Implants were placed immediately at time of lateral window, or after 9 mo using surgical guides Bio-Oss graft was used with lateral window Retrospectively evaluated clinically and radiographically for 24 mo	Dizziness Nausea Sinus membrane perforation	More dizziness and nausea with osteotome than lateral window, which disappeared within 2–4 wk 4 of 79 sinus perforation cases (2 osteotome and 2 lateral window)	No obvious maxillary sinus complications for 24 mo after sinus floor elevation using osteotome and lateral window, followed by implants placement Clinical assessment of individual risk and modifying factors before procedures

| A retrospective study of the effects on sinus complications of exposing dental implants to the maxillary sinus cavity[25] | Investigate whether dental implant exposure to the maxillary sinus cavity increased the risk of maxillary sinus complications | 9 patients 23 implants inserted into the maxillary sinus >4 mm No sinus membrane lift 6–10 mo evaluation using questionnaire and CT Astra implants and 1 Osstem implant used | Nasal congestion Obstruction Pathologic secretion Pain and tenderness in the sinus region | No clinical signs of sinusitis CT scans showed postoperative sinus mucus thickening around 14 of the 23 implants | This study showed that implant exposure to the maxillary sinus cavity can cause sinus mucus thickening around the implants Implant exposure to the sinus cavity might contribute to the development of maxillary sinusitis in patients with a predisposition for sinusitis Implant extension into the nasal cavity can give rise to rhinosinusitis (Raghoebar and colleagues) |

(continued on next page)

Table 1
(continued)

Article	Aim	Materials	Criteria	Results	Conclusion
A case of massive maxillary sinus bleeding after dental implant[26]	A case of maxillary sinus bleeding during dental implant	Maxillary sinus osteoplasty with a vascularized pedicled bone flap through a maxillary sinus approach General anesthesia	Signs of posterior nasal bleeding Swelling of the gingival 1 d after admission, the bleeding was not controlled Hemoglobin level measured 7.1 g/dL	The patient was discharged 3 d after surgery, and 6 mo after surgery, there were no signs of rebleeding with normal use of the dental implant	Surgery is needed in cases in which nasal bleeding is not conservatively controlled Cauterization of the bleeding site using a nasal endoscope is the most common operative technique Vascularized pedicled bone flap allows a shorter length of hospital stay and fewer outpatient clinic visits because it causes minimal swelling of the isthmus and minimal injury to the maxillary mucosa

| Fungal infection as a complication of sinus bone grafting and implants: a case report[27] | Report a case of a middle-aged male patient along with the clinical, radiographic, and histologic findings | 48-y-old man
10 cigarettes/d
Failed sinus bone grafting (irradiated cancellous bone) and osseointegration of implants (Nobel Biocare), which were placed after 6 mo of sinus graft
Surgical exposure of the maxillary sinus
Systemic prophylactic antibiotics used
Removal of infected bone graft
Sinus membrane elevation
Perforation sealed with bioresorbable membrane and fibrin glue (to stabilize the membrane)
Demineralized bone matrix paste with cancellous bone was grafted into the sinus and covered by Tutoplast pericardium
Postoperative systemic antibiotics, nonsteroidal antiinflammatory drugs for 10 d and antifungal drug
Implants placed after 8 mo | Increased radiopacity of the right maxillary sinus
Sphere-shaped foreign body mass composed of dark brown and red material curetted from maxillary sinus
Caused by *Aspergillus* and polypous mucosa | Newly grafted allograft in the sinus showed no specified inflammation or fungal hyphae | First case report of fungal sinusitis that developed after maxillary sinus bone grafting followed by implant placement
Surgical treatment of noninvasive fungal sinusitis produced good results, and no recurrence was observed |

(continued on next page)

Table 1
(continued)

Article	Aim	Materials	Criteria	Results	Conclusion
Oroantral communication as an osteotome sinus elevation complication[28]	Case report of an oroantral communication that developed as a complication to a sinus elevation surgery performed with the crestal approach	54-year-old woman History of sleep apnea and smoking (1 pack/d) Patient has a bridge from 2 to 4 with missing 3 Extraction of tooth 2 and freeze-dried bone allograft socket preservation After 3 mo, exploratory surgery was performed Amoxicillin and methylprednisolone for 7 d before surgery There were no bone fills inside the socket Freeze-dried bone allograft mixed with platelet-rich plasma to elevate the sinus using osteotome over tooth 3 space Collagen membrane used Postoperative instructions and chlorhexidine 0.12% used	6 d later the patient returned to the clinic and claimed the surgical site had "opened up" Water coming through her nose while drinking The sutures were broken and the flaps open	De-epithelization of buccal and lingual flaps, and rotating buccal flap mesially, to cover the site Postoperative instructions, and patient instructed to stop using continuous positive airway pressure mask Patient was followed every 2 wk for 2 mo, and the area appeared to be healed, with complete closure by the end of the first month After 4 y, patient presented with normal healing, no smoking, and a new lateral window sinus lift was performed to restore 4 successfully	Use of a positive pressure mask may have complicated a sinus elevation surgery. Other factors that may have contributed to this complication include smoking and delayed healing of the area

Potential adverse events of endosseous dental implants penetrating the maxillary sinus: long-term clinical evaluation[29]	Evaluate the nature and incidence of long-term maxillary sinus Adverse events related to endosseous implant placement with protrusion into the maxillary sinus	70 patients with 83 implants placed into maxillary sinus (<3 mm) with membrane perforation Minimum of 5 y follow-up Perioperative prophylactic clindamycin Straumann implants were placed after 1-stage procedure Postoperative antibiotics for 4 d Prosthetic rehabilitation after osseointegration from 2–6 mo	Clinical and radiographic assessment monitoring signs of sinusitis, and by asking the patients about any symptoms, including nasal bleeding, congestion or obstruction, nasal secretion, and pain or tenderness in the infraorbital region	12 patients had >1 implant penetrating the sinus 7 had bilateral perforation Implants were localized in premolar/molar area 2/83 implants diagnosed with peri-implantitis were treated without recurrence Radiologic follow-up showed a normal bone healing process in all patients	No sinus complication was observed after implant penetration into the maxillary sinus ($\leq$20 y) Absence of complications was related to maintenance of successful osseointegration

(continued on next page)

Table 1
(continued)

Article	Aim	Materials	Criteria	Results	Conclusion
The management of complications after displacement of oral implants in the paranasal sinuses: a multicenter clinical report and proposed treatment protocols[30]	Study retrospectively analyzed paranasal sinus complications after displacement of oral implants in the maxillary sinus treated according to clinical situation by functional endoscopic sinus surgery (FESS), an intraoral approach, or a combination of both procedures	27 patients (13 male; 14 female) Age: 27–73 y More than 5 y treatment of complications involving the paranasal sinuses after displacement of oral implants in the maxillary sinuses Patients were treated with FESS (functional endoscopic sinus surgery), intraoral approach to the sinus, or FESS associated with an intraoral approach	Implant displacement Implant displacement with or without reactive sinusitis or with or without associated oroantral communication	26 patients recovered completely 1 patient underwent reintervention with FESS and an intraoral approach 2 y after implant removal followed by complete recovery	The results show that a rational choice of surgical protocol for the treatment of complications involving the paranasal sinuses after displacement of implants in the maxillary sinuses may lead to reliable results
Effect of Schneiderian membrane perforation on posterior maxillary implant survival[31]	To assess the survival rate of implants placed in the posterior maxilla by intentionally perforating the Schneiderian membrane and protruding the implant up to 3 mm beyond the sinus floor in cases of reduced crestal bone height	56 patients with 63 implants intentionally penetrated the Schneiderian membrane engaging sinus floor cortical bone (Nobel Biocare) Implants were placed using 2-stage technique 1 y follow-up after implant restoration (12–14 wk) Postoperative antibiotics		1 implant failure 7 patients experienced mild epistaxis during the immediate postoperative period, with no associated implant loss 1 patient developed sinusitis secondary to the surgical procedure, which was treated by antibiotic therapy and the patient improved clinically, with no associated implant loss	Intentional perforation of the Schneiderian membrane using a 2-mm twist drill at the time of implant placement and protrusion of the implant up to 3 mm beyond the sinus floor does not alter the stability and outcome of dental implants, 1 y after restoration

Transcrestal sinus floor elevation with osteotomes: simplified technique and management of various scenarios[32]	Understand the structure of the maxillary sinus region Describe a simplified transcrestal sinus floor elevation technique Manage issues and factors that may be encountered when performing a sinus floor elevation	Implant success rate after osteotome sinus lift is 90.9%–92.8% Septa are present 31.7% at premolar area Pneumatization of the sinus occurs within 6 mo after tooth extraction <4 mm of bone subantral then a lateral window is recommended >5 mm of bone is needed to place an implant with osteotome sinus lift If only 4 mm of bone is present, then implant needs to be submerged under the gum >4 mm of subantral bone leads to 96% survival rate compared with only 84.7% when bone is <4 mm Simplified osteotome technique: used for medium and soft dense bone Assume there is only 4 mm subantral bone	Complications: most frequently encountered complication is Schneiderian Membrane perforation (38%) Infection 0.8% In case of extensive malleting, postoperative headache or benign paroxysmal positional vertigo can occur	Simplified technique to perform sinus floor elevation in medium dense bone has been presented Enhances patient comfort and reduces the need to mallet osteotomes

(continued on next page)

Table 1 (*continued*)

Article	Aim	Materials	Criteria	Results	Conclusion
		Using Straumann system and the corresponding osteotome			
		Periapical radiograph is taken, for subantral bone determination considering 14% error			
		2-mm drill used till 1 mm short of the subantral floor			
		Guide pin insertion			
		Then subsequent drills are used to widen the osteotomy			
		An osteotome corresponding to the last drill is used to upfracture the sinus floor			
		A metal stop is placed on the osteotome at 4 mm in this case and the tip of osteotome is dipped in saline			
		Few gentle malleting taps facilitate the infracture			

(continued on next page)

Some hemorrhage occurs once penetrating the sinus floor

Bone graft material could be used before infracture to act as cushion, although might reduce the tactile perception

After placing bone grafting material in the osteotomy, using an amalgam carrier, the same osteotome is used to push the bone substitute and elevate the membrane

This provides 2 mm of bone height

Repeat till desired length is reached

Bone forms at the sinus floor at a rate of 1 mm

Slanted sinus floor:

Drill is stopped 1 mm short of the most inferior sinus wall

Drills are increased in size normally, then, a small osteotome is used angled toward the thicker bone to break the bone

Table 1
(continued)

Article	Aim	Materials	Criteria	Results	Conclusion
		Any sinus perforation should be verified using the Valsalva maneuver Some clinicians recommend abortion and healing for 4 wk, then, redoing the procedure Implant platform should be placed supracrestal when there is minimum subantral bone to achieve supracrestal biological width			

Table 2		
The incidence of sinus membrane perforation during sinus augmentation therapy		
Author, Year	**Numbers of Sinus Augmentations**	**Perforations (%)**
Khoury,[37] 1999	216	23.5
Shlomi et al,[38] 2004	73	28
Ardekian et al,[39] 2014	110	32
Barone et al,[40] 2008	26	23–30
Hernandez-Alfaro et al,[41] 2008	474	21.9
Becker et al,[42] 2008	201	20.4
Pjetursson et al,[5] 2008	1300	19.5
Testori et al,[43] 2012	144	28
Nolan et al,[23] 2014	359	41

perforation during window preparation are significantly reduced by using a piezo surgical approach, rather than a conventional dental bur. Weitz and colleagues[46] reported a sinus membrane perforation incidence of 17.5% using a piezo surgical approach. Tactile sense is greatly improved with piezo surgery, as is the accuracy of the osteotomy. Initial membrane elevation runs the risk of a membrane tear occurring as a result of too much pressure being placed in 1 position and direction. To ameliorate this concern, it is recommended that the osteotomy window be wholly detached. A piezo surgical tip is then used, which pushes against the window before touching the membrane, imploding it slightly and creating a small space for insertion of the piezo surgery tip, which then begins membrane reflection. As subsequent curettes are inserted, the curette always applies pressure against the osteotomy window first, further imploding the window and creating space between the outer alveolar bone and the membrane, allowing for passive insertion of the curette. Toscano and colleagues[47] reported an incidence of sinus membrane perforation involving 3.6% after use of a piezo surgical approach to affect sinus augmentation therapy. Such an approach greatly decreases the chances of membrane perforation.[48] In contrast, Barone and colleagues[40] concluded that piezo surgery and conventional instrumentation showed no significant differences in the incidence of sinus membrane perforation.

All membrane reflection must be accomplished in a three-dimensional manner. Reflection should not only be in a medial direction. Medial, mesial, and distal reflections must occur in concert with each other, if perforations are to be avoided in the later stages of membrane reflection. Geminiani and colleagues[48] compared the incidence of sinus membrane perforations using piezo surgical and conventional handpiece approaches in a total of 130 sinus augmentation procedures (51 rotary instrument and 79 piezo surgery). Incidence of sinus membrane perforation of 27.5% was noted when a rotary instrument approach was used, compared with an incidence of sinus membrane perforation of 12.7% when a piezo surgical approach was used.

Treatment

If a membrane perforation occurs, the perforation must be classified and treated accordingly.

Is the presence of a sinus membrane perforation cause to either abort the planned augmentation procedure or modify a planned augmentation with simultaneous implant procedure so that only the augmentation is performed during the first surgical visit?

These questions are answered, and predictable treatment results obtained, through the use of a framework by which to deal with sinus membrane perforations and effect predictable sinus augmentation, with or without simultaneous implant placement.

Treatment of sinus membrane perforations involves the following steps:

- Classification of the perforation (**Fig. 2**)
- Management of the perforation
- Possible modification of the timing of implant placement, if used

On discovery of a sinus membrane perforation, the clinician must avoid manipulation of the membrane to ascertain the size of the tear, because such manipulation only worsens the tear. The buccal mucoperiosteal flap may have to be extended through lengthening of the mesial and distal vertical releasing incisions and their horizontal extensions, and further full-thickness flap reflection, to gain greater visualization and access to the prepared sinus window area. After additional mucoperiosteal flap reflection as required, the membrane perforation is evaluated, classified, and treated.[49]

Membrane perforations are first classified with respect to location. Class I perforations occur at any point along the most apical wall of the prepared sinus window. Class II perforations occur along the lateral or crestal aspects of the prepared sinus window and are further subdivided according to their position relative to the most mesial, distal, or crestal bony walls of the underlying sinus. Class III perforations occur at any location within the body of the prepared sinus window.

CLASS I SINUS MEMBRANE PERFORATIONS

The presence of a class I sinus membrane perforation poses no concerns with regard to either sequencing of therapy or the final treatment result, assuming appropriate perforation management. Sinus membrane elevation is easily accomplished. The apical displacement of the sinus membrane after its reflection results in the membrane folding over itself, sealing the class I sinus membrane perforation. A piece of collagen tape may be placed over the area. If simultaneous implant placement had been planned, such implant placement may then be carried out (**Fig. 3**).

CLASS II SINUS MEMBRANE PERFORATIONS

Both the repair of a class II sinus membrane perforation, and the need or lack of need to alter the proposed course of therapy, are dependent on the position of the membrane perforation in relation to the bordering walls of the subantral space to be

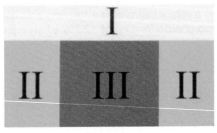

Fig. 2. Sinus perforation locations.

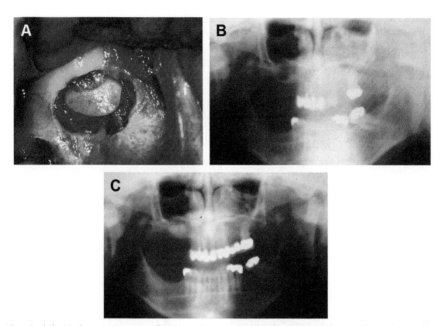

Fig. 3. (*A*) A class I sinus perforation is noted. (*B, C*) Preoperative and postoperative panoramic radiographs show successful bone augmentation after repair of the class I sinus membrane perforation.

augmented. If the initial sinus window was precisely prepared to approximate the bordering sinus cavity walls, repair of a class II sinus membrane perforation is more difficult, and has a greater impact on the course of therapy than if the initial sinus window preparation was undersized and did not approximate the bordering sinus cavity walls.

CLASS IIA SINUS MEMBRANE PERFORATIONS

A class IIA sinus membrane perforation may occur anywhere along the expanse of the lateral or coronal walls of the prepared sinus window, when the sinus cavity to be augmented extends a minimum of 4 to 5 mm beyond the position of the membrane perforation. For example, if the membrane perforation is on the mesial aspect of the sinus window, and the sinus extends at least 4 to 5 mm mesially beyond the prepared sinus window, this perforation is classified as IIA. In such a situation, care is taken after mucoperiosteal flap extension to gently extend the osteotomy further mesially using a piezo surgery tip, thus exposing intact sinus membrane mesial to the perforation. The reflecting instrument is extended over the membrane perforation to the intact sinus membrane area, thus bridging the tear and allowing gentle reflection of the intact sinus membrane and rotation of the membrane and the attached bony window medially and apically. A resorbable membrane is then placed over the area, sealing the membrane. If simultaneous implant therapy had been planned preoperatively, it can be accomplished at this time (**Fig. 4**).

CLASS IIB SINUS MEMBRANE PERFORATIONS

If the prepared aspect of the sinus window approximates the extension of the sinus cavity in this area, no additional space exists for performance of a further osteotomy

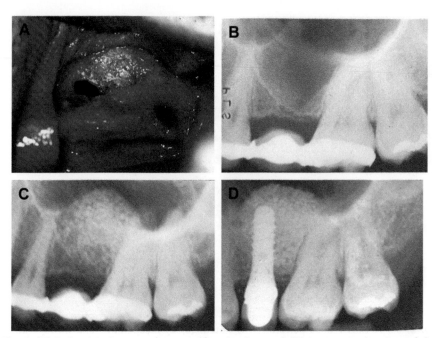

Fig. 4. (*A*) A class IIA sinus membrane perforation is noted. (*B*) A preoperative view of the sinus area that is to be augmented. (*C*) After repair of the class IIA sinus membrane perforation, successful augmentation has been carried out. (*D*) A radiograph taken after implant restoration shows stable augmented and crestal peri-implant bone.

to expose intact membrane lateral to the perforation. For example, when the mesial wall of the prepared sinus window approximates the mesial extent of the sinus to be augmented, it is impossible to remove additional bone mesial to the prepared sinus window in an effort to uncover intact sinus membrane for use during reflection. Attempts to reflect the remnants of the sinus membrane increase the size of membrane perforation, rendering it unmanageable. It is imperative that a new membrane be recreated, to provide the clinician with a containing element for reception of the planned regenerative materials. Insertion of collagen tape or other pliable, nonsecured materials in an attempt to form a containing element within the augmented sinus is unpredictable. Therefore, a resorbable membrane is shaped and inserted into the sinus window, with its ends extruding out of the window. The extruding aspects of the membrane are secured to the surrounding alveolar bone with 1 or 2 fixation tacks. A curette is used to gently mold the morphology of the membrane within the sinus cavity to be augmented, ensuring the creation of adequate space to receive and contain the augmentation materials. If preoperative planning called for simultaneous implant placement at the time of sinus augmentation, this course of therapy is abandoned. When faced with an extensive membrane perforation requiring the aforementioned reconstructive therapy, only augmentation is carried out during this surgical session. Implant placement occurs at a second visit, after maturation of regenerating hard tissues in the augmented sinus area.

CLASS III SINUS MEMBRANE PERFORATIONS

A class III membrane perforation is treated in an identical manner to that of a class IIB sinus membrane perforation (**Fig. 5**).

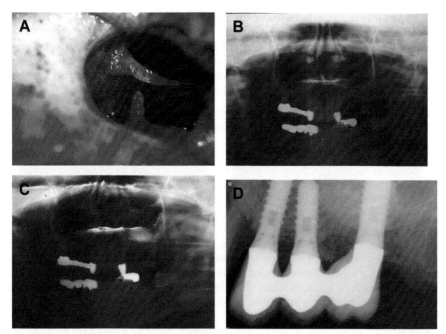

Fig. 5. (*A*) A class III sinus membrane perforation is noted. (*B*) A preoperative radiograph of the maxillary left sinus area, which is to be augmented. (*C*) After membrane repair, successful sinus augmentation has been carried out. (*D*) A radiograph taken 11 years after implant restoration shows stable regenerated and crestal peri-implant bone.

Postoperative medications after sinus augmentation therapy include augmentin 875 mg twice a day for 10 days (patients allergic to augmentin receive levaquin, 1 a day for 10 days), and etodolac 400 mg, 3 times a day for 5 days, unless medically contraindicated. Patients are instructed not to blow their noses for 14 days postoperatively.

Sinus Augmentation Therapy with Concomitant Bucco or Palatal Ridge Augmentation

Simultaneous sinus and ridge augmentation is a highly predictable procedure.[50–52] In addition to the concerns addressed earlier, complications may occur with regard to the ridge augmentation procedure.

Diagnostic complications
The most frequent diagnostic complication is an underestimation of the extent of regenerative therapy that must be performed, especially at the alveolar crest.

Technical complications
Inadequate flap design severely limits the clinician's ability to attain passive primary closure over the regenerative materials that are placed. If passive soft tissue primary closure cannot be attained and maintained, the regenerative results are less than ideal. Therefore, adequate soft tissue management is of paramount importance.

The sine qua non of successful guided bone regeneration therapy is appropriate flap management.[53,54] Although bone regeneration can be achieved without attaining and maintaining passive soft tissue primary closure over the regenerating site, the extent and morphology of the regenerated hard tissues often fall short of the desired ideal treatment outcome. In addition, the resultant soft tissue covering when passive soft tissue primary closure is not maintained is usually thinner than desired and represents a potential aesthetic compromise. Incisions should be made within keratinized tissue to ensure keratinized margins to the mucoperiosteal flaps, both to enhance soft tissue manipulation and to help avoid fraying of the mucoperiosteal flap margins. Incision design is recommended to be as follows.

- A horizontal midcrestal incision within keratinized tissue: this incision is made along the crest of the ridge and carried at least 6 to 8 mm distal to the area to be augmented, to provide appropriate access to the underlying atrophic ridge. The incision is carried to within 1 to 2 mm of the tooth anterior to the edentulous posterior region, but does not reach the adjacent tooth, to preserve a portion of the papilla and thus a soft tissue cover over the supporting bone on the distal aspect of the tooth.
- Releasing incisions: 4 releasing incisions are used. They are placed at the mesio-buccal, distobuccal, mesiopalatal, and distopalatal aspects of the midcrestal horizontal incision, extend beyond the mucogingival junction well into mucosa, and are crucial if appropriate flap reflection and defect visualization are to be achieved. All palatal releasing incisions are placed obliquely. An oblique incision may be placed approximately 30% less deeply into the palatal vault than a straight releasing incision, retaining the same degree of flap reflection and defect visualization.
- Horizontal extensions of the releasing incisions: horizontal releasing incisions are placed at the most apical extents of all buccal vertical releasing incisions in the maxilla. These horizontal releasing incisions may extend up to 10 mm, depending on the need for greater flap mobility. Such horizontal extensions are of no use throughout the palate, because the palatal flap cannot be coronally positioned.
- Full-thickness flap reflection: all flaps are reflected in a full-thickness manner, including the horizontal extensions at the apices of the vertical releasing incisions. No periosteal fenestration is used at any time. Adequate full-thickness flap reflection after appropriate releasing incision design results in greater flap mobility than periosteal fenestration. In addition, postoperative morbidity (ie, swelling) is less when full-thickness reflection is used compared with periosteal fenestration. These flap designs provide adequate flap mobility to attain and maintain passive soft tissue primary closure throughout the course of regeneration. When the previously outlined flap designs are not adequate to attain passive primary closure after placement of regenerative materials in the maxilla, a rotated palatal pedicle is used.

A full-thickness palatal mucoperiosteal flap is reflected. An incision is then made with a 15 blade mesiodistally on the internal aspect of the palatal flap, approximately 3 to 4 mm from the base of the mucoperiosteal flap. Using tissue forceps and a 15 blade, the flap is split internally toward its crestal aspect. The internal aspect of the flap is filleted and rotated crestally to lengthen the palatal flap by approximately 70%. Care is taken neither to perforate the flap at its most crestal aspect nor to render the residual isthmus of tissue so thin as to be in danger of sloughing during healing.

The efficacy of these flap designs in the attainment and maintenance of primary closure of soft tissue throughout the course of regeneration was assessed through the examination of almost 900 consecutive guided bone regeneration cases.[53–55]

Postoperative complications

Loss of soft tissue primary closure results in premature membrane exposure. When this complication occurs, the clinician must carefully assess the situation and attempt to maintain the area through the use of chlorhexidine gluconate rinses. If the extent of membrane exposure increases, or purulence is noted, the membrane must be removed. If membrane exposure occurs before 8 weeks, the regenerative results are severely compromised at best and often must be classified as a failure. Should such membrane removal occur after 8 weeks, significant bone regeneration is usually achieved.

Treatment
If the ridge augmentation did not result in adequate bone for ideal implant positioning, a new ridge augmentation procedure must be performed before implant placement. If adequate bucco or palatal bone regeneration has occurred to allow ideal implant positioning, the implants are inserted and the area is regrafted with particulate material and a covering membrane at the time of implant insertion, to attain the desired alveolar morphology.

Trephine and Osteotome Use, in Anticipation of Implant Placement

Diagnostic complications
Care must be taken to accurately assess the extent of the alveolar bone that is present crestal to the floor of the sinus and the ability to accomplish the desired extent of augmentation through an osteotome and trephine approach.

Technical complications
Two potential technical complications are encountered.

The first is evidence of the bony core within the trephine on trephine removal from the mouth. In such a situation, the core is gently removed from the trephine, inserted into the osteotomy, and imploded to the desired level.

The second complication is evidence of both the bony core and the corresponding sinus membrane within the trephine on trephine removal. Once again, this complex is gently removed from the trephine, reinserted at the osteotomy, and imploded to the desired level.

Neither complication significantly affects the regenerative outcome, assuming that care is taken when managing the complication.

Use of a Trephine and Osteotome Approach, with Simultaneous Implant Placement

Diagnostic complication
Care must be taken to accurately assess whether or not the implant of the appropriate length can be placed, and the ability to accomplish the desired augmentation through an osteotome and trephine approach. An implant should be placed only at the time a trephine and osteotome sinus augmentation procedure is performed if 2x–2 is an adequate length for the implant, with x being the preoperative height of the bone crestal to the floor of the sinus (**Figs. 6** and **7**).[56]

Technical complications
Three potential technical complications are encountered.

a. The first is evidence of the bony core within the trephine on trephine removal from the mouth. In such a situation, the core is replaced in the osteotomy, and the implant is then inserted as originally planned (**Fig. 8**).
b. The second complication is evidence of both the bony core and the corresponding sinus membrane within the trephine on trephine removal. In such a situation, the implant is not inserted as originally planned. Rather, the core is replaced in the os-teotomy to the desired level, the area is allowed to heal, and the implant is inserted in the second procedure.

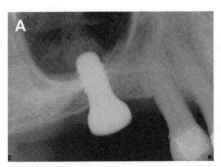
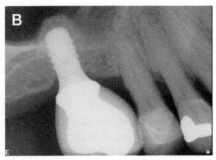

Fig. 6. (*A*) An implant is placed after an osteotome and trephine approach. (*B*) An 8-year postrestoration radiograph shows stability of both the crestal peri-implant bone and the bone around the implant apex.

Neither of these complications significantly affects the regenerative outcome, assuming care is taken when managing the complication.

c. Overinstrumentation of the osteotomy site before implant placement is a common occurrence, because the bone in the area is both delicate and less than abundant. This complication is managed through a modified technique. A trephine is used with a 2 mm internal diameter and a 2.8 mm external diameter to prepare an osteotomy within 1 mm of the floor of the sinus, at a maximum of 500 RPM. The prepared core of bone is imploded to a depth of 1 mm less than that of the initial trephine osteotomy. Flat-ended osteotomes are used to widen the osteotomy site to 1 bur size less than conventional preparation. For example, if a 4.8-mm-wide body Straumann implant is to be placed, osteotome widening of the site occurs to 3.5 mm. A 4.2-mm-wide bone tap is then used to a depth of 2 threads. A 4.8-mm-wide body Straumann implant is now placed at 30 RPM. The conventional diameter osteotomy attained to the depth of 2 threads of the bone tap allows placement of the implant without any wiggling and undesirable overenlarging of the entry to the osteotomy.

Trephine and Osteotome Use, Followed by a Second Trephine and Osteotome Procedure, with Simultaneous Implant Placement

Diagnostic complications
Inadequate diagnosis and treatment planning are the most prevalent concern with this double osteotome and trephined approach. Care must be taken to ensure that

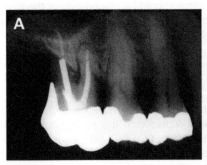
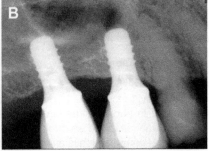

Fig. 7. (*A*) The second molar is missing and the first molar presents with an intrafurcal fracture. The tooth is extracted and implants are placed using an osteotome and trephine approach. (*B*) A radiograph taken 7 years after implant restoration shows stable peri-implant crestal bone.

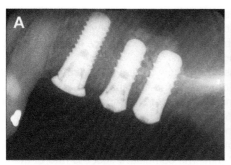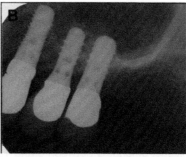

Fig. 8. (*A*) Implants have been placed after an osteotome and trephine approach. (*B*) A radiograph taken 14 years after implant restoration with individual abutments and crowns shows stable peri-implant crestal bone.

this is indeed the appropriate treatment modality for the given situation. If 4x–6 yields an implant of adequate length for the situation in question, with x being the preoperative bone crestal to the floor of the sinus, then the double osteotome and trephine technique is used. A core of bone is imploded to a depth of 1 mm less than the extent of alveolar bone coronal to the sinus floor. Graft material is placed in the osteotomy, and the site is allowed to heal. The area is re-entered approximately 10 weeks postoperatively. At that time, an osteotome and trephine approach is again used, with simultaneous implant placement. The length of the implant does not exceed 2x–2, where x is the residual alveolar bone crestal to the floor of the sinus, after the healing that has occurred after previous augmentation therapy.

The use of the proposed treatment algorithms for implant placement after, or in conjunction with, trephine and osteotome use, results in placement of shorter implants than is generally suggested. For example, if 5 mm of bone is present crestal to the floor of the sinus, use of the formula 2x–2 results in placement of an 8-mm-long implant. Is such an implant sufficient to withstand functional forces over time in the maxillary posterior region?

When ossseointegrating implants were introduced to the dental community, an assumption was made that longer implants (ie, implants with a greater surface area for potential osseointegration) would prove more advantageous, and present with a superior long-term prognosis when compared with shorter implants, in most if not all clinical situations. Early publications documenting the extensive use of machined screw Branemark implants seemed to bear out this belief. Osseointegrating implants documented in these studies were machined screw, hex headed implants placed in a countersunk manner.

Nevertheless, if success rates are attainable that are comparable with those of their longer counterparts, shorter implant use helps the clinician avoid vital structures, such as the sinus floor and the inferior alveolar canal. The use of shorter implants may also eliminate the need to perform augmentation therapy or simplify augmentation therapy when it is required.

A review of both finite element analysis (FEA) and the clinical literature supported the use of shorter implants in such situations. A total of 315 standard neck Straumann implants were placed in atrophic posterior mandibular areas and followed for up to 84 months in function, with a mean time in function of 36.2 months.[57] Four implants were mobile at uncovery, and 1 implant was lost during the first 12 months of function, yielding a cumulative success rate of 98.4%. The cumulative success rate of the shorter implants in function over the mean time of 36.2 months was 99.7% when the 4 implants mobile at uncovery are excluded, because implants mobile at uncovery cast no reflection up on the ability or inability of shorter implants to withstand functional forces over time. Shorter implants can be routinely used to replace missing maxillary posterior teeth with abutments and single crowns.

A total of 987 implants replaced missing maxillary molars and were restored with solid abutments and unsplinted single crowns.[58] The implants were followed for up to 84 months in function with a mean time in function of 29.3 months, yielding a cumulative success rate in function of 95.1%. Followed to the present day, and including implants placed since publication, a total of 2746 implants have been placed and restored with solid abutments and single crowns in intact arches, in maxillary molar positions, of lengths between 6 and 12 mm. The cumulative success rate of the implants in function is 96.2%.

As discussed earlier, implants of various lengths are often placed in conjunction with trephine and osteotome use to implode a core of the residual bone crestal to the floor of the sinus. Data that examine implants placed in such situations so far show that 306 implants 6, 7, or 8 mm long, placed at the time of trephine and osteotome use and restored with single crowns, were in function for up to 8 years with a mean time in function of 30.9 months and a cumulative success rate of 99.0%.[57] During the same time frame, the cumulative success rates of 10-mm-long and 11-mm-long implants placed at the time of trephine and osteotome use and restored with single crowns was 98.9%. The difference was not statistically significant. Followed to the present day, and including implants placed since publication, a total of 1119 implants have been placed and restored with single crowns, in maxillary molar positions, of lengths between 6 and 8 mm. The cumulative success rate in function is 99.4%.

Technical complications

The technical complications are the same as stated earlier.

a. The first is evidence of the bony core within the trephine on trephine removal from the mouth. In such a situation, the core is replaced in the osteotomy, and the implant is then inserted as originally planned.
b. The second complication is evidence of both the bony core and the corresponding sinus membrane within the trephine on trephine removal. In such a situation, the implant is not inserted as originally planned. Rather, the core is replaced in the osteotomy to the desired level, the area is allowed to heal, and the implant is inserted in the second procedure.

Neither of these complications significantly affects the regenerative outcome, assuming care is taken when managing the complication.

COMPLICATIONS FROM SEPTA

The most effective means by which to manage a septal complication is to avoid it. Certain steps must be taken in the presence of a septa.

Identify the Septum

Appropriate imaging for such septal identification must involve a formatted CT scan, thus allowing appropriate and complete visualization of the septal morphology and position.

Classify the Septum

There is no universally accepted septum classification system. Any such classification system must have direct clinical applications to be of use to the clinician. Such clinical application must include all innovative techniques for minimizing the impact of the septum on the course of therapy.[4]

Class I
Class I septa have no impact on the course of treatment because of its position with relation to the planned reconstructive therapy. Augmentation, with or without simultaneous implant placement, is carried out as initially planned.

Class II
Class II septa have minimal impact on the planned course of therapy and do not influence the timing of implant placement. Such septa fall into 1 of 3 categories:

- Class IIA: a septum is present in the area of planned reconstructive therapy. However, adequate buccopalatal dimension of the ridge, and adequate bone crestal to the floor of the sinus, are noted both mesial and distal to the septum, in planned positions of implant placements. In such a situation, trephines and osteotomes are used to prepare osteotomies mesial and distal to the septum, as described earlier. If immediate implant placement is planned, it is carried out at this time.
- Class IIB: adequate buccopalatal dimension of the alveolar bone is noted, and adequate bone is present crestal to the floor of the sinus mesial or distal of the septum for implant placement, and inadequate bone is present for planned implant placement on the other aspect of the septum (mesial or distal). An osteotome and trephine approach is used, with immediate implant placement as described earlier, in the area of adequate bone crestal to the floor of the sinus for ideal implant positioning. Sinus augmentation therapy is carried out where inadequate bone is present for use of an osteotome and trephine approach. Simultaneous implant placement may occur, depending on the amount of available bone crestal to the floor of the sinus. When performing a lateral wall sinus augmentation approach in the presence of a bony septum, membrane reflection need not extend wholly around the septum in a medial direction. Medial extension of membrane reflection should occur only to the extent needed to affect the desired augmentation therapy. Such an understanding significantly lessens the incidence of membrane perforation during reflection in the presence of a bony septum.
- Class IIC: adequate buccopalatal dimension of the alveolar ridge is noted. Inadequate bone is present mesial and distal to the bony septum for the use of an osteotome and trephine approach, with or without simultaneous implant placement. In such a situation, a lateral window osteotomy is carried out. This osteotomy often results in 2 distinct windows, on the mesial and distal aspects of the septum, respectively. Sinus membrane reflection is effected to the extent necessary for the desire augmentation therapy. If no membrane, or a class I or class IIA perforation is noted, the perforation is managed as described earlier, and simultaneous implant placement is carried out if indicated. However, should a class IIB or class III perforation be encountered, the course of therapy must be altered. The membrane is reflected as best as possible, and the septum is removed using a piezo surgical approach. The membrane is repaired as described earlier, the septum is lacerated and mixed with the augmentation material, and augmentation is carried out. No immediate implant placement occurs in such a scenario.

The presence of a bony septum is not a contraindication to reconstruction of the posterior maxilla. Such a septum should be viewed as a further challenge, which must be assessed, classified, and managed in a logical manner.

POSTOPERATIVE INFECTION

The most common postoperative complication after sinus lift procedure is postoperative sinusitis.[16,59,60] Because maxillary sinus neighbors several vital structures, such a complication may lead to more serious complications, such as cavernous sinus thrombosis. It seems that patients with a history of sinusitis are more prone to postoperative infection of the sinus. Testori and colleagues[61] reported that failure in the diagnosis of established chronic sinusitis before the sinus augmentation surgery may lead to acute graft material infection. Emphasis should be made on accurate preoperative diagnosis to rule out any apical pathology of teeth and preexisting sinusitis. Extraction of hopeless teeth and establishment of periodontal health are required before the execution of lateral window procedure. Measures to reduce the incidence of sinus infection should be strictly followed. Poor aseptic technique is the major cause for acute sinusitis after sinus augmentation procedure. Caution during sinus membrane elevation to minimize the chance of perforation, avoidance of the placement of implant into sinus, and aseptic surgical field should be strictly followed. Preformation of the Schneiderian membrane and contamination with saliva creates an ideal atmosphere for bacterial and sinus infection. If postoperative infection of the sinus is noticed, it should be aggressively treated. In case of localized swelling, an incision and drainage should be performed and wide-spectrum antibiotic should be used.

Failure to achieve primary closure after lateral window procedure facilitates the entrance of oral and environmental bacteria to the newly elevated sinus, especially when teeth that communicate with the sinus are extracted at the time of sinus lift.[61] Barone and colleagues[40,62] reported that the lateral ridge augmentation at the time of lateral window could increase infection incidence significantly compared with lateral window with no lateral augmentation. These investigators also attributed the infection to the absence of primary closure and subsequent graft and sinus infection.

Ostium blockage may occur after the migration of the graft particulates into the maxillary sinus through a Schneiderian perforation, overfilling the maxillary sinus in the apical direction, or postoperative infection or inflammation. Ostium blockage has a negative impact on the healing process, allowing more pathogenic bacteria to grow within the grafted sinus.[61] The development of a postoperative sinusitis can be a significant concern. Steps must be taken to assess the extent of the sinusitis, prescribe stronger antibiotics if necessary, and seek a consultation with an ear, nose, and throat (ENT) specialist if the antibiotics are not effective.

Bleeding

Excessive intraoperative bleeding is occasionally encountered during the lateral window procedure.[21,50] The main source of bleeding during the osseous lateral window preparation is the trauma to small blood vessels of intraosseous branches of the posterior superior alveolar artery (PSAA), which run in the lateral aspect of the maxilla. Severing the extraosseous branches of the PSAA and branches of the intraorbital artery may cause excessive bleeding during the flap elevation or releasing incisions. The incidence of excessive intraoperative bleeding is low and is reported to be 2%.[51] Application of pressure, use of bone wax, or cauterization of the vessels is the first choice of the management of excessive bleeding from these vessels. Crushing of vessels should be the last choice, because it may further fracture the thin wall of the lateral maxilla.

Implant Exposure to the Maxillary Sinus Cavity

Implant exposure or displacement into the maxillary sinus can cause sinus mucus thickening around the implant and can give rise to rhinosinusitis. Untreated sinus infection could lead to chronic sinusitis, which might be resistant to antibiotic therapy.[52] The chronic sinusitis could get worse if the implant was improperly pushed into the sinus cavity.[61]

Loss of Graft Containment into the Sinus

It is possible for the bone graft particulates to be forced into the sinus cavity. The graft material should be filled and packed sequentially against the anterior wall, the posterior wall, and medial wall of the lateral window, without forcing the graft material into the sinus (**Fig. 9**). The vestibular wall is the last to be filled.[61] In case of small Schneiderian membrane perforation, a collagen membrane can be laid on the perforation to ensure containment of the graft particulates. It is also recommended, in case of membrane perforation, mixing the graft particulates with calcium sulfate, which acts as a particle holder when it sets, and therefore, it prevents the graft material from displacement into the sinus.

Overfill

Overfill of the elevated sinus with graft material could cause the perforation of the Schneiderian membrane and loss of the graft material into the sinus cavity and could cause sinus infection.[63,64] In such a case, the patient usually reports feeling particles in the throat for a few days. Overfilling the sinus with bone graft apically may cause the physical obstruction of the ostium and subsequent sinus infection, congestion, or increase in the pressure within the sinus.[61] An uncommon indication of sinus infection or

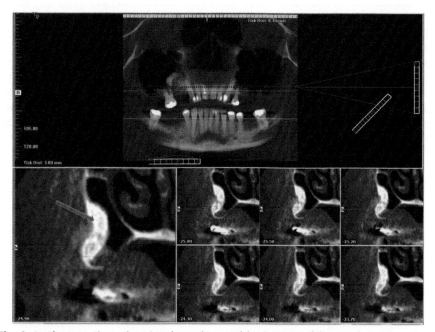

Fig. 9. Inadequate sinus elevation (*arrow*) caused by incorrect filling and packing of the bone grafting material into the medial and alveolar walls.

congestion is the leak of the graft material through the window, which is caused by increased pressure within the sinus cavity. Postoperative bleeding may also cause increase pressure in the sinus, pushing the graft material out of the lateral window. Blowing the nose and sneezing have a similar effect on the stability of graft material.[61]

Hematoma

Some uncontrolled intraoperative or postoperative bleeding may cause vestibular and facial hematoma and loss of the graft materials. PSAA and its anastomosis injury is usually the main reason for bleeding.[50] Amoxicillin (750 mg) with clavulanic acid (125 mg) for 10 days can be administered to the patient to prevent infection of the hematoma site.

Wound Dehiscence

Poor flap design and suturing technique and flap closure with no releasing incision may lead to wound dehiscence and subsequent infection. If this infection spreads out, a fistula development and oroantral communication occur. In this case, the graft material should be partially or completely removed, and a pedicle or gingival graft can be used to achieve primary closure.[37,52]

Oroantral Communication

If sinus infection is developed after the lateral window procedure and the ostium is blocked, an oroantral communication may occur. The patient usually complains of water coming through the nose while drinking. Referral to an ENT physician is warranted if infection is not controlled and oroantral communication is not closed (**Fig. 10**).

Pain

Tenderness in the sinus region and tenderness in the infraorbital region are common after the lateral window procedure and may last for 2 to 3 weeks. Adequate narcotic in combination with nonnarcotic analgesic can be administered.

Vertigo

Postoperative headache, dizziness, nausea, or benign paroxysmal positional vertigo has been reported in rare cases after the use of extensive malleting during the vertical approach of sinus augmentation. It is recommended to perform such procedures under conscious sedation and to use a gentle intermittent malleting technique.[32]

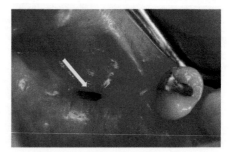

Fig. 10. An oroantral communication (*arrow*) that occurred soon after a sinus augmentation procedure. The patient had sinus infection with complete obstruction of the ostium.

SUMMARY

Sinus augmentation with or without simultaneous ridge augmentation therapy is a highly predictable treatment modality. However, its success depends on exquisite diagnosis, appropriate treatment planning, and impeccable technical execution.

REFERENCES

1. Jensen OT, Shulman LB, Block MS, et al. Report of the Sinus Consensus Conference of 1996. Int J Oral Maxillofac Implants 1998;13(Suppl):11–45.
2. Wallace SS, Froum SJ. Effect of maxillary sinus augmentation on the survival of endosseous dental implants. A systematic review. Ann Periodontol 2003;8(1): 328–43.
3. Del Fabbro M, Testori T, Francetti L, et al. Systematic review of survival rates for implants placed in the grafted maxillary sinus. Int J Periodontics Restorative Dent 2004;24(6):565–77.
4. Del Fabbro M, Rosano G, Taschieri S. Implant survival rates after maxillary sinus augmentation. Eur J Oral Sci 2008;116(6):497–506.
5. Pjetursson BE, Tan WC, Zwahlen M, et al. A systematic review of the success of sinus floor elevation and survival of implants inserted in combination with sinus floor elevation. J Clin Periodontol 2008;35(Suppl 8):216–40.
6. Chiapasco M, Casentini P, Zaniboni M. Bone augmentation procedures in implant dentistry. Int J Oral Maxillofac Implants 2009;24(Suppl):237–59.
7. Jensen S. Proceedings of the 4th consensus conference and literature review: sinus elevation procedures. In: Buser D, Chen S, Wismeijer D, editors. ITI Treatment Guide Volume 5: Sinus Elevation Procedures. Chicago: Quintessence; 2011. p. 7.
8. Lai HC, Zhuang LF, Lv XF, et al. Osteotome sinus floor elevation with or without grafting: a preliminary clinical trial. Clin Oral Implants Res 2010;21(5):520–6.
9. Kim JM, Sohn DS, Heo JU, et al. Minimally invasive sinus augmentation using ultrasonic piezoelectric vibration and hydraulic pressure: a multicenter retrospective study. Implant Dent 2012;21(6):536–42.
10. Albrektsson T, Dahl E, Enbom L, et al. Osseointegrated oral implants. A Swedish multicenter study of 8139 consecutively inserted Nobelpharma implants. J Periodontol 1988;59(5):287–96.
11. Bergstrom J, Eliasson S, Preber H. Cigarette smoking and periodontal bone loss. J Periodontol 1991;62(4):242–6.
12. Smiler DG, Johnson PW, Lozada JL, et al. Sinus lift grafts and endosseous implants. Treatment of the atrophic posterior maxilla. Dent Clin North Am 1992; 36(1):151–86 [discussion: 187–8].
13. Tawil G, Younan R, Azar P, et al. Conventional and advanced implant treatment in the type II diabetic patient: surgical protocol and long-term clinical results. Int J Oral Maxillofac Implants 2008;23(4):744–52.
14. Timmenga NM, et al. Maxillary sinusitis after augmentation of the maxillary sinus floor: a report of 2 cases. J Oral Maxillofac Surg 2001;59(2):200–4.
15. Timmenga NM, Raghoebar GM, Liem RS, et al. Effects of maxillary sinus floor elevation surgery on maxillary sinus physiology. Eur J Oral Sci 2003;111(3):189–97.
16. Timmenga NM, Raghoebar GM, Boering G, et al. Maxillary sinus function after sinus lifts for the insertion of dental implants. J Oral Maxillofac Surg 1997;55(9): 936–9 [discussion: 940].
17. Alkan A, Celebi N, Bas B. Acute maxillary sinusitis associated with internal sinus lifting: report of a case. Eur J Dent 2008;2(1):69–72.

18. Heitz-Mayfield LJ. Peri-implant diseases: diagnosis and risk indicators. J Clin Periodontol 2008;35(Suppl 8):292–304.

19. Brook I. Sinusitis of odontogenic origin. Otolaryngol Head Neck Surg 2006; 135(3):349–55.

20. Busenlechner D, Furhauser R, Haas R, et al. Long-term implant success at the Academy for Oral Implantology: 8-year follow-up and risk factor analysis. J Periodontal Implant Sci 2014;44(3):102–8.

21. Moreno Vazquez JC, Gonzalez de Rivera AS, Gil HS, et al. Complication rate in 200 consecutive sinus lift procedures: guidelines for prevention and treatment. J Oral Maxillofac Surg 2014;72(5):892–901.

22. Wen SC, Lin YH, Yang YC, et al. The influence of sinus membrane thickness upon membrane perforation during transcrestal sinus lift procedure. Clin Oral Implants Res 2014. [Epub ahead of print].

23. Nolan PJ, Freeman K, Kraut RA. Correlation between Schneiderian membrane perforation and sinus lift graft outcome: a retrospective evaluation of 359 augmented sinus. J Oral Maxillofac Surg 2014;72(1):47–52.

24. Al-Almaie S, Kavarodi AM, Al Faidhi A. Maxillary sinus functions and complications with lateral window and osteotome sinus floor elevation procedures followed by dental implants placement: a retrospective study in 60 patients. J Contemp Dent Pract 2013;14(3):405–13.

25. Jung JH, Choi BH, Jeong SM, et al. A retrospective study of the effects on sinus complications of exposing dental implants to the maxillary sinus cavity. Oral Surg Oral Med Oral Pathol Oral Radiol Endod 2007;103(5):623–5.

26. Hong YH, Mun SK. A case of massive maxillary sinus bleeding after dental implant. Int J Oral Maxillofac Surg 2011;40(7):758–60.

27. Sohn DS, Lee JK, Shin HI, et al. Fungal infection as a complication of sinus bone grafting and implants: a case report. Oral Surg Oral Med Oral Pathol Oral Radiol Endod 2009;107(3):375–80.

28. Anzalone JV, Vastardis S. Oroantral communication as an osteotome sinus elevation complication. J Oral Implantol 2010;36(3):231–7.

29. Abi Najm S, Malis D, El Hage M, et al. Potential adverse events of endosseous dental implants penetrating the maxillary sinus: long-term clinical evaluation. Laryngoscope 2013;123(12):2958–61.

30. Chiapasco M, Felisati G, Maccari A, et al. The management of complications following displacement of oral implants in the paranasal sinuses: a multicenter clinical report and proposed treatment protocols. Int J Oral Maxillofac Surg 2009;38(12):1273–8.

31. Nooh N. Effect of Schneiderian membrane perforation on posterior maxillary implant survival. J Int Oral Health 2013;5(3):28–34.

32. Greenstein G, Cavallaro J. Transcrestal sinus floor elevation with osteotomes: simplified technique and management of various scenarios. Compend Contin Educ Dent 2011;32(4):12, 14–20, [quiz: 22].

33. Lee HW, Lin WS, Morton D. A retrospective study of complications associated with 100 consecutive maxillary sinus augmentations via the lateral window approach. Int J Oral Maxillofac Implants 2013;28(3):860–8.

34. Schwartz-Arad D, Herzberg R, Dolev E. The prevalence of surgical complications of the sinus graft procedure and their impact on implant survival. J Periodontol 2004;75(4):511–6.

35. Urban IA, Nagursky H, Church C, et al. Incidence, diagnosis, and treatment of sinus graft infection after sinus floor elevation: a clinical study. Int J Oral Maxillofac Implants 2012;27(2):449–57.

36. Del Fabbro M, Wallace SS, Testori T. Long-term implant survival in the grafted maxillary sinus: a systematic review. Int J Periodontics Restorative Dent 2013; 33(6):773–83.
37. Khoury F. Augmentation of the sinus floor with mandibular bone block and simultaneous implantation: a 6-year clinical investigation. Int J Oral Maxillofac Implants 1999;14(4):557–64.
38. Shlomi B, Horowitz I, Kahn A, et al. The effect of sinus membrane perforation and repair with Lambone on the outcome of maxillary sinus floor augmentation: a radiographic assessment. Int J Oral Maxillofac Implants 2004;19(4): 559–62.
39. Ardekian L, Oved-Peleg E, Mactei EE, et al. The clinical significance of sinus membrane perforation during augmentation of the maxillary sinus. J Oral Maxillofac Surg 2006;64(2):277–82.
40. Barone A, Santini S, Marconcini S, et al. Osteotomy and membrane elevation during the maxillary sinus augmentation procedure. A comparative study: piezoelectric device vs. conventional rotative instruments. Clin Oral Implants Res 2008; 19(5):511–5.
41. Hernandez-Alfaro F, Torradeflot MM, Marti C. Prevalence and management of Schneiderian membrane perforations during sinus-lift procedures. Clin Oral Implants Res 2008;19(1):91–8.
42. Becker ST, Terheyden H, Steinriede A, et al. Prospective observation of 41 perforations of the Schneiderian membrane during sinus floor elevation. Clin Oral Implants Res 2008;19(12):1285–9.
43. Testori T, Weinstein RL, Taschieri S, et al. Risk factor analysis following maxillary sinus augmentation: a retrospective multicenter study. Int J Oral Maxillofac Implants 2012;27(5):1170–6.
44. von Arx T, Fodich I, Bornstein MM, et al. Perforation of the sinus membrane during sinus floor elevation: a retrospective study of frequency and possible risk factors. Int J Oral Maxillofac Implants 2014;29(3):718–26.
45. van den Bergh JP, ten Bruggenkate CM, Disch FJ, et al. Anatomical aspects of sinus floor elevations. Clin Oral Implants Res 2000;11(3):256–65.
46. Weitz DS, Geminiani A, Papadimitriou DE, et al. The incidence of membrane perforation during sinus floor elevation using sonic instruments: a series of 40 cases. Int J Periodontics Restorative Dent 2014;34(1):105–12.
47. Toscano NJ, Holtzclaw D, Rosen PS. The effect of piezoelectric use on open sinus lift perforation: a retrospective evaluation of 56 consecutively treated cases from private practices. J Periodontol 2010;81(1):167–71.
48. Geminiani A, Weitz DS, Ercoli C, et al. A comparative study of the incidence of Schneiderian membrane perforations during maxillary sinus augmentation with a sonic oscillating handpiece versus a conventional turbine handpiece. Clin Implant Dent Relat Res 2013. [Epub ahead of print].
49. Fugazzotto PA, Vlassis J. A simplified classification and repair system for sinus membrane perforations. J Periodontol 2003;74(10):1534–41.
50. Solar P, Geyerhofer U, Traxler H, et al. Blood supply to the maxillary sinus relevant to sinus floor elevation procedures. Clin Oral Implants Res 1999;10(1): 34–44.
51. Zijderveld SA, van den Bergh JP, Schulten EA, et al. Anatomical and surgical findings and complications in 100 consecutive maxillary sinus floor elevation procedures. J Oral Maxillofac Surg 2008;66(7):1426–38.
52. Moses JJ, Arredondo A. Sinus lift complications: avoiding problems and finding solutions. Dent Implantol Update 1997;8(9):70–2.

53. Fugazzotto PA. Maintaining primary closure after guided bone regeneration procedures: introduction of a new flap design and preliminary results. J Periodontol 2006;77(8):1452–7.

54. Fugazzotto PA. Maintenance of soft tissue closure following guided bone regeneration: technical considerations and report of 723 cases. J Periodontol 1999; 70(9):1085–97.

55. Fugazzotto PA. Report of 302 consecutive ridge augmentation procedures: technical considerations and clinical results. Int J Oral Maxillofac Implants 1998;13(3): 358–68.

56. Fugazzotto PA. Immediate implant placement following a modified trephine/ osteotome approach: success rates of 116 implants to 4 years in function. Int J Oral Maxillofac Implants 2002;17(1):113–20.

57. Fugazzotto PA. Shorter implants in clinical practice: rationale and treatment results. Int J Oral Maxillofac Implants 2008;23(3):487–96.

58. Fugazzotto PA, Beagle JR, Ganeles J, et al. Success and failure rates of 9 mm or shorter implants in the replacement of missing maxillary molars when restored with individual crowns: preliminary results 0 to 84 months in function. A retrospective study. J Periodontol 2004;75(2):327–32.

59. Tatum OH Jr, Lebowitz MS, Tatum CA, et al. Sinus augmentation. Rationale, development, long-term results. N Y State Dent J 1993;59(5):43–8.

60. Tidwell JK, Blijdorp PA, Stoelinga PJ, et al. Composite grafting of the maxillary sinus for placement of endosteal implants. A preliminary report of 48 patients. Int J Oral Maxillofac Surg 1992;21(4):204–9.

61. Testori T, editor. Maxillary sinus surgery and alternatives in treatment. Hanover Park (IL): Quintessence International; 2009. p. 191–217.

62. Barone A, Santini S, Sbordone L, et al. A clinical study of the outcomes and complications associated with maxillary sinus augmentation. Int J Oral Maxillofac Implants 2006;21(1):81–5.

63. Ulm CW, Solar P, Krennmair G, et al. Incidence and suggested surgical management of septa in sinus-lift procedures. Int J Oral Maxillofac Implants 1995;10(4): 462–5.

64. Aimetti M, Romagnoli R, Ricci G, et al. Maxillary sinus elevation: the effect of macrolacerations and microlacerations of the sinus membrane as determined by endoscopy. Int J Periodontics Restorative Dent 2001;21(6):581–9.

Persistent Pain and Neurosensory Disturbance After Dental Implant Surgery

Pathophysiology, Etiology, and Diagnosis

Mohanad Al-Sabbagh, DDS, MS[a],*, Jeffrey P. Okeson, DMD[b],
Mohd W. Khalaf, DDS[c], Ishita Bhavsar, BDS[a]

KEYWORDS

- Implant • Neurosensory • Neuropathic • Pain • Nerve injury • Sensation • Etiology
- Diagnosis

KEY POINTS

- There are multiple risk factors for the development of persistent postsurgical pain; however, the incidence of neurosensory disturbance after dental implant placement is relatively low.
- Many factors probably contribute to the development of a neurosensory deficit, including variations in implant techniques, the operator's skill, the proximity to the nerve canal, and even the psychological status of patient.
- Some studies suggest that certain patients may be genetically more susceptible to neurosensory changes after nerve injury.
- Identifying the clinical features of chronic pain conditions and neuropathies after implant placement can assist in establishing a differential diagnosis.

INTRODUCTION

All dental structures are innervated by the trigeminal nerve, and common dental procedures can result in injury to one of the many branches of this nerve. These procedures, including the determination of local anesthesia,[1] endodontic procedures (**Fig. 1**),[2,3] suture placement, soft-tissue manipulation (**Fig. 2**),[4] and third-molar extractions,[5,6] can cause injury to branches of the trigeminal nerve. The nerve most

[a] Division of Periodontology, Department of Oral Health Practice, University of Kentucky, College of Dentistry, 800 Rose Street, Lexington, KY 40536, USA; [b] Department of Oral Health Science, College of Dentistry, University of Kentucky, 800 Rose Street, Lexington, KY 40536, USA; [c] Orofacial Pain and Oral Medicine Division, Department of Head and Neck Surgery, Kaiser Permanente, 7300 Wyndham Street, Sacramento, CA 95823, USA
* Corresponding author.
E-mail address: malsa2@email.uky.edu

Dent Clin N Am 59 (2015) 131–142
http://dx.doi.org/10.1016/j.cden.2014.08.004   **dental.theclinics.com**
0011-8532/15/$ – see front matter © 2015 Elsevier Inc. All rights reserved.

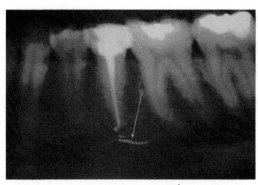

Fig. 1. Arrow in radiograph showing injury to the inferior alveolar nerve after the introduction of endodontic filling into the inferior alveolar canal.

commonly injured during dental procedures is the inferior alveolar nerve (64.4%), followed by the lingual nerve (28.8%).[7] Injuries to these nerves are most often associated with dental anesthesia.

In recent years, the great success of dental implants has led to wide acceptance of such treatment. However, nerve injury and neurosensory impairment can occur after implant placement, even after accurate evaluation and careful treatment (**Fig. 3**).[5] A recent study found that 73% of dentists have reported that their patients have experienced neurosensory impairment after surgical implant procedures.[4]

The published incidence of altered sensation after implant surgery is highly variable, ranging from 8.5% to 36%.[8,9] In addition, published reports vary greatly in the terminology used to describe patients' symptoms after nerve injury. Initially the term paresthesia was used to describe several forms of altered sensation reported by patients, including pain, warmth, cold, burning, numbness, and tingling.

The International Association for the Study of Pain[10] has more clearly defined some of the most common conditions associated with neurosensory alterations (**Table 1**). For example, anesthesia refers to complete loss of sensation; dysesthesia refers to an unpleasant form of altered sensation, such as burning, stinging, or stabbing; paresthesia refers to an altered sensation that is not necessarily unpleasant; allodynia refers to the pain produced by a nonpainful stimulus (light touch); and hyperesthesia is defined as an increased response to a painful stimuli. Although many types of neurosensory changes can occur, persistent pain after implant placement can be

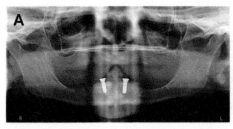
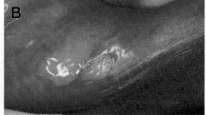

Fig. 2. (A) Radiograph showing implant placement with no evidence of injury to the inferior alveolar nerve. (B) Clinical presentation of lip biting 1 week after the implant procedure. The patient experienced analgesia attributable to flap manipulation to locate the mental foramina during the implant placement procedure.

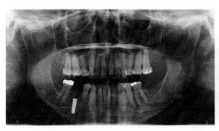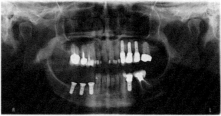

Fig. 3. Radiograph showing injury to the inferior alveolar nerve after implant placement. The implant appears to be completely intruding into the inferior alveolar nerve canal.

neuropathic. Very few data are available regarding the development of chronic persistent neuropathic pain after dental implant surgery.

Injury to a major nerve or a peripheral branch during surgery can result in postsurgical neuropathic pain, some of which can be chronic and persistent.[11] In 1991, Jemt[12] evaluated 2199 implant-supported fixed prostheses in 384 patients, and found that only 3 mandibular implants were removed because of pain within 1 year of placement. With the increasing frequency of dental implant procedures, it is likely that more patients will experience chronic neuropathic pain and altered sensation in the future.

Patients with nerve injury can experience a slight loss or a complete loss of sensation, or even debilitating chronic pain.[4] These symptoms can substantially hinder activities such as eating, drinking, speaking, and socializing, thereby greatly reducing the patient's quality of life.[13] Nerve injury and subsequent altered sensation after implant surgery may result in liability claims.[14,15] Therefore, the clinician must be able to recognize and evaluate factors that can lead to nerve injury associated with implant procedures.

Table 1
Definitions of common neurosensory deficits according to the International Association for the Study of Pain

Term	Definition
Pain	An unpleasant sensory and emotional experience associated with actual or potential tissue damage, or described in terms of such damage
Allodynia	Pain due to a stimulus that does not normally provoke pain
Analgesia	Absence of pain in response to stimulation that would normally be painful
Dysesthesia	An unpleasant abnormal sensation, whether spontaneous or evoked
Hyperalgesia	Increased pain from a stimulus that normally provokes pain
Hyperesthesia	Increased sensitivity to stimulation, excluding the special senses
Hypoalgesia	Diminished pain in response to a normally painful stimulus
Hypoesthesia	Decreased sensitivity to stimulation, excluding the special senses
Paresthesia	An abnormal sensation, whether spontaneous or evoked
Neuralgia	Pain in the distribution of a nerve or nerves
Neuritis	Inflammation of a nerve or nerves
Neuropathic pain	Pain caused by a lesion or disease of the somatosensory nervous system

Adapted from Merskey H, Bogduk N, editors. Classification of chronic pain, second edition, IASP Task Force on Taxonomy. Seattle (WA): IASP Press; 1994. p. 209–14.

BIOLOGY OF THE NERVE CELLS AND THEIR RESPONSE TO INJURY

The basic structure of the nerve trunk consists of nerve fibers that are collectively organized into fascicles. Each fascicle is surrounded by a layer of loose connective tissue, the perineural layer, which protects the nerve fibers from compressive forces.[16] Each nerve fiber is covered with well-organized tissue, called the endoneurial sheath, which consists of loose connective tissue and blood vessels. The most external surface surrounding the nerve trunk is composed of loose areolar connective tissue and is known as the epineurium.

A typical nerve fiber is composed of a cell body, dendrites, an axon, and axon terminals; this structure is surrounded by a myelin sheath and Schwann cells. The Schwann cells produce myelin, which plays an important role in facilitating nerve conduction. When a nerve fiber is subjected to mechanical injuries, it undergoes a series of structural and biochemical changes. Wallerian degeneration of the tissue distal to the injury begins,[13] and macrophages then infiltrate the site to phagocytose and degrade the debris associated with the damaged myelin sheath and axons.[13,17] Schwann cells proliferate to provide the metabolites needed for the regeneration of the nerve. The original neuron produces new axonal sprouts, which migrate toward the original endoneurial tube, thereby innervating the original tissue.

On occasion, collagen fiber is deposited and scar tissue forms within the endoneurial tube, obstructing the growth of a new axonal sprout and causing intermingling of the new axons.[13] This bundle of new neural tissue is called a neuroma. In addition, the new tissue can grow toward other endoneurial tubes to establish connections and innervate other tissues. In this way certain impulses are transmitted from peripheral nerves to the central nervous system.[17] The degree of complete nerve regeneration depends on the type and extent of the injury; therefore, recovery of sensation cannot always be expected after the nerve-regeneration process.

CLASSIFICATION OF NERVE INJURY

Seddon[18] described 3 types of nerve injury: neurapraxia, axonotmesis, and neurotmesis. Neurapraxia is associated with a temporary blockade of conduction as a result of minor nerve injury. Axonotmesis is a moderate to severe type of nerve injury whereby the basic structure of the nerve tissue is still intact. However, Wallerian degeneration can occur. Neurotmesis is the most severe type of nerve injury, involving complete transection of the nerve that results in permanent nerve injury.

More recently, Sunderland[16] described 5 types of nerve injuries; his classification is based on the anatomic structure of the nerve fibers. A first-degree nerve injury is associated with a temporary conduction block across the fiber without disruption of the anatomy of the axon. With this type of injury, nerve function usually returns to normal.

A second-degree nerve injury is associated with the loss of axon continuity; however, the endoneurial sheath remains intact. Compression or traction may cause transient ischemia, and recovery can be variable. However, regeneration of the axon within the endoneurial tube can occur.

A third-degree nerve injury results from trauma to the neural tissues that disrupts the continuity of the axon and the endoneurium, but leaves fasciculi intact. Regeneration of axons occurs after Wallerian degeneration, which is confined to within the fascicles. An intermingling of the fibers into other endoneurial tubes can occur if the endoneurial tube is occluded by scar tissue that may continue to hinder the regeneration of the axon. Complete recovery is usually not possible.

A fourth-degree nerve injury is associated with disruption of the axon, endoneurium, and fasciculi, but leaves loose connective tissue surrounding the nerve trunk.

Regeneration of the axon is prevented by the development of fibrous scar tissue. Second-, third-, and fourth-degree nerve injuries are similar to Seddon's axonotmesis, depending on the severity of the nerve injury. A fifth-degree nerve injury, the most severe form, consists of complete loss of nerve trunk continuity and is equivalent to Seddon's neurotmesis.

PATHOPHYSIOLOGY OF CHRONIC PAIN

The most common symptom reported after a surgical procedure is pain, which can be categorized as inflammatory, nociceptive, or neuropathic.[19] Immediately after a surgical procedure, pain is experienced because of soft-tissue manipulation, active inflammation, and injury to the peripheral tissues.[11,19] This type of inflammatory pain usually subsides as the tissue heals. Nociceptive pain occurs in response to noxious stimulation of sensory receptors by mechanical, thermal, or chemical provocation. Neuropathic pain can occur even in the absence of any noxious stimuli. It is usually associated with disease or a lesion within the nervous system.[19] The pathophysiology of chronic neuropathic pain involves both peripheral and central mechanisms.

Peripheral Mechanisms That Induce Chronic Pain

Several processes contribute to the development of chronic pain, including increased sensitivity, neuroma formation, ectopic impulse generation, and cross-talk between axons.[20] A neuroma is proliferating neural tissue consisting of fibroblasts and Schwann cells.[11] It is very sensitive to certain neurotransmitters such as norepinephrine, which can evoke spontaneous nerve impulses. This ectopic spontaneous firing sends a nociceptive input into the central nervous system, and this input can be interpreted as an abnormal pain sensation. The response of the nerve tissue depends on the severity of the nerve trauma. Neuroma formation has been associated with puncture, laceration, and stretch injuries to the nerves.[21] Published studies have reported an association between neuropathic complications of the implant procedures and neuroma formation.[11,21] Thus, neuroma formation is suggested to be one of the pathophysiologic features of neuropathic pain.[11,20]

The hallmark of the neuropathic pain is the sensation of pain in the absence of any stimulus. After peripheral nerve injuries, ectopic impulses are generated at various sites, including neuromas and the cell body of the injured neuron.[19] An increase in the number of postsynaptic neurotransmitter receptors after deafferentation of the injured nerve could result in this spontaneous impulse activity.[11] The ephaptic transmission is associated with the development of cross-talk between newly formed fibers or a neuroma and adjacent nerve axons. This activity involves the exchange of impulses between axons and a neuroma that can impose on the central nervous system.[11]

Central Mechanisms That Induce Neuropathic Pain

Changes in the processing of neural impulses in the brain and brainstem can contribute to the development of chronic pain. Continuous neuropathic pain may arise as a direct consequence of a lesion or disease affecting the somatosensory system.[22] Nerve injury can produce ongoing sensitization of central neurons, leading to persistent pain.[23] An injured peripheral nerve can initiate a cascade of neurochemical changes at the site of the injury and in the dorsal horn, or, in the case of the trigeminal nerve, in the spinal tract nucleus. These changes may lead to a reduction in the pain thresholds of afferent nerve terminals in the region of the injury, resulting in primary hyperalgesia.[11] At this point, the patient may begin to report spreading of the pain (expansion of the receptive field).

Central neurons respond to the nociceptive input by altering their function. These neurons begin to respond more quickly to the incoming stimulus, a condition known as central sensitization.[20] Central sensitization also leads to a phenomenon by which even non-nociceptive input carried by A-β fibers (ie, proprioception) is now perceived as painful, so that even light touch to the implant causes pain. The term used to describe this condition is allodynia. Once the dorsal horn cells have become sensitized, the entire processing of nociception can be altered. These changes can be long-lasting or even permanent. In such cases, pain continues even without further nociceptive input. In other words, the tooth or implant continues to be painful even though there is no local cause. The pain now becomes a centrally mediated neuropathic pain that can no longer be managed successfully by manipulating the peripheral tissues. When this condition occurs, pain is no longer the symptom of a disease; it actually is the disease. Genetic polymorphisms, gender, and age may be risk factors that influence whether a particular patient experiences persistent neuropathic pain.[19]

INCIDENCE OF NEUROSENSORY DEFICITS AFTER DENTAL IMPLANT SURGERY

According to several published studies, the incidence of altered sensation after surgical implant placement ranges from 8.5% to 36%.[8,9,11,24] This wide variability may be attributed to a variety of factors: variability in the techniques of implant placement, surgical skills, proximity of the nerve canal, variation in the psychological status of patient, and lack of documentation in evaluating neurosensory function.

Kiyak and colleagues[25] performed a study involving 39 patients who had undergone implant surgery; the investigators used questionnaires to assess patients' psychological response during treatment. Of the 27 patients who completed the study, 43.5% experienced facial paresthesia within 2 weeks after implant placement. Only 4.3% of these patients were expected to have some kind of sensory disturbance. Psychological assessment suggested that high levels of neuroticism or emotional stress may contribute to patient dissatisfaction; these factors should be considered during patient selection.

Astrand and colleagues[26] reported that 18 (39%) of 69 patients receiving dental implants experienced some sensory disturbances within 4 weeks after implant placement. One patient reported complete anesthesia. After 2 years, 9 patients continued to report some sensory disturbance, but the other 9 experienced complete recovery. The investigators concluded that most sensory disturbances resolve within 2 years.

Two prospective multicenter studies reported that paresthesia of the lips after implant placement occurred in 16 (10%) of 159 patients[27] and 19 of (7%) 133 patients.[28] Ten of the 16 and 16 of the 19 patients recovered completely from the paresthesia within 6 months to 1 year. Together, these 2 studies found that 3% of patients continued to have sensory alterations 2 years after implant placement. Other studies have reported persistent paresthesia of the lower lip that continued for more than 3 years in approximately 4% of cases.[29,30]

Ellies and Hawker[8] studied the incidence of altered sensation after dental implant procedures by using a retrospective questionnaire, and classified the condition either as a transient neurosensory deficit that resolved or a persistent neurosensory deficit that continued for more than 6 months after the procedure. Thirty-one patients (36%) experienced altered sensation after mandibular implant procedures and 11 patients (11%) reported persistent changes with no signs of resolution.[8] Patients reported the onset of altered sensation immediately following the procedure, and 90% of the patients with transient altered sensation experienced recovery within 6 months. Daily activities such as speaking, drinking, and eating were most frequently affected. The lip and chin were the most commonly affected orofacial sites. The incidence of persistent changes (11%) is higher than that reported by other studies. The reasons for this higher percentage may be the retrospective design of the study and the use of a questionnaire, which can introduce recall bias. Furthermore, the chronicity of persistent changes was ambiguously defined in this study. Hence, the incidence of altered sensation reported should be considered with caution.

A randomized controlled clinical trial by Wismeijer and colleagues[31] involved 103 edentulous patients with bone loss who were treated with dental implants. Because severe bone loss required placement of the implants closer than usual to the mental nerve, the study evaluated any alteration in sensation of the lower lip. Eleven of the patients (9.4%) experienced sensory disturbances in the lower the lip within 10 days after the procedure, and 10 patients (10.3%) were still experiencing sensory disturbances 1.5 years after the procedure. It should be noted that 27 of the patients reported some sensory disturbances before implant placement. Therefore, the sensory deficit noted in this study may not have been a direct consequence of the implant procedure. The investigators suggested that altered sensation could be attributed either to the close proximity of the implant to the mental nerve or to pressure caused by ill-fitting over dentures. It is important to interpret these findings with caution, because persistent changes included not only spontaneous neurosensory deficits caused by implant placement but also those possibly caused by the prosthesis.

Bartling and colleagues[9] studied the incidence of altered sensation in 94 patients after placement of mandibular dental implants. According to the treatment plan, the implants were to be located 2 mm above the inferior alveolar nerve canal, as determined by panoramic images, and 1 mm above the canal, as determined by computed tomography (CT) images. Based on these criteria, there was no radiographic evidence of nerve injury. The investigators found that 8.5% of the patients reported altered nerve sensation at their first visit after the placement of the implant. All subjects reported complete resolution of symptoms within 4 months (121 days). One subject reported complete anesthesia for 2 months but a return to normal sensation after that time. The results of this study suggest that injuries to the small intraosseous branches of the trigeminal nerve are less associated with persistent neuropathic disorders.

DIAGNOSIS

A diagnosis of persistent chronic pain is made after the exclusion of all other pathoses that may provoke pain in the affected area. Patient history, gender, age, medical status, dental history, diagnostic imaging studies, and clinical examination should be assessed for a diagnosis of chronic pain. The patient history provides the temporal relationship between injury, normal healing, and persistent pain after an adequate healing time.

When pain continues beyond the normal healing time, the clinician must rule out all potential local causative factors, such as infection or peri-implantitis (**Fig. 4**). When such conditions have been ruled out, a diagnosis of persistent neuropathic pain should be considered. A helpful clinical diagnostic method is neurosensory testing, which includes mapping of the area involved in paresthesia or pain (**Fig. 5**), discriminating between dull and sharp probes, and assessing for allodynia.[32] Validated questionnaires have been used in clinical settings to screen patients with chronic pain and neuropathies; such questionnaires may be an effective tool for diagnosing neuropathic pain.[33] These questionnaires use the clinical characteristics of the pain to distinguish neuropathic pain from other pain disorders, and have been demonstrated to have good validity.

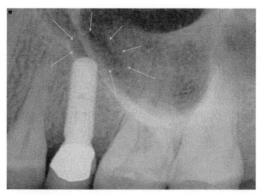

Fig. 4. Radiograph showing dormant long-standing infection around the apex of the implant (*arrows*) causing persistent pain.

Identifying the clinical features of chronic pain conditions and neuropathies after implant placement can assist in establishing a differential diagnosis. The development of paresthesia or anesthesia immediately after or soon after implant placement is a common characteristic of suspected nerve injury. Allodynia, hyperalgesia, or dysesthesia usually has a later onset. Renton and colleagues,[34] Gregg,[21] and Kraut and colleagues[35] have reported the late manifestations of allodynia, hyperalgesia, and dysesthesia in patients with nerve injuries after implant placement.

RISK FACTORS

A substantial proportion of persistent postsurgical pain is very likely to be neuropathic in origin.[36–38] Factors such as preoperative pain, concomitant pain conditions, and impairment in general physical functioning have been associated with persistent postsurgical pain.[39–42] Psychological factors such as anxiety and depression,[39] fear of surgery,[41,42] psychic vulnerability,[43] and catastrophizing[44] have also been reported as risk factors associated with the development of postsurgical chronic pain. In addition, social and economic factors have been associated with an increased likelihood of chronic pain.[37] Genetic risk factors for developing neuropathic pain in humans have been proposed.[19,45,46]

Several studies have reported that women are more likely than men to experience altered sensation and chronic pain.[8,37,47] According to the available case reports in

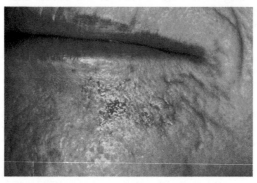

Fig. 5. Clinical presentation of mapped neuropathic area of the lower lip 1 week after injury to the inferior alveolar nerve during implant placement.

the literature, most patients who experienced a neurosensory deficit after implant placement were women older than 40 years.

Risk factors associated with the development of neuropathic pain include age greater than 40 years, smaller-sized mandibles, and bone resorption in response to hormone changes.[26] Gregg[21] reported that chronic neuropathic pain after implant placement is more prevalent in older patients who smoke. Other associated risk factors are resorbed ridges,[31] smoking,[21] and medical conditions such as diabetic polyneuropathies[48] and multiple sclerosis.[49] Patients who engage in activities such as reading, yoga, meditation, and exercise seem to deal better with neurosensory deficits, and young patients show greater improvement than older counterparts.[50]

It is interesting that in one study more than 70% of the patients who reported pain within 6 months after implant placement were not specifically warned of the potential for nerve injury.[51] This finding suggests a relationship between lack of informed consent and continued pain after implant surgery.

SUMMARY

There are multiple risk factors for the development of persistent postsurgical pain. However, the incidence of neurosensory deficits after dental implant placement is relatively low. Many factors probably contribute to the development of a neurosensory deficit, including variations in implant techniques, the operator's skill, the proximity to the nerve canal, and even the psychological status of patient. In addition, some studies suggest that certain patients may be genetically more susceptible to neurosensory changes after nerve injury.[52,53]

It is also important to realize that published studies of neurosensory deficits have not always separated painful conditions from nonpainful alterations. Although all neurosensory deficits have a negative impact on the patient, persistent neuropathic pain disorders are likely to have the greatest effect on quality of life. The dentist must focus on these conditions and determine how to minimize these adverse consequences.

Clinicians who perform implant surgery must be aware of these risk factors, and must consider each of them when making clinical decisions for their patients. Patients should also be informed of these risk factors so that they can actively participate in treatment selection. Further investigations are necessary not only to better understand the relationship between dental implant procedures and neurosensory deficits but also to better understand how to prevent these adverse consequences.

REFERENCES

1. Pogrel MA, Thamby S. Permanent nerve involvement resulting from inferior alveolar nerve blocks. J Am Dent Assoc 2000;131(7):901–7.
2. Grotz KA, Al-Nawas B, de Aguiar EG, et al. Treatment of injuries to the inferior alveolar nerve after endodontic procedures. Clin Oral Investig 1998;2(2):73–6.
3. Givol N, Rosen E, Bjorndal L, et al. Medico-legal aspects of altered sensation following endodontic treatment: a retrospective case series. Oral Surg Oral Med Oral Pathol Oral Radiol Endod 2011;112(1):126–31.
4. Misch CE, Resnik MR. Mandibular nerve neurosensory impairment after dental implant surgery: management and protocol. Implant Dent 2010;19(5):378–86.
5. Ziccardi VB, Assael LA. Mechanisms of trigeminal nerve injuries. Atlas Oral Maxillofac Surg Clin North Am 2001;9(2):1–11.
6. Bhat P, Cariappa KM. Inferior alveolar nerve deficits and recovery following surgical removal of impacted mandibular third molars. J Maxillofac Oral Surg 2012; 11(3):304–8.

7. Tay AB, Zuniga JR. Clinical characteristics of trigeminal nerve injury referrals to a university centre. Int J Oral Maxillofac Surg 2007;36(10):922–7.

8. Ellies LG, Hawker PB. The prevalence of altered sensation associated with implant surgery. Int J Oral Maxillofac Implants 1993;8(6):674–9.

9. Bartling R, Freeman K, Kraut RA. The incidence of altered sensation of the mental nerve after mandibular implant placement. J Oral Maxillofac Surg 1999;57(12):1408–12.

10. Merskey H, Bogduk N, editors. Classification of chronic pain, 2nd edition, IASP Task Force on Taxonomy. Seattle (WA): IASP Press; 1994. p. 209–14.

11. Delcanho RE. Neuropathic implications of prosthodontic treatment. J Prosthet Dent 1995;73(2):146–52.

12. Jemt T. Failures and complications in 391 consecutively inserted fixed prostheses supported by Branemark implants in edentulous jaws: a study of treatment from the time of prosthesis placement to the first annual checkup. Int J Oral Maxillofac Implants 1991;6(3):270–6.

13. Hegedus F, Diecidue RJ. Trigeminal nerve injuries after mandibular implant placement–practical knowledge for clinicians. Int J Oral Maxillofac Implants 2006;21(1):111–6.

14. Worthington P. Medicolegal aspects of oral implant surgery. Aust Prosthodont J 1995;9(Suppl):13–7.

15. Chaushu G, Taicher S, Halamish-Shani T, et al. Medicolegal aspects of altered sensation following implant placement in the mandible. Int J Oral Maxillofac Implants 2002;17(3):413–5.

16. Sunderland S. The anatomy and physiology of nerve injury. Muscle Nerve 1990; 13(9):771–84.

17. Fukuda K, Ichinohe T, Kaneko Y. Pain management for nerve injury following dental implant surgery at Tokyo Dental College Hospital. Int J Dent 2012; 2012:209474.

18. Seddon HJ. A classification of nerve injuries. Br Med J 1942;2(4260):237–9.

19. Costigan M, Scholz J, Woolf CJ. Neuropathic pain: a maladaptive response of the nervous system to damage. Annu Rev Neurosci 2009;32:1–32.

20. Okeson JP. Bell's oral and facial pain. 7th edition. Chicago: Quintessence Publishers; 2014.

21. Gregg JM. Neuropathic complications of mandibular implant surgery: review and case presentations. Ann R Australas Coll Dent Surg 2000;15:176–80.

22. Treede RD, Jensen TS, Campbell JN, et al. Neuropathic pain: redefinition and a grading system for clinical and research purposes. Neurology 2008;70(18):1630–5.

23. Sheen K, Chung JM. Signs of neuropathic pain depend on signals from injured nerve fibers in a rat model. Brain Res 1993;610(1):62–8.

24. Ellies LG. Altered sensation following mandibular implant surgery: a retrospective study. J Prosthet Dent 1992;68(4):664–71.

25. Kiyak HA, Beach BH, Worthington P, et al. Psychological impact of osseointegrated dental implants. Int J Oral Maxillofac Implants 1990;5(1):61–9.

26. Astrand P, Borg K, Gunne J, et al. Combination of natural teeth and osseointegrated implants as prosthesis abutments: a 2-year longitudinal study. Int J Oral Maxillofac Implants 1991;6(3):305–12.

27. van Steenberghe D, Lekholm U, Bolender C, et al. Applicability of osseointegrated oral implants in the rehabilitation of partial edentulism: a prospective multicenter study on 558 fixtures. Int J Oral Maxillofac Implants 1990;5(3):272–81.

28. Johns RB, Jemt T, Heath MR, et al. A multicenter study of overdentures supported by Branemark implants. Int J Oral Maxillofac Implants 1992;7(4):513–22.

29. Henry PJ, Tolman DE, Bolender C. The applicability of osseointegrated implants in the treatment of partially edentulous patients: three-year results of a prospective multicenter study. Quintessence Int 1993;24(2):123–9.
30. Higuchi KW, Folmer T, Kultje C. Implant survival rates in partially edentulous patients: a 3-year prospective multicenter study. J Oral Maxillofac Surg 1995;53(3): 264–8.
31. Wismeijer D, van Waas MA, Vermeeren JI, et al. Patients' perception of sensory disturbances of the mental nerve before and after implant surgery: a prospective study of 110 patients. Br J Oral Maxillofac Surg 1997;35(4):254–9.
32. Walk D, Sehgal N, Moeller-Bertram T, et al. Quantitative sensory testing and mapping: a review of nonautomated quantitative methods for examination of the patient with neuropathic pain. Clin J Pain 2009;25(7):632–40.
33. Bennett MI, Smith BH, Torrance N, et al. The S-LANSS score for identifying pain of predominantly neuropathic origin: validation for use in clinical and postal research. J Pain 2005;6(3):149–58.
34. Renton T, Yilmaz Z. Profiling of patients presenting with posttraumatic neuropathy of the trigeminal nerve. J Orofac Pain 2011;25(4):333–44.
35. Kraut RA, Chahal O. Management of patients with trigeminal nerve injuries after mandibular implant placement. J Am Dent Assoc 2002;133(10):1351–4.
36. Katz J, Seltzer Z. Transition from acute to chronic postsurgical pain: risk factors and protective factors. Expert Rev Neurother 2009;9(5):723–44.
37. Kehlet H, Jensen TS, Woolf CJ. Persistent postsurgical pain: risk factors and prevention. Lancet 2006;367(9522):1618–25.
38. Johansen A, Romundstad L, Nielsen CS, et al. Persistent postsurgical pain in a general population: prevalence and predictors in the Tromso study. Pain 2012; 153(7):1390–6.
39. Nikolajsen L, Ilkjaer S, Kroner K, et al. The influence of preamputation pain on postamputation stump and phantom pain. Pain 1997;72(3):393–405.
40. Perkins FM, Kehlet H. Chronic pain as an outcome of surgery. A review of predictive factors. Anesthesiology 2000;93(4):1123–33.
41. Peters ML, Sommer M, de Rijke JM, et al. Somatic and psychologic predictors of long-term unfavorable outcome after surgical intervention. Ann Surg 2007; 245(3):487–94.
42. Peters ML, Sommer M, van Kleef M, et al. Predictors of physical and emotional recovery 6 and 12 months after surgery. Br J Surg 2010;97(10):1518–27.
43. Jorgensen T, Teglbjerg JS, Wille-Jorgensen P, et al. Persisting pain after cholecystectomy. A prospective investigation. Scand J Gastroenterol 1991;26(1): 124–8.
44. Khan RS, Ahmed K, Blakeway E, et al. Catastrophizing: a predictive factor for postoperative pain. Am J Surg 2011;201(1):122–31.
45. Uchida H, Matsushita Y, Ueda H. Epigenetic regulation of BDNF expression in the primary sensory neurons after peripheral nerve injury: implications in the development of neuropathic pain. Neuroscience 2013;240:147–54.
46. Max MB, Wu T, Atlas SJ, et al. A clinical genetic method to identify mechanisms by which pain causes depression and anxiety. Mol Pain 2006;2:14.
47. Caumo W, Schmidt AP, Schneider CN, et al. Preoperative predictors of moderate to intense acute postoperative pain in patients undergoing abdominal surgery. Acta Anaesthesiol Scand 2002;46(10):1265–71.
48. Dyck PJ, Davies JL, Wilson DM, et al. Risk factors for severity of diabetic polyneuropathy: intensive longitudinal assessment of the Rochester Diabetic Neuropathy Study cohort. Diabetes Care 1999;22(9):1479–86.

49. Jensen TS, Rasmussen P, Reske-Nielsen E. Association of trigeminal neuralgia with multiple sclerosis: clinical and pathological features. Acta Neurol Scand 1982;65(3):182–9.
50. Pogrel MA, Jergensen R, Burgon E, et al. Long-term outcome of trigeminal nerve injuries related to dental treatment. J Oral Maxillofac Surg 2011;69(9):2284–8.
51. Renton T, Dawood A, Shah A, et al. Post-implant neuropathy of the trigeminal nerve. A case series. Br Dent J 2012;212(11):E17.
52. Young EE, Costigan M, Herbert TA, et al. Heritability of nociception IV: neuropathic pain assays are genetically distinct across methods of peripheral nerve injury. Pain 2014;155(5):868–80.
53. Dominguez CA, Strom M, Gao T, et al. Genetic and sex influence on neuropathic pain-like behavior after spinal cord injury in the rat. Eur J Pain 2012;16(10):1368–77.

Persistent Pain and Neurosensory Disturbance After Dental Implant Surgery
Prevention and Treatment

Mohanad Al-Sabbagh, DDS, MS[a],*, Jeffrey P. Okeson, DMD[b], Elizangela Bertoli, DDS, MS[c], Denielle C. Medynski, DMD[d], Mohd W. Khalaf, DDS[e]

KEYWORDS

- Implant • Neurosensory • Neuropathic pain • Nerve injury • Prevention
- Management

KEY POINTS

- Although the success rates associated with implants are good, adverse events can occur.
- Disruption of normal sensation and pain can be consequence of implant placement.
- Clinicians must be aware of these adverse consequences and avoid them whenever possible; avoidance can be best achieved by careful advanced planning before implants are placed.
- When neurosensory alterations or pain results, pharmacologic management can be helpful.
- Microsurgical repair of damaged nerve tissue should be considered.

INTRODUCTION

Nerve injury associated with implant placement may occur during injections of local anesthetic, osteotomy preparation, or implant placement. One of the most common complications associated with nerve injury during implant surgery is altered sensation.[1] Patients often experience complete or partial loss of sensation, such as

[a] Division of Periodontology, Department of Oral Health Practice, University of Kentucky, College of Dentistry, 800 Rose Street, Lexington, KY 40536, USA; [b] Department of Oral Health Science, College of Dentistry, University of Kentucky, 800 Rose Street, Lexington, KY 40536, USA; [c] Division of Restorative Dentistry, Department of Oral Health Practice, University of Kentucky, College of Dentistry, 800 Rose Street, Lexington, KY 40536, USA; [d] UCSF Center for Orofacial Pain, 513 Parnassus Avenue, S-738, San Francisco, CA 94143-0476, USA; [e] Private Practice, Orofacial Pain and Oral Medicine Division, Department of Head and Neck Surgery, Kaiser Permanente, 7300 Wyndham Street, Sacramento, CA 95823, USA
* Corresponding author.
E-mail address: malsa2@email.uky.edu

Dent Clin N Am 59 (2015) 143–156
http://dx.doi.org/10.1016/j.cden.2014.08.005
0011-8532/15/$ – see front matter © 2015 Elsevier Inc. All rights reserved.

perceptions of touch, pressure, or temperature. These symptoms may seriously affect a patient's ability to perform daily activities, such as drinking and eating, and may also lead to traumatic biting of soft tissues (lips or cheeks) during mastication. In addition to these symptoms, some patients may also experience severe pain that can be debilitating.

Persistent pain after implant placement can be neuropathic in nature. Neuropathic pain (NP) is defined as "pain initiated or caused by primary lesion or dysfunction in the nervous system."[2] In addition, NP may be associated with paresthesia, dysesthesia (burning, stinging, or stabbing sensations), sensory deficits, allodynia, and hyperesthesia.[3]

As described in the article by Al-Sabbagh and colleagues elsewhere in this issue, the pathophysiology of NP is complex and has not yet been completely elucidated. Treatment is complicated by the fact that NP does not normally respond well to conventional analgesics and opioids.[3,4] Currently, many therapeutic approaches are being explored, but to date none has been consistently helpful. Because NP is often intense, debilitating, and resistant to treatment, practitioners should be familiar with the basic mechanisms that contribute to NP disorders (see article by Al-Sabbgh and colleagues) so that they can plan procedure more carefully and often prevent these complications. Also, understanding that certain risk factors predispose patients to NP can help minimize its occurrence.

INITIAL THERAPEUTIC CONSIDERATIONS AND PREVENTION OF NERVE INJURY

When a nerve injury is suspected, clinicians must be able to recognize the cause, type, and extent of the injury. Local anesthetic blocks have been reported to cause trauma to nerves.[5] It has been reported that 25% to 29% of local anesthetic injections that cause nerve injuries result in a permanent change to the nerve tissue.[6] Avoiding multiple injections can help prevent iatrogenic nerve injury related to local anesthetics. The treatment of patients with nerve injury includes antiinflammatory medications (steroids or nonsteroidal antiinflammatory drugs [NSAIDs]) to reduce the neural inflammation, along with counseling and reassurance.[6]

It is important to appreciate the need for local anesthetic blocks even when surgical procedures are performed with patients under sedation. Preemptive analgesia with local anesthetics, opioids, antiinflammatories, and glucocorticoids has been associated with reduced postoperative pain, less postoperative use of analgesics, and shorter hospital stays.[7,8] Lee and colleagues[9] tested whether perineural injections of dexamethasone and bupivacaine exerted preemptive analgesic effects in a nerve injury model. They found that mechanical allodynia did not develop and that preoperative infiltration of dexamethasone and bupivacaine exerted a substantially better analgesic effect than did infiltration of dexamethasone or bupivacaine alone. Bupivacaine has been shown to reduce postoperative pain and to block sensory input beyond the duration action of the local anesthetic.[10]

Another consideration that may lead to nerve tissue injury is the heat produced by an implant drill. The pressure, speed, sharpness, time of use, and irrigation system of the drill are often directly linked to the production increased heat during implant placement.[11] The neural tissue is sensitive and easily damaged by heat stimuli. Increased temperature has been associated with a reduction in the ability of bone tissue to repair and regenerate.[11] It can also enhance osteoclastic activity, thereby resulting in the failure of the osseointegration process.[11]

Continuous contact between implant drill and bony wall occurs during the implant osteotomy procedure. Sometimes the implant drill can slip because of the presence of softer bone in the direction of drilling; such slipping can cause mechanical trauma to the structures, in particular the nerves. Therefore, the risk of nerve injury can be reduced by careful evaluation of the thickness and density of the bone mass surrounding the nerve and by the use of less force during implant drilling as the bur approaches the canal.[12]

Continuous irrigation of the bur helps reduce heat generation and prevents clogging by debris during implant osteotomy procedures. The presence of certain chemicals in the irrigating solutions has been associated, however, with chemical nerve injury, particularly when the osteotomy is prepared close to the nerve canal. The use of sodium hypochlorite solution is not recommended for irrigating the implant bed because it can result in an alkalemic nerve injury.[13]

Both the buccal and the lingual plates play an important role in determining the reference point for all of the measurements required during the implant osteotomy procedure. Bone loss in the alveolar ridge after tooth extraction usually occurs in the buccal aspect, resulting in an uneven ridge in which the lingual side is higher than the buccal side. Clinicians should keep this in mind when establishing a reference point. The lingual side generally provides more available vertical bone measurements than the buccal. Therefore, the amount of bone available and the location of the nerve canal should be precisely measured with a cone-beam CT (CBCT) scan. As a preventive measure for nerve injury, a CBCT scan is useful for appreciating the 3-D relationship of the implant and the surrounding structures, including the nerve canals and foramina (**Fig. 1**). This image provides 3-D measurements that help clinicians avoid unnecessary iatrogenic nerve trauma. It has been reported that nerve injuries are less likely to occur when CBCT scans are used to evaluate the site before implant placement.[14]

Even after careful evaluation and measurements, nerve injury can occur during implant placement. A safety zone of approximately 2 to 3 mm between implant apex and nerve canal helps minimize direct nerve trauma during implant procedures (**Fig. 2**). Direct mechanical injury to the nerve by implant intrusion can cause either encroachment of the implant into the nerve canal or complete transection of the nerve. Such severe nerve injury induces retrograde degeneration proximally and leads to cell body degeneration. It has been reported that injuries at the ramus region (proximal site) are more serious than those that occur at the area of the mental foramen (distal site).[15]

If the apex of an implant is placed close to the nerve canal, secondary injuries to the nerve may occur (**Fig. 3**). These injuries include chipping of the roof of the inferior alveolar nerve (IAN) canal; this injury can result in the accumulation of debris and the development of compression injuries to the IAN.[13] Compression injuries can produce altered sensation after implant placement and can be treated by immediate removal of the implant to relieve the compression. As discussed previously, the perineurium layer protects the nerve fibers from compression or stretch injuries. When pressure

B

A

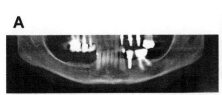
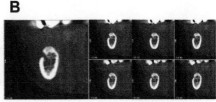

Fig. 1. (*A*) IAN and mental foramina can't be traced on the panoramic image. (*B*) CT scan provides information on the amount of available bone and the location of the IAN canal and mental foramina.

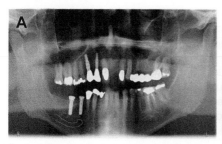
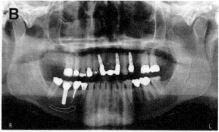

Fig. 2. (A) Radiograph showing a safety zone of approximately 2 to 3 mm between the implant apex and the IAN canal. (B) Safety zone helps minimize direct nerve trauma during implant procedures.

and elongation of more than 30% occur, however, severe damage to the axon is possible.[16] Occasionally, severe nerve injuries can lead to anesthesia with loss of function accompanied by radiating pain. Neuropathic and myofascial pain is associated with positioning of the implant in the vicinity of the nerves. Rodríguez-Lozano and colleagues[17] reported a patient who experienced NP 6 months after implant placement. They also reported that NP patients may not respond to implant removal and may require a consultation with a pain specialist or a multidisciplinary clinic. Such cases may result from alterations within the central dorsal horn, such as central sensitization associated with the nerve injury. When such sensitization occurs, further surgical procedures in the area, such as removing the implant, may only exaggerate the NP.

In conclusion, surgical procedures associated with the placement of dental implants have been associated with several types of nerve injuries, even when skilled clinicians use careful, well-planned procedures.[18] Some of the common sources of nerve injuries are local anesthetic injections, flap reflection, suturing, soft tissue swelling, and pressure around nerves. Because resolution of nerve injury is unpredictable and NP is often resistant to treatment, careful planning in advance of treatment is the most effective treatment strategy.[9]

TREATMENT OPTIONS

Effective treatment depends not only on the nature and degree of the nerve injury but also on the ability of clinicians to evaluate the trauma. In most cases, the injury is likely

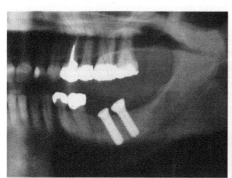
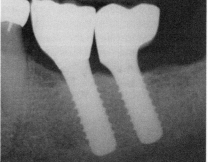

Fig. 3. Radiograph on the left showing the apex of the implant was placed close to the IAN canal. Patient experienced hypoalgesia of the lower lip that was successfully treated with high doses of NSAIDs. Radiograph on the right showing implants were successfully restored and put into function without any clinical symptoms.

related to mandibular dental implants. The treatment of patients with iatrogenic nerve injuries related to dental implants should be aimed at managing symptoms as soon as they become evident. Decisions about the type of nerve injury and the timing of treatment are vital to the outcome of patients. The management of NP involves primarily pharmacotherapy. Invasive and irreversible approaches should generally be avoided. A comprehensive evaluation should include psychological and behavioral aspects. This type of pain is often best managed by a multidisciplinary team composed of orofacial pain dentists, neurologists, neurosurgeons, psychologists, and other specialists as appropriate.[3]

Pharmacologic Management

Immediately after the surgical procedure, the inflammatory process begins. This process includes the activation of several cytokines, chemokines, and inflammatory mediators, such as interleukin 1β and tumor necrosis factor α. If the nerve has been traumatized during the surgical procedure, these inflammatory mediators contribute to the development of NP by activating the neurons and their nociceptors.[19] Therefore, antiinflammatory drugs are usually recommended for patients with nerve injuries, and case reports have recommended NSAIDs for such patients.[13,20] Khawaja and Renton[13] reported a patient who experienced paresthesia after implant placement. The clinician prescribed ibuprofen, 800 mg; amoxicillin, 500 mg (both 3 times a day); and prednisolone, 50 mg once daily, for 5 days, tapered to 10 mg for next 5 days. Although the investigators reported pain reduction, the implant was immediately removed. Therefore, it is difficult to determine the reason for the success. Misch and Resnik[15] recommended the use of steroids in addition to high doses of NSAIDs, such as ibuprofen (600–800 mg) 3 times daily for 3 weeks, but no supportive data were presented (**Fig. 4**).

Corticosteroids, commonly used antiinflammatory drugs, are often recommended for patients with neurosensory deficits after nerve injury. Reports have suggested that these drugs can help prevent the formation of neuromas; therefore, higher dosages have been recommended within the first week after the nerve injury.[15] It has been suggested[21] that patients with persistent dysesthesia after dental implant procedures should be given a series of injections containing a mixture of dexamethasone, 4 mg/mL, and 2% lidocaine with 1:100,000 epinephrine (50:50 mixture) into the most painful area. These injections should be repeated until the pain symptoms disappear. Misch and Resnik[15] suggested that if known trauma (observed nerve injury) or compression of the nerve occurs during the implant osteotomy, 1 to 2 mL of

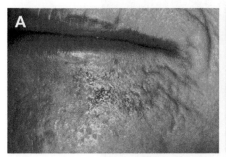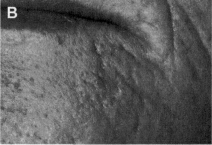

Fig. 4. (*A*) Clinical presentation of mapped neuropathic area after injury to the IAN after implant placement. Patient was experiencing analgesia of the lower lip. (*B*) Clinical presentation of mapped area after 4 months of treatment with steroids in addition to high doses of NSAIDs.

dexamethasone (4 mg/mL) should be applied topically for 1 to 2 minutes to minimize neural inflammation and soft tissue swelling that can compress the nerve. In addition, an oral regimen of dexamethasone should be administered for 6 days.

Other pharmacologic medications that have been recommended for patients with nerve injuries are antidepressants and anticonvulsants. Park and colleagues[22] evaluated the response of 85 patients with trigeminal nerve injury after implant surgery to antidepressive and anticonvulsant drugs. Patients reported a 24.8% reduction in pain after 12 weeks of anticonvulsant and antidepressant medications; however, the study had no control group (**Fig. 5**).

Pharmacotherapy for NP includes a variety of agents. The authors recommend that clinicians study a systematic review of drug trials so that they can better manage NP.[3]

Pharmacologic therapy for NP includes the following:

a. Tricyclic antidepressants drugs, such as amitriptyline, desipramine, and nortriptyline. The analgesic effects of these drugs are believed independent of the antidepressant effect. The main mechanism of action of these drugs is to inhibit the reuptake of monoamines and to blockade sodium channels; they also exert anticholinergic effects. Common adverse effects include somnolence, dry mouth, constipation, and weight gain.

b. Serotonin and norepinephrine reuptake inhibitors, such as duloxetine and venlafaxine, are also used to manage NP.[23] Commonly reported adverse effects are nausea and hypertension at high dosages.

c. Anticonvulsants drugs, such as gabapentin and pregabalin, are also used for the management of NP. The main mechanism of action is the decrease of central sensitization and nociceptive transmission. Common adverse side effects include sedation, dizziness, peripheral edema, and weight gain.

d. Local anesthetics are often used as a diagnostic tool for orofacial pain and may even have therapeutic value in some instances of NP because of their membrane stabilization potential. Local anesthetics suppress sympathetic sprouting, which is associated with NP. The effectiveness of lidocaine suppression of nerve growth factor has been demonstrated.[24]

e. Topical medications, such as lidocaine or benzocaine, can be helpful in reducing local pain. Often, other medications, such as amitriptyline, carbamazepine, and ketamine, can be added to the mixture by a compounding pharmacy. Capsaicin has also been used. Many of these topical medications can be helpful, but well-controlled clinical trials have not demonstrated their effectiveness.

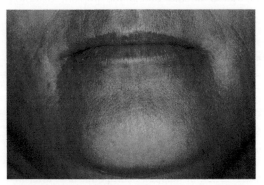

Fig. 5. Clinical presentation of mapped neuropathic area 1 year after injury to the IAN after implant placement. Patient was experiencing dysesthesia that was treated successfully with anticonvulsant medications.

f. Opioids are normally discouraged for the management of NP. Typically, opioids are not effective in treating this type of pain, and, because NP is often chronic, the likelihood of habituation and abuse is great. Opioids should be considered only when all other medications have failed and then only under the supervision of a long-term pain management team. A more thorough review of the pharmacologic management of NP pain can be found in other resources.[25]

Considerations for Surgical Removal of the Implant

Implant in close proximity to the canal or a major nerve

Many case reports have shown that close proximity between implant fixtures and major nerves or canals can lead to neurosensory impairments that manifest themselves as paresthesia or anesthesia (numbness). Substantial improvement in sensation has also been reported after early implant removal and pharmacologic treatment. In these cases, violation of an inferior alveolar canal (IAC) may not be visible on CT or panoramic tomography scans.[13,26]

If an implant appears to be in close approximation to the neurovascular bundle, the most important therapy during the surgery is to either reposition or remove the implant. Additional information regarding nerve canal violation is attained by a postsurgical radiograph or CT scan.

Implant encroaching on the canal or a major nerve

Anesthesia or paresthesia is evident at the early stage of nerve injury; allodynia, dysesthesia, and hyperalgesia are present in the later period of injury.[13,27–29] Of patients included in these reports, only one reported improvement in sensation after apicoectomy of the impinging implant.[29] Berberi and colleagues[28] reported that immediate removal of the implant and initiation of pharmacologic treatment resulted in remarkable improvement in tongue sensation after lingual nerve injury. In contrast, Khawaja and Renton[13] reported that removing the implant 4 days after placement and initiating pharmacologic treatment did not substantially improve the symptoms or bring about neurosensory recovery. Gregg[27] did not remove the implant but administered pharmacologic treatment alone; no substantial improvement occurred. Results achieved by early removal of the implant were equivocal in cases of implant encroachment. The results of pharmacologic intervention in managing symptoms after the placement of implants were also equivocal.

If an implant appears to be encroaching on the canal, the implant should be backed out; a shorter implant may be placed at the same site. No published reports suggest, however, that either backing out implants or placing shorter implants completely resolves altered sensation. Nonetheless, current opinion suggests that such treatment can greatly enhance a patient's ability to cope with altered sensation. On the other hand, if a patient experiences altered sensation with no known surgical trauma to the nerve (closed nerve injury), the decision to remove the offending dental implant depends on its osseointegration status. A case report by Park and colleagues[26] described a patient with hyperesthesia and paresthesia of the lip and chin after an implant procedure. An 8-week course of dexamethasone was prescribed but did not reduce the painful symptoms. Removal of the offending implant, however, relieved the paresthesia immediately. Therefore, after the administration of pharmacologic therapy, it is important to monitor the neurosensory status of patients. If the symptoms do not improve, other methods of treatment should be considered.

Persistent pain after implant placement

A few case reports have described persistent pain after implant. In those cases, neither CT scans nor panoramic tomography showed violation to a major nerve or canal. These reports also determined that the complaints of pain were attributed to injury to a peripheral nerve or to the proximity of the implant fixture to an IAC. Dramatic improvement of symptoms was reported after implant removal and pharmacologic treatment. In these cases, the implant was removed within 39 days after placement. In these case reports, none of the patients reported paresthesia or anesthesia.[20,21,30]

In a case series, Khawaja and Renton[13] questioned whether the length of time between implant placement and its removal had an effect on NP. In the 2 cases they discussed, the implants were removed within 24 hours, with marked improvement in the symptoms of neurosensory deficit. In 2 other cases, the implants were removed 2 to 4 days after placement, with no reduction in neuropathy. The investigators concluded that the best results in reducing symptoms are achieved when implants associated with IAN injuries are removed early (within 36 hours). They also recommended that clinicians should initiate the assessment of neurosensory changes as early as possible by contacting patients within 6 hours after the surgical procedure, after local anesthesia has been metabolized.[13] These case reports indicate that, in cases of known injury, surgically removing the implant within 24 hours of its placement and administering pharmacologic therapy may help reduce the damage to the nerve. Consistent with the findings of Khawaja and Renton[13] are those of a recent study[31] in which patients whose implants were removed within 30 hours after placement showed marked resolution of neuropathy within a few weeks. In contrast, when implants were removed 3 to 90 days after placement, no resolution of the neurosensory symptoms was noticed. The investigators concluded that implants should be removed within 24 hours of placement if patients exhibit immediate signs of neuropathy; such early removal maximizes the chances of resolution.

The process of osseointegration typically requires 2 to 4 months. If an implant is completely osseointegrated, the management of nerve injury depends on the extent of the nerve damage, the amount of pain, and patient desire for treatment. As discussed previously, reassurance, counseling, pharmacologic management, follow-up, and surgical procedure are some of the treatment options. Some patients accept the symptoms of nerve injury, whereas others find it difficult to cope with accept the symptoms. Therefore, the treatment associated with osseointegrated implants depends on a patient's motivation. If an implant requires removal, measures should to be taken to minimize the amount of circumferential bone tissue that is removed adjacent to the implant.[32] Removal is followed by a bone grafting procedure aimed at allowing regeneration of bone in that area, which may be a potential site for a future implant. Some reports suggest that removing an implant after osseointegration does not help reduce the symptoms of neuropathy.[31] Clinicians and patients should also be aware that removal of the implant may even exacerbate the pain because of the possibility of additional nerve injury and the exacerbation of already hyperexcitable central neurons. Large sensory deficits that involve larger areas suggest a more serious nerve injury; in such cases, surgical intervention may prove less effective. When NP cannot be resolved by pharmacology, surgical procedure, or both, patients may have difficulty coping with the pain. Such patients should be encouraged to be seek help from a chronic pain management team.

Rodríguez-Lozano and colleagues[17] reported a patient who experienced NP 6 months after the placement of 8 maxillary dental implants. Because there was no anatomic involvement between the implants and any nerve, the decision was made not to remove the implants. Such patients should be given education about the mechanisms of NP and should initiate appropriate medications. If this conservative treatment fails, a referral to a pain management team with understanding of orofacial pain is appropriate.

Levitt[29] described "cutting back the apex of the implant" as a treatment of implant-induced nerve impingement. The investigators recommended that this procedure should be considered if osseointegration of the implant has occurred.[29] In this case report, apicoectomy of the implant resolved the symptoms of paresthesia within 1 month, a finding suggesting that this procedure is effective alternative treatment of osseointegrated implants associated with neuropathy.

Elian and colleagues[33] reported a case in which an osseointegrated implant placed in close proximity to the mental foramen produced repeated swelling and suppuration with typical signs of periimplantitis. The implant remained in place for 4.5 years, and the patient continued to report paresthesia during this time. When the implant was finally removed, the patient reported a reduction of 40% in the sensory disturbances, and the symptoms improved even more over the next few months. After the implant site had healed, a second implant was placed in the vicinity, resulting in no sensory alterations. The investigators concluded that removal of implants associated with nerve injury can relieve neuropathy even 50 months after implant placement. Furthermore, a second implant in the same region does not necessarily lead to the redevelopment of sensory disturbances. These results must be interpreted with caution, because the outcome of one case report cannot be extrapolated to all patients. Clinicians should be aware of complications and should make the best decision for each patient in conjunction with a multidisciplinary team.

Considerations for Microsurgical Repair

Several microsurgical procedures have been suggested for nerve injuries after the placement of dental implants (**Table 1**). Surgical repair may be considered for patients who experience prolonged sensory alteration and pain and who demonstrate little or no response to any of the aforementioned treatments. Such patients should be informed of the likelihood of success and the risk factors associated with the procedure. Armed with this knowledge, patients should be involved in determining the need for the procedure. Patients who agree to such procedures are typically experiencing pain that has become so debilitating that it is producing a substantial reduction in quality of life.[34]

When a nerve injury has been observed (open injury), such as a perceived nerve transection or an exposed nerve during the surgical procedure, the authors recommend that a clinician immediately repair the nerve (primary repair). The process of immediate repair can be postponed for 1 to 2 weeks if a patient requires a referral to a trained microsurgeon.

In some instances, a nerve injury is not observed by the operator. This type of injury is called a closed injury. Signs associated with such injuries are often experienced soon after the procedure. Determining the site and the extent of nerve trauma after a closed nerve injury is challenging; therefore, nerve exploration and microsurgical

Table 1	
List of common microneurosurgical procedures	
Procedure	**Description**
External decompression	Removal of foreign material or bone around the nerve
Internal neurolysis	Nerve exploration and decompression
Excision of neuroma	Removal of neuroma
Neurorrhaphy	Microsurgical anastomosis of the proximal and distal end of a transected nerve
Nerve graft	Nerve reconstruction with an allogenic or autogenous nerve graft

repair are recommended. When signs of nerve injury occur after implant placement, patients should be referred to a microsurgeon within 3 months of the injury. No evidence-based standard protocol exists, however, for the comprehensive assessment and treatment of these patients[35,36] because the appropriate time between the nerve injury and microsurgical repair is often debated and has been inconsistently reported in the dental literature. It is likely that the time between injury and repair plays an important role in predicting the outcome of the treatment.[37] Several published reports suggest that early treatment achieves an outcome.[38] Another report suggests, however, that there is no association between time of repair and achievement of successful outcome.[39]

Robinson and colleagues[39] concluded that late repair can still provide an optimal outcome and that most patients consider it worthwhile. These investigators suggested that the reason for inconsistency in results between early and late repair is related to factors, such as the mechanism (partial or complete) and the magnitude of the injury. The conclusion is that patients who show some response to other treatments can be monitored for more than 3 months. If an acceptable response is not achieved, these patients may still be considered candidates for microsurgery.[39]

Pogrel[38] reported that approximately 50% of patients (28 of 51) who underwent microsurgical repair exhibited some improvements in sensation. They found a slight discrepancy between the success of IAN repair and lingual nerve repair; IAN repair was associated with a better outcome. This difference in outcome was attributed to the anatomy of the nerve, which facilitates regeneration, and to its location within the bony canal. The investigators recommended that microsurgical repair should be performed within 10 weeks after injury if the best results are to be obtained. Gender was not associated with any statistically significant difference in outcome. Sites of longstanding nerve injury may contain neuromas that must be excised during the surgical repair. Such excision leads to large gaps in the nerve tissue and can directly affect the surgical outcome. In addition, direct anastomosis requires nerve mobilization. Therefore, according to Pogrel,[38] the outcome of early repair is more favorable than that of late repair.

In a study involving 20 patients, Rutner and colleagues[40] reported no statistically significant correlation between outcome after microsurgical repair of the lingual nerve and the time after injury (2.5–7 months). Overall, 50% of their patients reported improvements in neurosensory functions. The investigators concluded that a moderate to substantial outcome can be expected when microsurgical repair of lingual nerve injuries is performed early.

Susarla and colleagues[37] demonstrated a statistically significant correlation between a positive outcome in neurosensory function after nerve repair and a decrease in the frequency of oral dysfunction 1 year postoperatively. Moreover, they found a direct correlation between increase in patient satisfaction and improvements in neurosensory function. Oral dysfunction may increase when patients experience no improvement after microsurgical repair. If this outcome occurs, patients should be referred to a multidisciplinary team that includes pain specialists, psychologists, and perhaps even a speech therapist.

Strauss and colleagues[36] reported that 90.2% of patients who underwent microsurgical repair of the IAN exhibited substantial improvement in neurosensory function when surgical repair was performed within 6.6 months of the nerve injury. Nerve injuries occurring more than 1 year earlier can be associated with distal nerve atrophy or scarring, which may result in a permanent sensory deficit because the outcome of the microsurgical procedure is less predictable.

A retrospective study by Susarla and colleagues[41] showed that patients who underwent early microsurgical repair of the lingual nerve (within 90 days) were 2.3 times more likely to achieve functional sensory recovery within 1 year postoperatively than were those who underwent late repair (more than 90 days). Similar results were shown with IAN repair. Furthermore, when there was clinical evidence of an intraoperative neuroma, patients often had not experienced functional sensory recovery at 1 year after microsurgical repair. The reason that complete functional sensory recovery did not occur was the need to excise the neuroma; such excision results in an increase in the gap between the proximal and distal nerve tissues. In addition, scar tissue often forms and prevents regeneration of the nerve tissue. The investigators concluded that microsurgical repair of the trigeminal nerve usually increases the likelihood of recovery of sensory function within 1 year after surgery.

Hillerup[42] reported that significant recovery occurred within 6 months after microsurgical repair of the IAN. Ziccardi and colleagues[43] reported that patients undergoing microsurgical repair more than 6 months after injury could show some sensory recovery but not as much as those who were treated earlier than 6 months after injury. They concluded that patients can be followed-up for 6 months if they show some signs of sensory improvement. Some patients experience a favorable outcome after late repair, but the results are not as good as those experienced by patients who are treated earlier.

Bagheri and colleagues[44] reviewed the outcome of 222 patients after lingual nerve microsurgical repair and reported that 201 (90.5%) showed recovery of sensory functions. Moreover, 94% of the 133 patients treated early (within 6 months of injury) experienced substantial improvement in neurosensory function. Of the 89 patients who were treated late (after 6 months of injury), 85.4% showed some improvement but not as much as the patients treated early. The likelihood of improvement in neurosensory function was 2.68 times higher with early treatment than with late treatment. For each additional month between injury and repair, there was a 5.85% decrease in the odds of achieving improvement. Consistent with this study, another study[45] demonstrated that the risk of not achieving a positive functional sensory return is 1.23 times (23%) greater for each month of delay between the date of injury and the date of surgical procedure. If the injury and the surgical repair occur more than 9 months apart, the risk of not achieving the return of sensory function is 4.67 times higher.[45]

Furthermore, Bagheri and colleagues[44] reported that the chances of attaining neurosensory function are better for patients younger than 45 years and that the odds of gaining recovery decrease by 5.5% for every year of age above 45. They concluded that the most successful recovery after microsurgical nerve repair was achieved when the repair occurred within 9 months after injury, particularly with younger patients (less than 45 years).

Pogrel and colleagues[46] found similar results. They reported that many patients described long-term problems associated with speaking, eating, relationships, depression, appearance, and employment issues that adversely affected their lives. The investigators concluded that young patients with long-term discomfort can experience improvement over time by participating in coping mechanisms, such as prayer, ice and heat packs, pressure on the teeth, exercise, yoga, meditation, chewing gum, relaxation and acupuncture, massage, herbal medication, and prescription medications, such as antidepressants.

Bhageri and colleagues[47] recommend that microsurgical repair should be executed as soon as possible after nerve injury so that functional recovery of sensation can be achieved. They reported that the likelihood of a positive outcome decreases substantially if the procedure occurs more than 12 months after placement and decreases by 3% every year thereafter.

Taken together, the available evidence leads to concluding that most patients undergoing microsurgical repair of the trigeminal nerve regain acceptable sensation and experience improvement in function.

Microsurgical repair also, however, carries with it the risk of negative outcome. For example, a patient with sensory loss and intermittent pain may experience complete loss of sensation and persistent pain. Furthermore, the time interval between injury and repair should be minimal if a successful outcome is to be achieved, but some degree of sensory improvement can be expected even with late microsurgical repair.

SUMMARY

Dental implants have become a routine part of restoring dental status for many patients. Although the success rates associated with implants are very good, adverse events can occur. Disruption of normal sensation and pain can be a consequence of implant placement. Clinicians must be aware of these adverse consequences and must avoid them whenever possible. This avoidance can be best achieved by careful advanced planning before implants are placed. When neurosensory alterations or pain results, pharmacologic management can be helpful. Microsurgical repair of damaged nerve tissue should be considered. Patients should be informed of these potential adverse effects and should provide informed consent before any surgical procedure is undertaken.

REFERENCES

1. Alhassani AA, AlGhamdi AS. Inferior alveolar nerve injury in implant dentistry: diagnosis, causes, prevention, and management. J Oral Implantol 2010;36(5):401–7.
2. Bogduk N, Merskey H. Classification of chronic pain: descriptions of chronic pain syndromes and definitions of pain terms. 2nd edition. Seattle (WA): IASP Press; 1994. p. 222.
3. Spencer CJ, Gremillion HA. Neuropathic orofacial pain: proposed mechanisms, diagnosis, and treatment considerations. Dent Clin North Am 2007;51(1):209–24, viii.
4. Fear C. Neuropathic pain: clinical features, assessment and treatment. Nurs Stand 2010;25(6):35–40.
5. Pogrel MA, Thamby S. Permanent nerve involvement resulting from inferior alveolar nerve blocks. J Am Dent Assoc 2000;131(7):901–7.
6. Renton T, Janjua H, Gallagher JE, et al. UK dentists' experience of iatrogenic trigeminal nerve injuries in relation to routine dental procedures: why, when and how often? Br Dent J 2013;214(12):633–42.
7. Dahl JB, Kehlet H. The value of pre-emptive analgesia in the treatment of postoperative pain. Br J Anaesth 1993;70(4):434–9.
8. Wall PD. The prevention of postoperative pain. Pain 1988;33(3):289–90.
9. Lee JB, Choi SS, Ahn EH, et al. Effect of perioperative perineural injection of dexamethasone and bupivacaine on a rat spared nerve injury model. Korean J Pain 2010;23(3):166–71.
10. Gordon SM, Dionne RA, Brahim J, et al. Blockade of peripheral neuronal barrage reduces postoperative pain. Pain 1997;70(2–3):209–15.
11. Tehemar SH. Factors affecting heat generation during implant site preparation: a review of biologic observations and future considerations. Int J Oral Maxillofac Implants 1999;14(1):127–36.
12. Basa O, Dilek OC. Assessment of the risk of perforation of the mandibular canal by implant drill using density and thickness parameters. Gerodontology 2011; 28(3):213–20.

13. Khawaja N, Renton T. Case studies on implant removal influencing the resolution of inferior alveolar nerve injury. Br Dent J 2009;206(7):365–70.
14. Maqbool A, Sultan AA, Bottini GB, et al. Pain caused by a dental implant impinging on an accessory inferior alveolar canal: a case report. Int J Prosthodont 2013; 26(2):125–6.
15. Misch CE, Resnik R. Mandibular nerve neurosensory impairment after dental implant surgery: management and protocol. Implant Dent 2010;19(5):378–86.
16. Hubbard JH. The quality of nerve regeneration. Factors independent of the most skillful repair. Surg Clin North Am 1972;52(5):1099–108.
17. Rodríguez-Lozano FJ, Sanchez-Perez A, Moya-Villaescusa MJ, et al. Neuropathic orofacial pain after dental implant placement: review of the literature and case report. Oral Surg Oral Med Oral Pathol Oral Radiol Endod 2010;109(4):e8–12.
18. Worthington P. Injury to the inferior alveolar nerve during implant placement: a formula for protection of the patient and clinician. Int J Oral Maxillofac Implants 2004;19(5):731–4.
19. Costigan M, Scholz J, Woolf CJ. Neuropathic pain: a maladaptive response of the nervous system to damage. Annu Rev Neurosci 2009;32:1–32.
20. Al-Ouf K, Salti L. Postinsertion pain in region of mandibular dental implants: a case report. Implant Dent 2011;20(1):27–31.
21. Wright EF. Persistent dysesthesia following dental implant placement: a treatment report of 2 cases. Implant Dent 2011;20(1):20–6.
22. Park JH, Lee SH, Kim ST. Pharmacologic management of trigeminal nerve injury pain after dental implant surgery. Int J Prosthodont 2010;23(4):342–6.
23. Attal N. Therapeutic advances in pharmaceutical treatment of neuropathic pain. Rev Neurol (Paris) 2011;167(12):930–7.
24. Takatori M, Kuroda Y, Hirose M. Local anesthetics suppress nerve growth factor-mediated neurite outgrowth by inhibition of tyrosine kinase activity of TrkA. Anesth Analg 2006;102(2):462–7.
25. Okeson JP. Bell's oral and facial pains. 7th edition. Chicago: Quintessence Publishers; 2014. p. 181–200.
26. Park YT, Kim SG, Moon SY. Indirect compressive injury to the inferior alveolar nerve caused by dental implant placement. J Oral Maxillofac Surg 2012;70(4): e258–9.
27. Gregg JM. Neuropathic complications of mandibular implant surgery: review and case presentations. Ann R Australas Coll Dent Surg 2000;15:176–80.
28. Berberi A, Le Breton G, Mani J, et al. Lingual paresthesia following surgical placement of implants: report of a case. Int J Oral Maxillofac Implants 1993; 8(5):580–2.
29. Levitt DS. Apicoectomy of an endosseous implant to relieve paresthesia: a case report. Implant Dent 2003;12(3):202–5.
30. Queral-Godoy E, Vazquez-Delgado E, Okeson JP, et al. Persistent idiopathic facial pain following dental implant placement: a case report. Int J Oral Maxillofac Implants 2006;21:136–40.
31. Renton T, Dawood A, Shah A, et al. Post-implant neuropathy of the trigeminal nerve. A case series. Br Dent J 2012;212(11):E17.
32. Bagheri SC, Meyer RA. Management of mandibular nerve injuries from dental implants. Atlas Oral Maxillofac Surg Clin North Am 2011;19(1):47–61.
33. Elian N, Mitsias M, Eskow R, et al. Unexpected return of sensation following 4.5 years of paresthesia: case report. Implant Dent 2005;14(4):364–7.
34. Meyer RA, Ruggiero LS. Guidelines for diagnosis and treatment of peripheral trigeminal nerve injuries. Oral Maxillofac Surg Clin North Am 2001;13(2):383–92.

35. Ziccardi VB, Assael LA. Mechanisms of trigeminal nerve injuries. Atlas Oral Maxillofac Surg Clin North Am 2001;9(2):1–11.

36. Strauss ER, Ziccardi VB, Janal MN. Outcome assessment of inferior alveolar nerve microsurgery: a retrospective review. J Oral Maxillofac Surg 2006;64(12): 1767–70.

37. Susarla SM, Lam NP, Donoff RB, et al. A comparison of patient satisfaction and objective assessment of neurosensory function after trigeminal nerve repair. J Oral Maxillofac Surg 2005;63(8):1138–44.

38. Pogrel MA. The results of microneurosurgery of the inferior alveolar and lingual nerve. J Oral Maxillofac Surg 2002;60(5):485–9.

39. Robinson PP, Loescher AR, Smith KG. A prospective, quantitative study on the clinical outcome of lingual nerve repair. Br J Oral Maxillofac Surg 2000;38(4):255–63.

40. Rutner TW, Ziccardi VB, Janal MN. Long-term outcome assessment for lingual nerve microsurgery. J Oral Maxillofac Surg 2005;63(8):1145–9.

41. Susarla SM, Kaban LB, Donoff RB, et al. Functional sensory recovery after trigeminal nerve repair. J Oral Maxillofac Surg 2007;65(1):60–5.

42. Hillerup S. Iatrogenic injury to the inferior alveolar nerve: etiology, signs and symptoms, and observations on recovery. Int J Oral Maxillofac Surg 2008; 37(8):704–9.

43. Ziccardi VB, Rivera L, Gomes J. Comparison of lingual and inferior alveolar nerve microsurgery outcomes. Quintessence Int 2009;40(4):295–301.

44. Bagheri SC, Meyer RA, Khan HA, et al. Retrospective review of microsurgical repair of 222 lingual nerve injuries. J Oral Maxillofac Surg 2010;68(4):715–23.

45. Erakat MS, Chuang SK, Shanti RM, et al. Interval between injury and lingual nerve repair as a prognostic factor for success using type I collagen conduit. J Oral Maxillofac Surg 2013;71(5):833–8.

46. Pogrel MA, Jergensen R, Burgon E, et al. Long-term outcome of trigeminal nerve injuries related to dental treatment. J Oral Maxillofac Surg 2011;69(9):2284–8.

47. Bagheri SC, Meyer RA, Cho SH, et al. Microsurgical repair of the inferior alveolar nerve: success rate and factors that adversely affect outcome. J Oral Maxillofac Surg 2012;70(8):1978–90.

Peri-implant Diseases

A Review of Treatment Interventions

 CrossMark

Georgios E. Romanos, DDS, PhD, Prof. Dr. med. dent[a],*, Fawad Javed, BDS, PhD[b],
Rafael Arcesio Delgado-Ruiz, DDS, MSc, PhD[c], José Luis Calvo-Guirado, DDS, MS, PhD[d]

KEYWORDS

- Guided bone regeneration • Laser • Nonsurgical • Peri-implantitis
- Peri-implant mucositis • Surgical • Treatment

KEY POINTS

- Risk factors of peri-implant mucositis and peri-implantitis are comparable to those of gingivitis and periodontitis.
- The ideal management of peri-implant diseases focuses on infection control, detoxification of implant surfaces, regeneration of lost tissues, and plaque control regimens via mechanical debridement.
- Implantoplasty (modification in implant surface topography), when used in combination with resective surgery, has been reported to significantly reduce the clinical parameters of peri-implantitis.
- A new technique, laser-assisted peri-implantitis protocol, is under investigation.
- There is lack of standardized treatment protocols for peri-implant disease.

Several studies[1–6] have reported that dental implants are functionally stable and have long-term success rates, and are therefore increasingly being used in the oral rehabilitation of partially and completely edentulous individuals. However, with the increasing number of patients receiving dental implants, the prevalence of inflammatory conditions around a dental implant has also escalated.[7] The consensus report from the 6th European Workshop on Periodontology has defined peri-implantitis as the presence of inflammation of the peri-implant mucosa and simultaneously loss of supporting bone.[8] In addition, it has also been described as a site-specific infection that

Conflict of Interest and Financial Disclosure: None declared.

[a] Department of Periodontology, School of Dental Medicine, Stony Brook University, 106 Rockland Hall, Stony Brook, NY 11794-8700, USA; [b] Engineer Abdullah Bugshan Research Chair for Growth Factors and Bone Regeneration, 3D Imaging and Biomechanical Laboratory, College of Applied Medical Sciences, King Saud University, Derriyah, P.O. Box 60169, Riyadh 11545, Saudi Arabia; [c] Department of Prosthodontics and Digital Technology, School of Dental Medicine, Stony Brook University, 1103 Westchester Hall, Stony Brook, NY 11794-8712, USA; [d] Faculty of Medicine and Dentistry, Hospital Morales Meseguer, University of Murcia, 2° Planta Clínica Odontológica Calle Marques de los Velez S/n, Murcia 30007, Spain
* Corresponding author.
E-mail address: Georgios.Romanos@stonybrook.edu

Dent Clin N Am 59 (2015) 157–178
http://dx.doi.org/10.1016/j.cden.2014.08.002
0011-8532/15/$ – see front matter © 2015 Elsevier Inc. All rights reserved.

exhibits features comparable to those of chronic adult periodontitis.[9] In indexed literature, there is a variance in the prevalence of peri-implantitis. Mombelli and colleagues[10] estimated the prevalence of peri-implantitis to be in the order of 10% implants and 20% patients during 5 to 10 years after implant placement; and Koldsland and colleagues[11] reported the prevalence to range between 11.3% and 47.1% in their study population. Moreover, in a recent study on Belgian adults, the prevalence of peri-implant mucositis and peri-implantitis was 31% and 37%, respectively.[12] It has been suggested that peri-implant mucositis and peri-implantitis are analogous to gingivitis and periodontitis, respectively.[13] However, it is pertinent to mention that biologic differences exist between natural teeth and implants. Therefore, the progression of infection around implants and natural teeth is also divergent. Moreover, tissues around implants are more prone to plaque-associated infections that spread into the alveolar bone.[14]

The ideal management of peri-implant diseases focuses on infection control, detoxification of implant surfaces, regeneration of lost tissues, and plaque-control regimens via mechanical debridement (with or without raising a surgical flap).[15,16] However, a variety of other therapeutic modalities also have been proposed for the management of peri-implantitis. These treatment strategies encompass use of antiseptics and/or antibiotics, laser therapy, guided bone regeneration, and photodynamic therapy.[16–23] The aim of this article was to review indexed literature with reference to the various therapeutic interventions proposed for the management of peri-implant diseases.

PERI-IMPLANT DISEASES: PERI-IMPLANT MUCOSITIS AND PERI-IMPLANTITIS

Peri-implant diseases are categorized into 2 types: peri-implant mucositis and peri-implantitis. Peri-implant mucositis is characterized by inflammation of the soft tissues surrounding the implant without any signs of bone loss (**Fig. 1**).[8] The clinical signs of peri-implant mucositis include bleeding on probing (BOP) and/or suppuration, which are usually associated with probing depth (PD) of at least 4 mm with no evidence of radiographic loss of bone.[24,25] It has been reported that inflammatory cell lesions in sites with peri-implant mucositis are dominated by T cells and have an apical extension that is restricted to the barrier epithelium.[26] Peri-implant mucositis is usually reversible (when early diagnosis and removal of etiology are implemented)[27,28]; however, it is considered as a precursor to peri-implantitis.[8]

The term "peri-implantitis" was introduced in literature more than 3 decades ago.[9] This term was modified in the 1990s to describe an inflammatory process around an implant that includes both soft tissue inflammation and progressive loss of supporting bone beyond biological remodeling (**Figs. 2** and **3**). In general, the clinical definition of

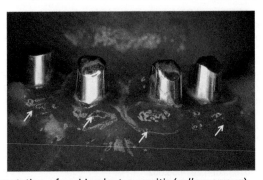

Fig. 1. Clinical presentation of peri-implant mucositis (*yellow arrows*).

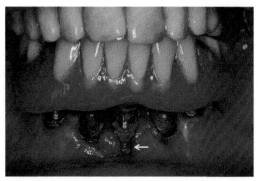

Fig. 2. Clinical presentation of peri-implantitis with extensive calculus deposition (*arrow*) around dental implants.

peri-implantitis has varied among studies. For example, in studies by Roos-Jansåker and colleagues,[29,30] peri-implantitis was described as a condition in which implants with varying degrees of bone loss are accompanied by a PD of at least 4 mm, BOP, and purulent discharge on gentle probing. However, in a systematic review by Berglundh and colleagues,[31] peri-implantitis was defined by PD of more than 6 mm and in combination with BOP and clinical attachment loss or bone loss of at least 2.5 mm (**Fig. 4**).

RISK FACTORS OF PERI-IMPLANT DISEASES

Risk factors of peri-implant mucositis and peri-implantitis are comparable to those of gingivitis and periodontitis.[27,32] The following risk factors have been associated with the etiology of peri-implant diseases.

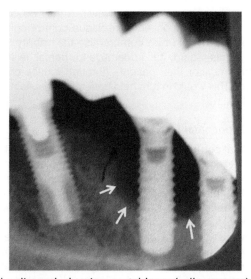

Fig. 3. A peri-apical radiograph showing crestal bone (*yellow arrows*) loss around dental implants.

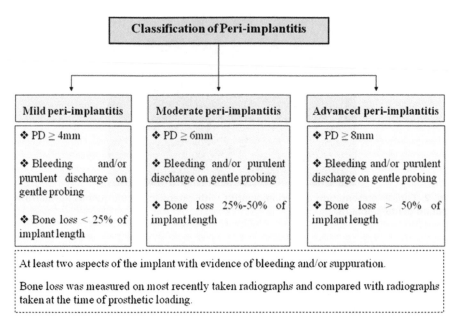

Fig. 4. Classification of peri-implantitis. (*Modified from* Froum SJ, Rosen PS. A proposed classification for peri-implantitis. Int J Periodontics Restorative Dent 2012;32:533–40.)

Poor Plaque Control

Implant geometry and surface characteristics may obligate patients to adopt non-conventional plaque-control regimens, such as interdental brushing and flossing in addition to traditional tooth-brushing techniques. The primary focus of these nonconventional plaque-control protocols is to maintain the periodontal health of the remaining dentition, thereby minimizing the possibilities of plaque accumulation and formation of periodontal and/or peri-implant pockets. However, it may be challenging for some patients to get accustomed to nonconventional plaque-control regimens (as stated previously) without ado. This may in turn compromise their ability in executing plaque control (see **Fig. 2**). In this regard, it is imperative for dental health care providers to educate and regularly monitor their patients (through routine check-ups) to ensure proper plaque control. This would in turn help patients in maintaining their periodontal and/or peri-implant health.[33]

Previous History of Periodontal Disease

It has been claimed that peri-implantitis is a common finding in patients with a history of periodontitis.[34,35] Results from a systematic review and meta-analysis showed that the relative risk for peri-implantitis was significantly higher in patients with a previous history of periodontitis compared with patients without a history of periodontal disease.[34] However, in a recent study, Meyle and colleagues[36] investigated the long-term clinical and radiographic parameters of osseointegrated implants in nonsmoking patients with a previous history of chronic periodontitis. The results showed that patients with a previous history of periodontitis regularly attending an oral hygiene maintenance program displayed implant survival rates up to 100% after 5 and 10 years. Similarly, in a systematic review, Pesce and colleagues[37] concluded that there is a lack of consensus regarding the role of periodontitis in the etiology of peri-implantitis.

Nevertheless, because several periodontopathogens (such as *Aggregatibacter actinomycetemcomitans*, *Prevotella intermedia*, and *Porphyromonas gingivalis*) associated with the etiology of periodontitis also have been isolated from peri-implant sulci of patients with peri-implantitis,[38–41] it is arduous to disregard the hypothesis that peri-implantitis is more common in patients with a history of periodontitis.

Stagnation of Residual Material in/Around the Gingivae Following Implant Prosthesis Cementation

A conventional approach toward restoration of dental implants using fixed prosthesis is the use of cement-retained restorations. In the absence of occlusal screw access openings, cement-retained restorations are useful in enhancing the number of occlusal contacts and simultaneously improving aesthetics.[42] However, inadequate removal of excessive cement at the time of implant cementation may lead to a complication: cement-induced peri-implantitis.[42] The probability of cement to remain in the peri-implant sulcus is high when margins of the restoration are placed 1.5 to 3 mm subgingivally.[43] Stagnation of residual cement in peri-implant sulcus has been associated with peri-implant tissue inflammation, BOP and/or suppuration, increased PD, evidence of bone loss on radiographs, and patient discomfort.[44] Shallow intracrevicular placement of the gingival margins reduces the occurrence of peri-implant inflammation and related complications.

Occlusal Overloading

Occlusal overloading is a major cause of biomechanical implant complications, including fracture and/or loosening of the implant (**Fig. 5**). Occlusal overloading in combination with plaque accumulation may also disturb the intricate bond between the implant surface and bone leading to peri-implantitis and, if left untreated, implant failure.[45–47] However, conflicting results also have been reported.[48,49] In a study on

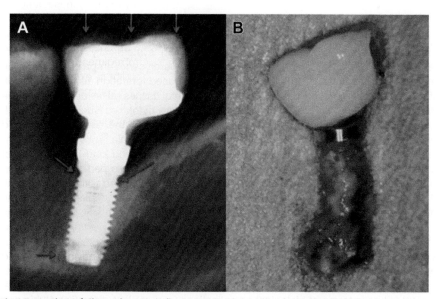

Fig. 5. Implant failure due to inflammation and occlusal overload. (*A*) Red arrows are showing the crown-implant relation and the bone loss. (*B*) The extracted implant surrounded by inflammatory tissue and plaque.

dogs, there was no loss of osseointegration and/or peri-implantitis following a period of 8 months of excessive occlusal load on titanium (Ti) implants.[49] Occlusal overloading may be prevented by performing comprehensive examinations, treatment planning, well-defined surgical and prosthetic treatments, and regular maintenance. However, Pesce and colleagues[37] reported in a recent systematic review that there is a lack of clinical evidence to support a cause-effect relationship between peri-implantitis and occlusal overload.

Habitual Tobacco Smoking

Tobacco smoking is a significant risk factor for periodontitis and peri-implant diseases,[50–53] and pathogenesis of periodontitis closely resembles that of peri-implantitis.[54] Tobacco smoking has been associated with an increased expression of receptor of advanced glycation end products (RAGE) in gingival tissues.[53,55] Experimental results by Katz and colleagues[55] showed an increased expression of RAGE in gingival epithelial cells of smokers as compared with nonsmokers. Moreover, it also has been reported that nornicotine (a metabolite of nicotine) upregulates RAGE expression in the gingivae of smokers. This stimulates the secretion of cytokines and reactive oxygen species, which enhance alveolar bone loss.[55,56] Furthermore, there is a synergistic effect of tobacco smoking and carriage of interleukin (IL)-1 gene polymorphism that results in increased risk of peri-implantitis.[57,58]

Galindo-Moreno and colleagues[59] reported that the rates of marginal bone loss around implants are significantly associated with smoking. Studies[60–64] have reported that rates of implant failure range between 6.5% and 20.0% among smokers compared with nonsmokers. In smokers, implant failures occur more often in the maxilla as compared with implants placed in the mandible[61,63,65]; most likely due to the presence of poor-quality trabecular bone in the maxilla.[66] Results from a recent systematic review and meta-analysis also reported a significantly higher risk of peri-implantitis in smokers as compared with nonsmokers.[67]

Diabetes

It is well acknowledged that periodontal inflammatory conditions are worse in patients with poorly controlled diabetes as compared with systemically healthy individuals.[4,50,68,69] This is primarily because chronic hyperglycemia impairs tissue repair and host defense mechanisms. In addition, an increased formation and accumulation of advanced glycation end-products in the periodontal tissues raises cellular oxidative stress and increases the production of proinflammatory cytokines (such as IL-6, IL-1β, IL-18, matrix metalloproteinase [MMP]-8 and MMP-9) in the serum, saliva, and gingival crevicular fluid of patients with chronic hyperglycemia.[68,70–73] These proinflammatory cytokines may jeopardize the osseointegration and long-term survival of implants in patients with chronic hyperglycemia. However, it is pertinent to mention that degree of glycemic control (in patients previously diagnosed with diabetes) may play a role in a successful osseointegration and survival of implants in diabetic patients.[4]

Genetic Factors

A correlation between IL-1 gene polymorphism and peri-implantitis has been reported by some studies.[74–76] However, in a systematic review, Dereka and colleagues[77] reported no apparent association between specific genetic polymorphism and dental implant failure in terms of biological complications (peri-implant diseases). Hultin and colleagues,[78] Rogers and colleagues,[79] and Campos and colleagues[80] also reported no association between gene polymorphism and peri-implantitis. Although the association of genetic factors with peri-implantitis cannot be completely disregarded, further studies are warranted to assess the role of genetics as a potential risk factor of peri-implantitis.

INCIDENCE AND PREVALENCE OF PERI-IMPLANT DISEASES

There is a lack of information regarding the incidence of peri-implant mucositis and peri-implantitis, as the interpretation of data is difficult. In this regard, the incidence of peri-implantitis may be underestimated. Renvert and colleagues[81] investigated the incidence of peri-implantitis over a period of 13 years between 2 dental implant systems (TiOBlast AstraTech [AT] and machine-etched Brånemark Nobel Biocare [NB] system, Gothenburg, Sweden, respectively). In this study,[81] the incidences of peri-implantitis for AT implants were 26.2% and 7.1% between years 1 and 7; and 30.4% and 11.5% for NB implants between years 7 and 13. There was no significant difference in the incidence of peri-implantitis over a period of 13 years between the 2 implant systems.[81] The investigators considered a history of periodontitis as a risk for future incidence of peri-implantitis.[81] The consensus report of the 7th European Workshop on Periodontology[82] also emphasized that there is a need to develop new and more efficient preventive and treatment approaches for periodontal disease. This report[82] also accentuated such preventive and treatment protocols should be based on recent advances in understanding of host modulation and inflammation resolution with direct management of the microbiota.

To our knowledge, only a limited number of studies have assessed the prevalence of peri-implant disease.[83–88] Moreover, we observed that the prevalence reported in these studies varied between patients and implant systems. For example, in the 5-year follow-up results by Fransson and colleagues,[88] the prevalence of peri-implant diseases was reported to be 92%, whereas in the study by Scheller and colleagues,[83] the prevalence of peri-implant diseases at 5-year follow-up was 24%. Zitzmann and Berglundh[8] reported the prevalence of peri-implantitis to vary between 12% and 43% of implants. This variation may be associated with a lack of standardization in the patient selection and criteria for diagnosing peri-implant mucositis and peri-implantitis among these studies. Therefore, a precise estimation of the prevalence of peri-implant disease remains debatable.

CLASSIFICATION OF PERI-IMPLANTITIS

To our knowledge from indexed literature, there is no globally accepted classification of peri-implantitis. However, Froum and Rosen[89] recently proposed a classification that differentiated peri-implantitis according the severity of inflammation and extent of bone loss around the implant. This classification was based on 3 different clinical stages of peri-implantitis: (1) early peri-implantitis, (2) moderate peri-implantitis, and (3) advanced peri-implantitis (see **Fig. 4**).[89] Early peri-implantitis was defined by PD of at least 4 mm and radiographic bone loss of less than 25% of the total implant length. Moderate peri-implantitis was defined by PD of at least 6 mm and radiographic bone loss of 25% to 50% of the total implant length, whereas advanced peri-implantitis was defined by PD of at least 8 mm with more than 50% of radiographic bone loss with reference to implant length. In this classification, BOP and/or suppuration on 2 or more aspects of the implant were selected as the markers of inflammation. The investigators conjectured that their proposed classification would help strengthen communication between clinical practitioners and researchers and help attain a better understanding of peri-implantitis[89]; however, further evidence-based clinical studies are needed to authenticate this classification.

ASSESSMENT OF END POINTS AMONG STUDIES ON THE TREATMENT OF PERI-IMPLANTITIS

End points are commonly used to determine the effectiveness of a clinical treatment. In studies addressing the treatment of peri-implantitis, "true end points" are preferred over "surrogate end points," because they are able to depict a considerable proportion of the effect of treatment on an outcome of interest, such as implant failure.[90–92] In a systematic review, Faggion and colleagues[91] explored indexed literature to determine the type of end points reported regarding peri-implantitis therapy and their frequency of use. Studies included in this systematic review[91] chiefly reported implant failure as a consequence of peri-implantitis therapy and not as an objective of an investigation. The investigators concluded that there is a lack of consensus regarding the efficacy of treatment of peri-implantitis for reducing the risk of implant failure.[27] A similar conclusion was reported by Lee.[92]

ETIOLOGY AND PATHOGENESIS OF PERI-IMPLANTITIS

Microbial colonization is the chief predisposing factor in the etiology of peri-implantitis. Subgingival microbes (such as *Aggregatibacter actinomycetemcomitans, Prevotella intermedia, P gingivalis,* and *Treponema denticola*) associated with the etiology of periodontitis are similar to those of peri-implantitis.[78] In addition, it also has been reported that patterns of plaque formation and accumulation on implant surfaces are comparable to those seen on teeth.[93]

The pathogenesis of peri-implantitis is similar to that of periodontitis.[94] Microbes in plaque stagnated on implant surface(s) release chemotactic peptides that attract neutrophils toward the peri-implant pocket(s). Moreover, cytokines are released into the peri-implant crevicular fluid as a result of microbial damage to epithelial cells, which attract more leukocytes (predominantly neutrophils) toward the affected site.[95] If neutrophils become overloaded with microbes, they degranulate and the toxic enzymes released from neutrophils cause tissue damage and gingival inflammation.[94] If the inflammation persists, it may progress to marginal gingiva and ultimately cause bone loss, a classical feature of peri-implantitis.[94] Stromal cells (such as granulation tissue fibroblasts) also may participate in the pathogenesis of peri-implantitis by upregulating vascularity and matrix breakdown, thereby promoting migration/maintenance of infiltrates (proinflammatory cytokines) into the inflamed site.[96]

MANAGEMENT OF PERI-IMPLANTITIS

A variety of treatment protocols have been proposed for the management of peri-implantitis.[97] The management of peri-implantitis can be divided into (1) nonsurgical management and (2) surgical management; surgical management encompass resective and regenerative treatment.[97–100] However, there is lack of standardized treatment protocols for peri-implant disease. The following text comprehensively reviews the different therapeutic protocols that have been proposed for the management of peri-implant diseases.

Nonsurgical Management of Peri-implant Diseases

Nonsurgical (closed debridement) treatment of peri-implant disease involves the mechanical removal of plaque and calculus (using mechanical instruments, such as scalers and curettes) from the implant surfaces (**Fig. 6**).[101] The significance of antibiotics and/or antiseptic oral rinses (including chlorhexidine [CHX]) as adjuncts to mechanical debridement remains debatable.[23,101,102] Renvert and colleagues[98] systematically reviewed

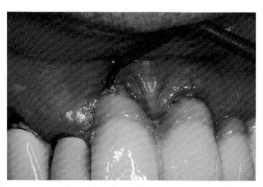

Fig. 6. Nonsurgical treatment of peri-implant diseases using hand instruments.

indexed literature that assessed the nonsurgical management of peri-implant mucositis and peri-implantitis. They reported that nonsurgical mechanical debridement alone is effective in the treatment of peri-implant mucositis. The adjunct use of antiseptic oral rinses in combination with nonsurgical mechanical debridement improved the treatment outcome of peri-implant mucositis as compared with the use of nonsurgical mechanical debridement alone.[98] In a study on cynomolgus monkeys, Trejo and colleagues[101] reported mechanical debridement with or without the adjunct use of CHX is effective in the treatment on experimental peri-implant mucositis. In addition, histologic results by Trejo and colleagues[101] showed minimal inflammation in groups treated by mechanical debridement (regardless of CHX use) as compared with the control group (no treatment group). However, Schwarz and colleagues[103] reported limited effect of nonsurgical mechanical debridement on the treatment of peri-implant diseases irrespective of type of adjunct treatment used.[103] Similar results were reported by Karring and colleagues.[104] Clinical results by Khoury and Buchmann[105] showed a temporary improvement in PD following nonsurgical treatment of peri-implant diseases. This could possibly have occurred due to an incomplete decontamination of implant surfaces during the nonsurgical treatment approach.

Although mechanical implant surface debridement constitutes the basic element for treatment of peri-implant diseases, other factors, such as implant positioning, geometry, and surface characteristics, may influence the overall outcomes of mechanical treatment of infected implants.[106] There is a need for further randomized controlled trials assessing treatment modalities of nonsurgical management of peri-implant mucositis and peri-implantitis.

Surgical Management of Peri-implant Diseases

Surgical management of peri-implantitis is usually recommended in patients with severe forms of peri-implant diseases (PD >5 mm and bone loss) (**Fig. 7**).[89,105,107] Three-year follow-up results from a clinical trial showed that surgical treatment of peri-implantitis was significantly more effective in reducing PD as compared with nonsurgical therapy.[105] However, there are no long-term clinical trials in indexed literature that have compared nonsurgical with surgical interventions for peri-implantitis.[108]

The surgical treatment approach is performed when an acute infection has resolved and appropriate oral hygiene of the patient is achieved. Guided bone regeneration (GBR) is a surgical approach in which a particulate graft material (such as allograft, xenograft, or alloplast) is directly placed into the osseous defect and covered with a barrier membrane (such as collagen membrane or expanded polytetrafluoroethylene

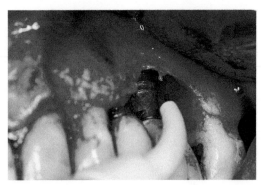

Fig. 7. Surgical treatment of peri-implant diseases using flap surgery and diode (810 nm) laser decontamination.

[ePtFE] membrane).[109–111] Schou and colleagues[110,111] investigated the efficacy of GBR by using autogenous bone graft and ePTFE membrane in the treatment of peri-implantitis in cynomolgus monkeys. In these studies,[105,106] experimental peri-implantitis was induced in the jaws of monkeys after 3 months of the placement of Ti plasma-sprayed implants. Plaque-control protocols were executed and implants were divided into 4 different surgical treatment groups that comprised: (1) placement of autogenous bone grafts over the defect and covered by membranes, (2) covering the defect with autogenous bone grafts alone, (3) covering the defect with membrane alone, or (4) access flap procedure as a control group. Euthanasia was performed after 6 months, and jaw segments were assessed by quantitative digital subtraction radiography. The results showed that bone levels corresponding to levels that existed before induction of peri-implantitis were achieved in cases in which autogenous bone graft particles were placed over the defect and covered with membrane as compared with other groups.[110,111]

The use of growth factors as adjuncts to conventional GBR protocols also has been reported to enhance osseointegration and promote new bone formation around induced peri-implant defects as compared with when GBR is performed without adjunct growth factor therapy.[112–115] Although studies[89,91,116] have reported that surgical management of peri-implant diseases yields promising results, long-term controlled studies are needed to validate the efficacy of these surgical treatments.

Lasers in the Treatment of Peri-implant Diseases

Some studies[17,19,117–119] have recommended the use of lasers as an adjunct to the conventional nonsurgical treatment of peri-implantitis. It has been shown that carbon dioxide (CO_2) and 980-nm diode lasers do not affect implant surfaces during irradiation of implant surfaces as compared with other lasers, such as Neodymium-doped Yttrium-Aluminum-Garnet (Nd:YAG) and Erbium:YAG laser.[119,120] In a case-series involving 15 patients, Romanos and Nentwig[19] investigated the efficacy of CO_2 laser in the decontamination of failing implants. Clinical and radiologic parameters were evaluated at baseline and approximately after 2 years. The results showed almost complete bone fill in the peri-implant defects and the study concluded that decontamination of the implant surfaces with the CO_2 laser is an effective treatment for the management of peri-implantitis.[19] Roncati and colleagues[117] compared the effect of using a 810-nm diode laser as adjunct to conventional nonsurgical and nonsurgical debridement alone (control) in the treatment of peri-implantitis. The 5-year follow-up outcomes showed nonsurgical debridement with adjunctive 810-nm diode laser therapy is a more effective treatment strategy for the management of peri-implantitis as compared with nonsurgical debridement alone.[117] Likewise, results from another study[121] reported osteoblastic attachment to implant surfaces and bone formation is higher in irradiated as compared with nonirradiated implant surfaces.

Recently, a new technique termed laser-assisted peri-implantitis protocol (LAPIP) is under investigation. The LAPIP technique is an implant-specific modification of the laser-assisted new attachment protocol (LANAP). LAPIP and LANAP protocols use a laser-ablation step to eradicate inflamed sulcular tissues (using Nd:YAG laser) and decontaminate the implant/root surface followed by nonsurgical periodontal therapy (scaling and root planing). The LAPIP works on the concept of creation of a blood clot, which allows the defect area to heal apico-coronally by preventing the downgrowth of gingival epithelium. However, there are no controlled trials in indexed literature regarding the efficacy of LAPIP for the management of peri-implantitis.

Photodynamic Therapy in the Treatment of Peri-implant Diseases

The concept of photodynamic therapy (PDT) is based on the application of light (generally red light with wavelength ranging between 630 and 700 nm) on a chemical dye (photosensitizer [PS]), which leads to the production of singlet oxygen molecules under aerobic conditions (**Fig. 8**).[122] These molecules have been reported to cause oxidative damage to the target cells, such as microbial and tumor cells.[123] PDT has been shown to be a noninvasive and practical and feasible treatment option for periodontitis and cancer.[124,125] Although clinical[126–128] and experimental[129–131] studies have investigated the efficacy of PDT in the management of peri-implantitis, there seems to be a lack of consensus among clinicians and researchers in nominating PDT as a treatment of choice for peri-implantitis. The factors associated with this discrepancy include variation in the study design, duration/frequency of treatment, selection criteria of control group and the laser-related parameter, such as type of laser PS. Thus, further long-term randomized controlled trials are needed to assess the role of PDT in the treatment of peri-implantitis.

Decontamination of Implant Surfaces

It has been reported that implant surface roughness influences the healing process by promoting osteogenesis and cell surface interactions.[132–135] However, implant surface roughness has a significant impact on the quantity and quality of the plaque formed.[136] In addition, bacterial adhesion in the grooves and pits of rough-surfaced

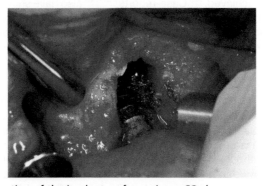

Fig. 8. Decontamination of the implant surface using a CO_2 laser.

implants may be difficult to remove. A variety of implant surface decontamination/detoxification techniques have been proposed; all of which aim to facilitate healing and render the implant surface biocompatible.

Mechanical decontamination

Implantoplasty (modification in implant surface topography) when used in combination with resective surgery has been reported to significantly reduce the clinical parameters of peri-implantitis, such as PD, sulcus bleeding, and suppuration.[137] Romeo and colleagues[137,138] showed 100% survival rate in implants decontaminated with implantoplasty compared with controls (implants decontaminated without implantoplasty). In addition, mechanical debridement of peri-implant granulation tissue using Teflon curettes and abrasive sodium carbonate air powder reduces inflammation and pathogenic microbes within 3 months of treatment.[139,140] According to Persson and colleagues,[141] cotton pellets soaked in normal saline may be sufficient to decontaminate microrough implant surfaces.

Chemical decontamination

The most common chemical agents used or detoxification of implant surfaces are 10% hydrogen peroxide (H_2O_2) and CHX.[137,138] However, epithelial cell growth has been reported to be higher on H_2O_2-treated implant surfaces as compared with CHX-treated surfaces.[142] It has been shown in vitro that rubbing a cotton pellet soaked with 3% H_2O_2 for 1 minute significantly decreases the microbial counts on implant surfaces as compared with untreated implant surfaces.[143]

Citric acid (CA) also has been used for the detoxification of the implant surfaces. In an in vitro study,[89] application of CA (pH1 with cotton pellet for 1 minute) was shown to significantly reduce microbial counts on Ti alloy grit-blasted surfaces compared with untreated controls. In another study, CA-soaked cotton pellets were rubbed on Ti cylindrical units contaminated with *P gingivalis* endotoxin for 1 minute and for 2 minutes on machined, Ti plasma-sprayed, and hydroxyapatite (HA)-coated implants. One-minute application of CA caused reduction in endotoxin by 85.8%, 27.0%, and 86.8% for machined, Ti plasma-sprayed, and HA-coated implants, respectively; whereas, 2-minute CA application caused reductions in endotoxin by 90.0%, 36.4%, and 92.1% for machined, Ti plasma-sprayed, and HA-coated implants, respectively. It can therefore be concluded that CA is a useful decontamination agent for machined and HA-coated implant surfaces as compared with Ti plasma-sprayed implant surfaces.[144]

Tetracycline is a bactericidal antibiotic that inhibits protein synthesis. In an experimental study by Hall and colleagues,[145] chronic bony defects induced around implants were cleaned with tetracycline. After 4 months of follow-up, 1.77 mm of reosseointegration was achieved.[145] Case-reports[146–148] also have shown that application of 50 mg/mL tetracycline for 5 minutes on implant surfaces after mechanical decontamination and followed by guided bone regeneration arrests the lesion and facilitates bone refill in the defect.

Use of lasers

To our knowledge from indexed literature, there is a lack of consensus on the type and settings of lasers that are most favorable for bacterial decontamination of titanium implant surfaces. Various lasers including Erbium-doped yttrium-aluminium-garnet (Er:YAG) and CO_2 lasers have been used for implant surface decontamination.[149–151] The Er:YAG laser has been shown to be effective in removing the oral biofilm from implant surfaces without jeopardizing the implant surface.[152] Likewise, the CO_2 laser also has been reported to be safe and it does not hinder osteoblastic attachment to implant surfaces. However, a major risk while using CO_2 and Er:YAG lasers is the temperature increase above the critical threshold (10°C) after 10 seconds of continuous irradiation. The Nd:YAG laser is contraindicated for the decontamination of implant surfaces because it produces morphologic changes in the implant surfaces, such as melting, cracks, and crater formation due to overheating.[153]

Antibiotics in the Treatment of Peri-implant Diseases

It is known that bacteria associated with peri-implantitis are similar to those related to periodontal disease.[38–41] Antibiotics when used as adjuncts in the treatment of peri-implant diseases have been reported to decrease microbial and peri-implant inflammatory parameters over a period of 12 months.[154] It is tempting to hypothesize that administration of local or systemic antibiotics with traditional peri-implantitis therapeutic regimens eliminates bacteria to a greater extent than when such treatments are performed alone. Several studies[20,154–159] have shown that traditional treatments of peri-implantitis when used with adjunct antibiotic therapy reduce gingival bleeding, suppuration, and PD. However, in most of these studies,[20,154–157,159] there was no placebo or control group. Khoury and Buchmann[105] tested the efficacy of 3 surgical approaches in the management of peri-implant diseases. In this study,[105] all patients were administered with antibiotics 4 weeks preoperatively for 1 week and later starting 1 day and finishing 7 days postoperatively. The results showed that the outcomes of the 3 surgical techniques (with preoperative and postoperative antibiotic cover) were comparable.[105] Moreover, results from a systematic review reported that the significance of using antibiotics as adjuncts to conventional peri-implantitis therapies remains debatable.[23]

Because there is heterogeneity of studies, which have used experimental combinations of different decontamination methods, it is exigent to establish a single standardized protocol for implant decontamination for the treatment of peri-implantitis. However, further information regarding implant surface decontamination is published elsewhere.[160]

PROPOSED GUIDELINES FOR THE MANAGEMENT OF PERI-IMPLANTITIS

Authors of the present review propose the following sequential guidelines for the management of peri-implantitis: (1) elevation of a full-thickness mucoperiosteal flap; (2) mechanical debridement of implant surface(s) using hand instruments (such as curettes) followed by decontamination using CO_2 laser (2-Watt, pulsed-mode or continuous wave); (3) guided bone regeneration using particular graft material and resorbable membrane; and (4) closure of the defect using resorbable sutures.

SUMMARY

There seems to be a lack of consensus over the treatment protocol that would yield the best outcomes in terms of management of peri-implant diseases in humans. Regardless of which therapeutic treatment protocol is adopted for the management of peri-implant diseases, a proficient diagnosis, patient compliance (plaque-control), control of possible risk factors, and skillful decontamination of implant surfaces influence the overall outcome of the treatment.

REFERENCES

1. Romanos GE, Gaertner K, Aydin E, et al. Long-term results after immediate loading of platform-switched implants in smokers versus nonsmokers with full-arch restorations. Int J Oral Maxillofac Implants 2013;28:841–5.

2. Romanos GE, Aydin E, Gaertner K, et al. Long-term results after subcrestal or crestal placement of delayed loaded implants. Clin Implant Dent Relat Res 2013. http://dx.doi.org/10.1111/cid.12084.

3. Javed F, Al-Hezaimi K, Al-Rasheed A, et al. Implant survival rate after oral cancer therapy: a review. Oral Oncol 2010;46:854–9.

4. Javed F, Romanos GE. Impact of diabetes mellitus and glycemic control on the osseointegration of dental implants: a systematic literature review. J Periodontol 2009;80:1719–30.

5. Javed F, Almas K. Osseointegration of dental implants in patients undergoing bisphosphonate treatment: a literature review. J Periodontol 2010;81:479–84.

6. Romanos GE, Gaertner K, Nentwig GH. Long-term evaluation of immediately loaded implants in the edentulous mandible using fixed bridges and platform shifting. Clin Implant Dent Relat Res 2013. http://dx.doi.org/10.1111/cid.12032.

7. Tonetti MS. Risk factors for osseodisintegration. Periodontol 2000 1998;17:55–62.

8. Zitzmann NU, Berglundh T. Definition and prevalence of peri-implant diseases. J Clin Periodontol 2008;35:286–91.

9. Mombelli A, van Oosten MA, Schurch E Jr, et al. The microbiota associated with successful or failing osseointegrated titanium implants. Oral Microbiol Immunol 1987;2:145–51.

10. Mombelli A, Muller N, Cionca N. The epidemiology of peri-implantitis. Clin Oral Implants Res 2012;23(Suppl 6):67–76.

11. Koldsland OC, Scheie AA, Aass AM. Prevalence of peri-implantitis related to severity of the disease with different degrees of bone loss. J Periodontol 2010;81:231–8.

12. Marrone A, Lasserre J, Bercy P, et al. Prevalence and risk factors for peri-implant disease in Belgian adults. Clin Oral Implants Res 2013;24:934–40.

13. Belibasakis GN. Microbiological and immuno-pathological aspects of peri-implant diseases. Arch Oral Biol 2014;59:66–72.

14. Lindhe J, Berglundh T, Ericsson I, et al. Experimental breakdown of peri-implant and periodontal tissues. A study in the beagle dog. Clin Oral Implants Res 1992; 3:9–16.

15. Bautista L, Huynh-Ba G. In patients with peri-implantitis, access flap surgery may be more effective than mechanical debridement in terms of clinical attachment gain although both treatments lead to improved clinical parameters (UT CAT #2432). Tex Dent J 2013;130:1112.

16. Schou S, Berglundh T, Lang NP. Surgical treatment of peri-implantitis. Int J Oral Maxillofac Implants 2004;19(Suppl):140–9.

17. Javed F, Hussain HA, Romanos GE. Re-stability of dental implants following treatment of peri-implantitis. Interv Med Appl Sci 2013;5:116–21.

18. Romanos GE, Gupta B, Yunker M, et al. Lasers used in dental implantology. Implant Dent 2013;22:282–8.

19. Romanos GE, Nentwig GH. Regenerative therapy of deep peri-implant infrabony defects after CO2 laser implant surface decontamination. Int J Periodontics Restorative Dent 2008;28:245–55.

20. Renvert S, Lessem J, Dahlen G, et al. Topical minocycline microspheres versus topical chlorhexidine gel as an adjunct to mechanical debridement of incipient peri-implant infections: a randomized clinical trial. J Clin Periodontol 2006;33: 362–9.

21. Bassetti M, Schar D, Wicki B, et al. Anti-infective therapy of peri-implantitis with adjunctive local drug delivery or photodynamic therapy: 12-month outcomes of a randomized controlled clinical trial. Clin Oral Implants Res 2014;25:279–87.

22. Javed F, Romanos GE. Does photodynamic therapy enhance standard antibacterial therapy in dentistry? Photomed Laser Surg 2013;31:512–8.
23. Javed F, Alghamdi AS, Ahmed A, et al. Clinical efficacy of antibiotics in the treatment of peri-implantitis. Int Dent J 2013;63:169–76.
24. Khammissa RA, Feller L, Meyerov R, et al. Peri-implant mucositis and peri-implantitis: clinical and histopathological characteristics and treatment. SADJ 2012;67:122, 124–126.
25. Jankovic S, Aleksic Z, Dimitrijevic B, et al. Prevalence of human cytomegalovirus and Epstein-Barr virus in subgingival plaque at peri-implantitis, mucositis and healthy sites. A pilot study. Int J Oral Maxillofac Surg 2011;40: 271–6.
26. Zitzmann NU, Berglundh T, Marinello CP, et al. Experimental peri-implant mucositis in man. J Clin Periodontol 2001;28:517–23.
27. Pontoriero R, Tonelli MP, Carnevale G, et al. Experimentally induced peri-implant mucositis. A clinical study in humans. Clin Oral Implants Res 1994;5:254–9.
28. Salvi GE, Aglietta M, Eick S, et al. Reversibility of experimental peri-implant mucositis compared with experimental gingivitis in humans. Clin Oral Implants Res 2012;23:182–90.
29. Roos-Jansåker AM, Lindahl C, Renvert H, et al. Nine- to fourteen-year follow-up of implant treatment. Part II: presence of peri-implant lesions. J Clin Periodontol 2006;33:290–5.
30. Roos-Jansåker AM, Lindahl C, Renvert H, et al. Nine- to fourteen-year follow-up of implant treatment. Part I: implant loss and associations to various factors. J Clin Periodontol 2006;33:283–9.
31. Berglundh T, Persson L, Klinge B. A systematic review of the incidence of biological and technical complications in implant dentistry reported in prospective longitudinal studies of at least 5 years. J Clin Periodontol 2002;29(Suppl 3): 197–212 [discussion: 232–3].
32. Leonhardt A, Berglundh T, Ericsson I, et al. Putative periodontal pathogens on titanium implants and teeth in experimental gingivitis and periodontitis in beagle dogs. Clin Oral Implants Res 1992;3:112–9.
33. Serino G, Strom C. Peri-implantitis in partially edentulous patients: association with inadequate plaque control. Clin Oral Implants Res 2009;20:169–74.
34. Sgolastra F, Petrucci A, Severino M, et al. Periodontitis, implant loss and peri-implantitis. A meta-analysis. Clin Oral Implants Res 2013. http://dx.doi.org/10. 1111/clr.12319.
35. Swierkot K, Lottholz P, Flores-de-Jacoby L, et al. Mucositis, peri-implantitis, implant success, and survival of implants in patients with treated generalized aggressive periodontitis: 3- to 16-year results of a prospective long-term cohort study. J Periodontol 2012;83:1213–25.
36. Meyle J, Gersok G, Boedeker RH, et al. Long term analysis of osseointegrated implants in non-smoker patients with a previous history of periodontitis. J Clin Periodontol 2014. http://dx.doi.org/10.1111/jcpe.12237.
37. Pesce P, Menini M, Tealdo T, et al. Peri-implantitis: a systematic review of recently published papers. Int J Prosthodont 2014;27:15–25.
38. Vargas-Reus MA, Memarzadeh K, Huang J, et al. Antimicrobial activity of nanoparticulate metal oxides against peri-implantitis pathogens. Int J Antimicrob Agents 2012;40:135–9.
39. Tamura N, Ochi M, Miyakawa H, et al. Analysis of bacterial flora associated with peri-implantitis using obligate anaerobic culture technique and 16S rDNA gene sequence. Int J Oral Maxillofac Implants 2013;28:1521–9.

40. Irshad M, Scheres N, Crielaard W, et al. Influence of titanium on in vitro fibro-blast-*Porphyromonas gingivalis* interaction in peri-implantitis. J Clin Periodontol 2013;40:841–9.

41. Liu P, Liu Y, Wang J, et al. Detection of *Fusobacterium nucleatum* and fadA adhesin gene in patients with orthodontic gingivitis and non-orthodontic peri-odontal inflammation. PLoS One 2014;9:e85280.

42. Pette GA, Ganeles J, Norkin FJ. Radiographic appearance of commonly used cements in implant dentistry. Int J Periodontics Restorative Dent 2013;33:61–8.

43. Linkevicius T, Vindasiute E, Puisys A, et al. The influence of margin location on the amount of undetected cement excess after delivery of cement-retained implant restorations. Clin Oral Implants Res 2011;22:1379–84.

44. Lang NP, Kiel RA, Anderhalden K. Clinical and microbiological effects of subgin-gival restorations with overhanging or clinically perfect margins. J Clin Periodontol 1983;10:563–78.

45. Naert I, Duyck J, Vandamme K. Occlusal overload and bone/implant loss. Clin Oral Implants Res 2012;23(Suppl 6):95–107.

46. Klinge B, Meyle J. Peri-implant tissue destruction. The Third EAO Consensus Conference 2012. Clin Oral Implants Res 2012;23(Suppl 6):108–10.

47. Chambrone L, Chambrone LA, Lima LA. Effects of occlusal overload on peri-implant tissue health: a systematic review of animal-model studies. J Periodontol 2010;81:1367–78.

48. Chang M, Chronopoulos V, Mattheos N. Impact of excessive occlusal load on successfully-osseointegrated dental implants: a literature review. J Investig Clin Dent 2013;4:142–50.

49. Heitz-Mayfield LJ, Schmid B, Weigel C, et al. Does excessive occlusal load affect osseointegration? An experimental study in the dog. Clin Oral Implants Res 2004;15:259–68.

50. Javed F, Nasstrom K, Benchimol D, et al. Comparison of periodontal and socio-economic status between subjects with type 2 diabetes mellitus and non-diabetic controls. J Periodontol 2007;78:2112–9.

51. Rinke S, Ohl S, Ziebolz D, et al. Prevalence of periimplant disease in partially edentulous patients: a practice-based cross-sectional study. Clin Oral Implants Res 2011;22:826–33.

52. Javed F, Al-Askar M, Samaranayake LP, et al. Periodontal disease in habitual cigarette smokers and nonsmokers with and without prediabetes. Am J Med Sci 2013;345:94–8.

53. Javed F, Al-Rasheed A, Almas K, et al. Effect of cigarette smoking on the clin-ical outcomes of periodontal surgical procedures. Am J Med Sci 2012;343:78–84.

54. Heitz-Mayfield LJ, Lang NP. Comparative biology of chronic and aggressive periodontitis vs. peri-implantitis. Periodontol 2000 2010;53:167–81.

55. Katz J, Yoon TY, Mao S, et al. Expression of the receptor of advanced glycation end products in the gingival tissue of smokers with generalized periodontal disease and after nornicotine induction in primary gingival epithelial cells. J Periodontol 2007;78:736–41.

56. Katz J, Caudle RM, Bhattacharyya I, et al. Receptor for advanced glycation end product (RAGE) upregulation in human gingival fibroblasts incubated with nor-nicotine. J Periodontol 2005;76:1171–4.

57. Laine ML, Leonhardt A, Roos-Jansaker AM, et al. IL-1RN gene polymorphism is associated with peri-implantitis. Clin Oral Implants Res 2006;17:380–5.

58. Gruica B, Wang HY, Lang NP, et al. Impact of IL-1 genotype and smoking status on the prognosis of osseointegrated implants. Clin Oral Implants Res 2004;15: 393–400.
59. Galindo-Moreno P, Leon-Cano A, Ortega-Oller I, et al. Marginal bone loss as success criterion in implant dentistry: beyond 2 mm. Clin Oral Implants Res 2014. http://dx.doi.org/10.1111/clr.12324.
60. Sanchez-Perez A, Moya-Villaescusa MJ, Caffesse RG. Tobacco as a risk factor for survival of dental implants. J Periodontol 2007;78:351–9.
61. De Bruyn H, Collaert B. The effect of smoking on early implant failure. Clin Oral Implants Res 1994;5:260–4.
62. Gorman LM, Lambert PM, Morris HF, et al. The effect of smoking on implant survival at second-stage surgery: DICRG Interim Report No. 5. Dental Implant Clinical Research Group. Implant Dent 1994;3:165–8.
63. Bain CA, Moy PK. The association between the failure of dental implants and cigarette smoking. Int J Oral Maxillofac Implants 1993;8:609–15.
64. Wallace RH. The relationship between cigarette smoking and dental implant failure. Eur J Prosthodont Restor Dent 2000;8:103–6.
65. Haas R, Haimbock W, Mailath G, et al. The relationship of smoking on peri-implant tissue: a retrospective study. J Prosthet Dent 1996;76:592–6.
66. Klokkevold PR, Han TJ. How do smoking, diabetes, and periodontitis affect outcomes of implant treatment? Int J Oral Maxillofac Implants 2007;22(Suppl): 173–202.
67. Sgolastra F, Petrucci A, Severino M, et al. Smoking and the risk of peri-implantitis. A systematic review and meta-analysis. Clin Oral Implants Res 2014. http://dx.doi.org/10.1111/clr.12333.
68. Javed F, Al-Askar M, Al-Hezaimi K. Cytokine profile in the gingival crevicular fluid of periodontitis patients with and without type 2 diabetes: a literature review. J Periodontol 2012;83:156–61.
69. Javed F, Sundin U, Altamash M, et al. Self-perceived oral health and salivary proteins in children with type 1 diabetes. J Oral Rehabil 2009;36:39–44.
70. Takeda M, Ojima M, Yoshioka H, et al. Relationship of serum advanced glycation end products with deterioration of periodontitis in type 2 diabetes patients. J Periodontol 2006;77:15–20.
71. Koromantzos PA, Makrilakis K, Dereka X, et al. Effect of non-surgical periodontal therapy on C-reactive protein, oxidative stress, and matrix metalloproteinase (MMP)-9 and MMP-2 levels in patients with type 2 diabetes: a randomized controlled study. J Periodontol 2012;83:3–10.
72. Ohnishi T, Bandow K, Kakimoto K, et al. Oxidative stress causes alveolar bone loss in metabolic syndrome model mice with type 2 diabetes. J Periodontal Res 2009;44:43–51.
73. Costa PP, Trevisan GL, Macedo GO, et al. Salivary interleukin-6, matrix metalloproteinase-8, and osteoprotegerin in patients with periodontitis and diabetes. J Periodontol 2010;81:384–91.
74. Kao RT, Curtis DA, Richards DW, et al. Increased interleukin-1 beta in the crevicular fluid of diseased implants. Int J Oral Maxillofac Implants 1995;10:696–701.
75. Panagakos FS, Aboyoussef H, Dondero R, et al. Detection and measurement of inflammatory cytokines in implant crevicular fluid: a pilot study. Int J Oral Maxillofac Implants 1996;11:794–9.
76. Lin YH, Huang P, Lu X, et al. The relationship between IL-1 gene polymorphism and marginal bone loss around dental implants. J Oral Maxillofac Surg 2007;65: 2340–4.

77. Dereka X, Mardas N, Chin S, et al. A systematic review on the association between genetic predisposition and dental implant biological complications. Clin Oral Implants Res 2012;23:775–88.

78. Hultin M, Gustafsson A, Hallstrom H, et al. Microbiological findings and host response in patients with peri-implantitis. Clin Oral Implants Res 2002;13: 349–58.

79. Rogers MA, Figliomeni L, Baluchova K, et al. Do interleukin-1 polymorphisms predict the development of periodontitis or the success of dental implants? J Periodontal Res 2002;37:37–41.

80. Campos MI, Santos MC, Trevilatto PC, et al. Evaluation of the relationship between interleukin-1 gene cluster polymorphisms and early implant failure in non-smoking patients. Clin Oral Implants Res 2005;16:194–201.

81. Renvert S, Lindahl C, Rutger Persson G. The incidence of peri-implantitis for two different implant systems over a period of thirteen years. J Clin Periodontol 2012;39:1191–7.

82. Tonetti MS, Chapple IL. Biological approaches to the development of novel periodontal therapies–consensus of the Seventh European Workshop on Periodontology. J Clin Periodontol 2011;38(Suppl 11):114–8.

83. Scheller H, Urgell JP, Kultje C, et al. A 5-year multicenter study on implant-supported single crown restorations. Int J Oral Maxillofac Implants 1998;13: 212–8.

84. Polizzi G, Grunder U, Goene R, et al. Immediate and delayed implant placement into extraction sockets: a 5-year report. Clin Implant Dent Relat Res 2000;2:93–9.

85. Baelum V, Ellegaard B. Implant survival in periodontally compromised patients. J Periodontol 2004;75:1404–12.

86. Karoussis IK, Bragger U, Salvi GE, et al. Effect of implant design on survival and success rates of titanium oral implants: a 10-year prospective cohort study of the ITI Dental Implant System. Clin Oral Implants Res 2004;15:8–17.

87. Bragger U, Karoussis I, Persson R, et al. Technical and biological complications/failures with single crowns and fixed partial dentures on implants: a 10-year prospective cohort study. Clin Oral Implants Res 2005;16:326–34.

88. Fransson C, Wennstrom J, Berglundh T. Clinical characteristics at implants with a history of progressive bone loss. Clin Oral Implants Res 2008;19:142–7.

89. Froum SJ, Rosen PS. A proposed classification for peri-implantitis. Int J Periodontics Restorative Dent 2012;32:533–40.

90. Hujoel PP, DeRouen TA. A survey of endpoint characteristics in periodontal clinical trials published 1988-1992, and implications for future studies. J Clin Periodontol 1995;22:397–407.

91. Faggion CM Jr, Listl S, Tu YK. Assessment of endpoints in studies on peri-implantitis treatment—a systematic review. J Dent 2010;38:443–50.

92. Lee DW. Validated surrogate endpoints needed for peri-implantitis. Evid Based Dent 2011;12:7.

93. Berglundh T, Lindhe J, Marinello C, et al. Soft tissue reaction to de novo plaque formation on implants and teeth. An experimental study in the dog. Clin Oral Implants Res 1992;3:1–8.

94. Kinane DF. Aetiology and pathogenesis of periodontal disease. Ann R Australas Coll Dent Surg 2000;15:42–50.

95. Javed F, Al-Hezaimi K, Salameh Z, et al. Proinflammatory cytokines in the crevicular fluid of patients with peri-implantitis. Cytokine 2011;53:8–12.

96. Bordin S, Flemmig TF, Verardi S. Role of fibroblast populations in peri-implantitis. Int J Oral Maxillofac Implants 2009;24:197–204.

97. Romanos GE, Weitz D. Therapy of peri-implant diseases. Where is the evidence? J Evid Based Dent Pract 2012;12:204–8.

98. Renvert S, Roos-Jansaker AM, Claffey N. Non-surgical treatment of peri-implant mucositis and peri-implantitis: a literature review. J Clin Periodontol 2008;35: 305–15.

99. de Waal YC, Raghoebar GM, Huddleston Slater JJ, et al. Implant decontamination during surgical peri-implantitis treatment: a randomized, double-blind, placebo-controlled trial. J Clin Periodontol 2013;40:186–95.

100. Renvert S, Polyzois I, Claffey N. Surgical therapy for the control of peri-implantitis. Clin Oral Implants Res 2012;23(Suppl 6):84–94.

101. Trejo PM, Bonaventura G, Weng D, et al. Effect of mechanical and antiseptic therapy on peri-implant mucositis: an experimental study in monkeys. Clin Oral Implants Res 2006;17:294–304.

102. Sahm N, Becker J, Santel T, et al. Non-surgical treatment of peri-implantitis using an air-abrasive device or mechanical debridement and local application of chlorhexidine: a prospective, randomized, controlled clinical study. J Clin Periodontol 2011;38:872–8.

103. Schwarz F, Jepsen S, Herten M, et al. Influence of different treatment approaches on non-submerged and submerged healing of ligature induced peri-implantitis lesions: an experimental study in dogs. J Clin Periodontol 2006;33:584–95.

104. Karring ES, Stavropoulos A, Ellegaard B, et al. Treatment of peri-implantitis by the Vector system. Clin Oral Implants Res 2005;16:288–93.

105. Khoury F, Buchmann R. Surgical therapy of peri-implant disease: a 3-year follow-up study of cases treated with 3 different techniques of bone regeneration. J Periodontol 2001;72:1498–508.

106. Stein AE, McGlmphy EA, Johnston WM, et al. Effects of implant design and surface roughness on crestal bone and soft tissue levels in the esthetic zone. Int J Oral Maxillofac Implants 2009;24:910–9.

107. Mombelli A, Lang NP. The diagnosis and treatment of peri-implantitis. Periodontol 2000 1998;17:63–76.

108. Heitz-Mayfield LJ, Mombelli A. The therapy of peri-implantitis: a systematic review. Int J Oral Maxillofac Implants 2014;29(Suppl):325–45.

109. Li X, Wang X, Zhao T, et al. Guided bone regeneration using chitosan-collagen membranes in dog dehiscence-type defect model. J Oral Maxillofac Surg 2014; 72:304.e1–14.

110. Schou S, Holmstrup P, Skovgaard LT, et al. Autogenous bone graft and ePTFE membrane in the treatment of peri-implantitis. II. Stereologic and histologic observations in cynomolgus monkeys. Clin Oral Implants Res 2003;14:404–11.

111. Schou S, Holmstrup P, Jorgensen T, et al. Autogenous bone graft and ePTFE membrane in the treatment of peri-implantitis. I. Clinical and radiographic observations in cynomolgus monkeys. Clin Oral Implants Res 2003;14:391–403.

112. Javed F, Al-Askar M, Al-Rasheed A, et al. Significance of the platelet-derived growth factor in periodontal tissue regeneration. Arch Oral Biol 2011;56: 1476–84.

113. Simion M, Rocchietta I, Monforte M, et al. Three-dimensional alveolar bone reconstruction with a combination of recombinant human platelet-derived growth factor BB and guided bone regeneration: a case report. Int J Periodontics Restorative Dent 2008;28:239–43.

114. Kaigler D, Avila G, Wisner-Lynch L, et al. Platelet-derived growth factor applications in periodontal and peri-implant bone regeneration. Expert Opin Biol Ther 2011;11:375–85.

115. Jung RE, Glauser R, Scharer P, et al. Effect of rhBMP-2 on guided bone regeneration in humans. Clin Oral Implants Res 2003;14:556–68.

116. Roos-Jansaker AM, Lindahl C, Persson GR, et al. Long-term stability of surgical bone regenerative procedures of peri-implantitis lesions in a prospective case-control study over 3 years. J Clin Periodontol 2011;38:590–7.

117. Roncati M, Lucchese A, Carinci F. Non-surgical treatment of peri-implantitis with the adjunctive use of an 810-nm diode laser. J Indian Soc Periodontol 2013;17:812–5.

118. Romanos G, Ko HH, Froum S, et al. The use of CO(2) laser in the treatment of peri-implantitis. Photomed Laser Surg 2009;27:381–6.

119. Romanos GE, Everts H, Nentwig GH. Effects of diode and Nd:YAG laser irradiation on titanium discs: a scanning electron microscope examination. J Periodontol 2000;71:810–5.

120. Ayobian-Markazi N, Karimi M, Safar-Hajhosseini A. Effects of Er:YAG laser irradiation on wettability, surface roughness, and biocompatibility of SLA titanium surfaces: an in vitro study. Lasers Med Sci 2013. http://dx.doi.org/10.1007/s10103-013-1361-y.

121. Crespi R, Barone A, Covani U, et al. Effects of CO2 laser treatment on fibroblast attachment to root surfaces. A scanning electron microscopy analysis. J Periodontol 2002;73:1308–12.

122. Siddiqui SH, Awan KH, Javed F. Bactericidal efficacy of photodynamic therapy against Enterococcus faecalis in infected root canals: a systematic literature review. Photodiagnosis Photodyn Ther 2013;10:632–43.

123. Sperandio FF, Huang YY, Hamblin MR. Antimicrobial photodynamic therapy to kill Gram-negative bacteria. Recent Pat Antiinfect Drug Discov 2013;8:108–20.

124. Figueiredo Souza LW, Souza SV, Botelho AC. Randomized controlled trial comparing photodynamic therapy based on methylene blue dye and fluconazole for toenail onychomycosis. Dermatol Ther 2014;27:43–7.

125. Kolbe MF, Ribeiro FV, Luchesi VH, et al. Photodynamic therapy during supportive periodontal care: clinical, microbiological, immunoinflammatory, and patient-centered performance in a split-mouth RCT. J Periodontol 2014. http://dx.doi.org/10.1902/jop.2014.130559.

126. Esposito M, Grusovin MG, De Angelis N, et al. The adjunctive use of light-activated disinfection (LAD) with FotoSan is ineffective in the treatment of peri-implantitis: 1-year results from a multicentre pragmatic randomised controlled trial. Eur J Oral Implantol 2013;6:109–19.

127. Schar D, Ramseier CA, Eick S, et al. Anti-infective therapy of peri-implantitis with adjunctive local drug delivery or photodynamic therapy: six-month outcomes of a prospective randomized clinical trial. Clin Oral Implants Res 2013;24:104–10.

128. Deppe H, Mucke T, Wagenpfeil S, et al. Nonsurgical antimicrobial photodynamic therapy in moderate vs severe peri-implant defects: a clinical pilot study. Quintessence Int 2013;44:609–18.

129. Eick S, Markauskaite G, Nietzsche S, et al. Effect of photoactivated disinfection with a light-emitting diode on bacterial species and biofilms associated with periodontitis and peri-implantitis. Photodiagnosis Photodyn Ther 2013;10:156–67.

130. Hayek RR, Araujo NS, Gioso MA, et al. Comparative study between the effects of photodynamic therapy and conventional therapy on microbial reduction in ligature-induced peri-implantitis in dogs. J Periodontol 2005;76:1275–81.

131. Marotti J, Tortamano P, Cai S, et al. Decontamination of dental implant surfaces by means of photodynamic therapy. Lasers Med Sci 2013;28:303–9.

132. Javed F, Romanos GE. The role of primary stability for successful immediate loading of dental implants. A literature review. J Dent 2010;38:612–20.

133. Tabassum A, Meijer GJ, Wolke JG, et al. Influence of surgical technique and surface roughness on the primary stability of an implant in artificial bone with different cortical thickness: a laboratory study. Clin Oral Implants Res 2010;21:213–20.

134. Javed F, Ahmed HB, Crespi R, et al. Role of primary stability for successful osseointegration of dental implants: factors of influence and evaluation. Interv Med Appl Sci 2013;5:162–7.

135. Javed F, Almas K, Crespi R, et al. Implant surface morphology and primary stability: is there a connection? Implant Dent 2011;20:40–6.

136. Teughels W, Van Assche N, Sliepen I, et al. Effect of material characteristics and/or surface topography on biofilm development. Clin Oral Implants Res 2006; 17(Suppl 2):68–81.

137. Romeo E, Ghisolfi M, Murgolo N, et al. Therapy of peri-implantitis with resective surgery. A 3-year clinical trial on rough screw-shaped oral implants. Part I: clinical outcome. Clin Oral Implants Res 2005;16:9–18.

138. Romeo E, Lops D, Chiapasco M, et al. Therapy of peri-implantitis with resective surgery. A 3-year clinical trial on rough screw-shaped oral implants. Part II: radiographic outcome. Clin Oral Implants Res 2007;18:179–87.

139. Maximo MB, de Mendonca AC, Renata Santos V, et al. Short-term clinical and microbiological evaluations of peri-implant diseases before and after mechanical anti-infective therapies. Clin Oral Implants Res 2009;20:99–108.

140. Duarte PM, de Mendonca AC, Maximo MB, et al. Effect of anti-infective mechanical therapy on clinical parameters and cytokine levels in human peri-implant diseases. J Periodontol 2009;80:234–43.

141. Persson LG, Ericsson I, Berglundh T, et al. Osseintegration following treatment of peri-implantitis and replacement of implant components. An experimental study in the dog. J Clin Periodontol 2001;28:258–63.

142. Ungvari K, Pelsoczi IK, Kormos B, et al. Effects on titanium implant surfaces of chemical agents used for the treatment of peri-implantitis. J Biomed Mater Res B Appl Biomater 2010;94:222–9.

143. Zablotsky MH, Diedrich DL, Meffert RM. Detoxification of endotoxin-contaminated titanium and hydroxyapatite-coated surfaces utilizing various chemotherapeutic and mechanical modalities. Implant Dent 1992;1:154–8.

144. Dennison DK, Huerzeler MB, Quinones C, et al. Contaminated implant surfaces: an in vitro comparison of implant surface coating and treatment modalities for decontamination. J Periodontol 1994;65:942–8.

145. Hall EE, Meffert RM, Hermann JS, et al. Comparison of bioactive glass to demineralized freeze-dried bone allograft in the treatment of intrabony defects around implants in the canine mandible. J Periodontol 1999;70:526–35.

146. Suh JJ, Simon Z, Jeon YS, et al. The use of implantoplasty and guided bone regeneration in the treatment of peri-implantitis: two case reports. Implant Dent 2003;12:277–82.

147. Tinti C, Parma-Benfenati S. Treatment of peri-implant defects with the vertical ridge augmentation procedure: a patient report. Int J Oral Maxillofac Implants 2001;16:572–7.

148. Park JB. Treatment of peri-implantitis with deproteinised bovine bone and tetracycline: a case report. Gerodontology 2012;29:145–9.

149. Kamel MS, Khosa A, Tawse-Smith A, et al. The use of laser therapy for dental implant surface decontamination: a narrative review of in vitro studies. Lasers Med Sci 2013. http://dx.doi.org/10.1007/s10103-013-1396-0.

150. Geminiani A, Caton JG, Romanos GE. Temperature increase during CO(2) and Er:YAG irradiation on implant surfaces. Implant Dent 2011;20:379–82.

151. Geminiani A, Caton JG, Romanos GE. Temperature change during non-contact diode laser irradiation of implant surfaces. Lasers Med Sci 2012;27:339–42.

152. Kreisler M, Kohnen W, Marinello C, et al. Bactericidal effect of the Er:YAG laser on dental implant surfaces: an in vitro study. J Periodontol 2002;73:1292–8.

153. Kreisler M, Gotz H, Duschner H. Effect of Nd:YAG, Ho:YAG, Er:YAG, CO2, and GaAlAs laser irradiation on surface properties of endosseous dental implants. Int J Oral Maxillofac Implants 2002;17:202–11.

154. Mombelli A, Lang NP. Antimicrobial treatment of peri-implant infections. Clin Oral Implants Res 1992;3:162–8.

155. Heitz-Mayfield LJ, Salvi GE, Mombelli A, et al. Anti-infective surgical therapy of peri-implantitis. A 12-month prospective clinical study. Clin Oral Implants Res 2012;23:205–10.

156. Renvert S, Lessem J, Dahlen G, et al. Mechanical and repeated antimicrobial therapy using a local drug delivery system in the treatment of peri-implantitis: a randomized clinical trial. J Periodontol 2008;79:836–44.

157. Salvi GE, Persson GR, Heitz-Mayfield LJ, et al. Adjunctive local antibiotic therapy in the treatment of peri-implantitis II: clinical and radiographic outcomes. Clin Oral Implants Res 2007;18:281–5.

158. Buchter A, Meyer U, Kruse-Losler B, et al. Sustained release of doxycycline for the treatment of peri-implantitis: randomised controlled trial. Br J Oral Maxillofac Surg 2004;42:439–44.

159. Mombelli A, Feloutzis A, Bragger U, et al. Treatment of peri-implantitis by local delivery of tetracycline. Clinical, microbiological and radiological results. Clin Oral Implants Res 2001;12:287–94.

160. Romanos GE. Advanced laser surgical dentistry. Chicago: Quintessence Publ, in press.

Biologic Markers of Failing Implants

Pinar Emecen-Huja, DDS, PhD[a],*, Iquebal Hasan, BDS[b], Craig S. Miller, DMD, MS[c]

KEYWORDS

- Peri-implantitis • Microbiological markers • Biological markers

KEY POINTS

- The diagnosis of peri-implantitis benefits from clinical, radiographic, microbiological, and biological information.
- Practitioners and patients can use biomarkers to identify risk of disease, disease activity, disease progression, and response to therapy.
- Peri-implantitis is a biofilm-induced condition. The microbial composition of peri-implantitis lesions is mixed, nonspecific, and less diverse than that of periodontitis but includes *Fusobacterium*, *Prevotella*, *Porphyromonas*, *Streptococcus*, *Campylobacter*, and *Neisseria* species.
- Failed implants are often associated with enteric bacteria, spirochetes, and opportunistic bacteria (ie, *Staphylococcus aureus*).
- Protein biomarkers detected in peri-implant crevicular fluid provide insight into the underlying biology of the disease and specificity regarding the stage of the disease.

INTRODUCTION

As a result of clinical translational research, biomarkers are becoming increasingly available. They supplement clinical and radiographic information, allowing clinicians to make better decisions. Patients can also use biomarkers to obtain information about their health status and the need for dental care. Although biomarkers are most commonly used to decide whether a patient has a disease, their usefulness is more expansive. As **Fig. 1** shows, biomarkers are important for identifying severity of disease, ongoing activity of disease, disease progression, and response to therapy. With respect to periodontal disease, salivary analytes interleukin 1 beta (IL-1β), matrix metalloprotease 8 (MMP-8), and macrophage inflammatory protein-1 alpha (MIP-1α)

[a] Division of Periodontics, Department of Oral Health Practice, College of Dentistry, University of Kentucky, D-440 Dental Science Building, 800 Rose Street, Lexington, KY 40536, USA; [b] Department of Oral Health Practice, College of Dentistry, University of Kentucky, MN320, Lexington, KY 40536-0297, USA; [c] Department of Oral Health Practice, College of Dentistry, University of Kentucky, MN324, Lexington, KY 40536-0297, USA
* Corresponding author.
E-mail address: pinar.emecenhuja@uky.edu

Dent Clin N Am 59 (2015) 179–194
http://dx.doi.org/10.1016/j.cden.2014.08.007
0011-8532/15/$ – see front matter Published by Elsevier Inc.

dental.theclinics.com

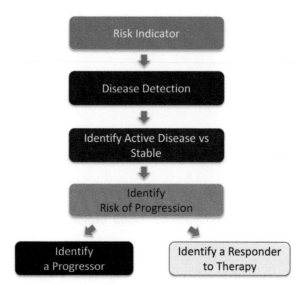

Fig. 1. Potential roles of biomarkers.

have recently been shown to serve in these roles. For example, high salivary concentrations of these analytes are associated with periodontal disease,[1–3] whereas high salivary concentration of MIP-1α is also a predictor of risk, that is, predictive of alveolar bone loss 6 to 9 months before radiographic evidence is apparent.[4] Oral fluid biomarkers can also be used to indicate response to therapy and have recently been shown to be useful in this role.[5] Together, the identification of biomarkers that have clinical utility for risk identification, disease detection, and identification of disease progression and response to therapy is the basis for establishing personalized care in the modern health care age and serve as the context for this article on peri-implantitis and failing dental implants. Specifically, this article discusses the milieu of microbes and proteins, that constitute the underlying biology of implant osseointegration and disease progression that can serve as indicators of implant health or failure.

DEFINITIONS

Peri-implantitis is a potentially progressive condition involving infection, inflammation, connective tissue destruction, and bone resorption.[6] The condition is characterized by microbial infection, deep probing depths, bleeding on probing, suppuration, and radiographic bone loss.[7–9] Risk factors include cigarette smoking, poor oral hygiene, and a previous history of periodontitis.[10] Peri-implantitis does not necessarily mean that the implant will fail. The implant can be salvaged if peri-implantitis is diagnosed early, if risk factors are reduced or eliminated, and if the site is treated appropriately.[11] In contrast, implant failure is defined as the inability of the host tissue to establish or maintain osseointegration, which is clinically diagnosed by mobility of the implant (**Fig. 2**).

Implant failures are classified as early or late, depending on the time of placement and the implant's functionality. Early failure occurs before prosthetic rehabilitation and before the implant is placed into function. Early failures generally result from surgical trauma, overheating of the bone during implant surgery, insufficient bone surrounding the implant, early loading of the implant, or perioperative bacterial

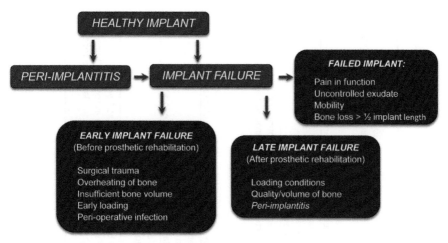

Fig. 2. Implant failure: definitions, etiology, and clinical features.

infection. Late failure occurs after prosthetic rehabilitation and indicates that established osseointegration has not been maintained. Late failures can further be classified as early or delayed depending on whether implant failure is observed before or after the first year of loading. Delayed late failures are generally associated with changes in loading conditions, the quality and volume of bone relations, and peri-implantitis.[12,13]

A failed implant is a clinical diagnosis defined by one or more of the following criteria: pain in function, presence of uncontrolled exudate, mobility, or radiographic alveolar bone loss more than half the length of the implant. Clinicians generally recommend removal of a failed implant[14]; however, because implant failure is a process requiring time, a clinician can experience the dilemma of a failing implant, characterized by progressive loss of alveolar bone support. In this instance, the clinician must decide what action to take and whether clinical, radiographic, or biological information can help in the decision-making process that could ultimately prevent the loss of the implant. Clinicians should be aware that a failing implant is associated with the accumulation of microbial plaque and bacterial infection around the implant. These microbes elicit many biological mediators, and it is conceivable that the milieu of microbial and biological molecules that surround and emanate from the sulcus of the implant can distinguish a healthy implant from one associated with peri-implantitis.

MICROBIOLOGICAL MARKERS OF FAILING DENTAL IMPLANTS

Peri-implantitis accounts for 10% to 50% of implant failures after the first year of loading.[12] Microorganisms play an important role in peri-implantitis; therefore, the identification of peri-implantitis-associated microbiota or bacteria is crucial for an understanding of peri-implantitis pathogenesis and of the bacteria that could serve as microbial biomarkers of this condition. **Table 1** summarizes the results of studies conducted during the last 3 decades that have analyzed the microbiota of peri-implantitis sites. Details regarding these studies are discussed below.

Bacterial Colonization and Microbial Composition Around Healthy Implants

Longitudinal studies of biofilm formation around dental implants have shown that bacterial colonization occurs immediately after implant placement (within 30 minutes).[15]

Table 1
Longitudinal studies of microbial colonization around teeth and implants

Authors	Follow-up	Implants (Patients)	Method	Results
Salvi et al,[19] 2008	12 mo	17 I 17 T (n = 13)	DNA-H	Sum of bacterial counts at T sites was higher than at I sites. *Pm, Lb, Cs,* and *Pi* were most prevalent at I sites at 12 mo (>30 × 10^5 cells). *Sg, Fn* ssp. *polymorphum,* and *vincentii* were most prevalent at T sites at 12 mo (>50 × 10^5 cells). *F* spp, *Strep* spp, *Pm,* and *Sa* were higher at I sites. Few differences in bacterial species between tooth and implant at 12 mo.
Furst et al,[15] 2007	3 mo	17 I 17 T (n = 14)	DNA-H	Bacterial colonization around implants starts at 30 min. *Pg, Td,* and *Tf* were present at implant sites at 12 wk. *Sa* was present at 15% of the implant sites at 12 wk.
Quirynen et al,[17] 2006	18 mo	NR (n = 42)	DNA-H culture	Red (5%) and orange (20%) complex bacteria were present around the implant at 1 wk. Red (8%) and orange (33%) complex bacteria were present around the implant at 3 mo. The subgingival microbiota was similar at I and T sites at 3 mo.
Leonhardt et al,[22] 2002	10 y	57 I 261 T (n = 15)	Culture	*Pg, Pi, Aa, C* ssp, and *Cr* were detected at baseline and at 10-yr follow-up at T and I sites. These bacterial species are members of the normal resident microbiota.
Hultin et al,[21] 2000	10 y	43 I 31 T (n = 15)	DNA probe	No marked differences were found between T and I at 10 yr. *Td, Si,* and *Pm* were the most common bacteria at I and T sites. *Aa, Pg, Td,* and *Tf* were found at implant sites with > 2-mm bone loss.
van Winkelhoff et al,[20] 2000	12 mo	NR (n = 20)	Culture	Prevalence of bacteria was similar at I and T sites at 6 mo. Implant failure was associated with high levels of *Pg.* *Aa* was not detectable around I sites.
Sbordone et al,[18] 1999	3 y	42 I 25 T (n = 25)	Culture	*Pg and C* ssp were the most prevalent bacteria around implants at 1 yr. Significantly fewer motile rods were found at implant sites than at teeth at 1 yr. No statistically significant difference in periodontopathogens at implant and tooth sites.

Abbreviations: Aa, Aggregatibacter actinomycetemcomitans; Cr, Campylobacter rectus; Cs, Campylocytophaga sputigena; C ssp, Capnocytophaga subspecies; DNA-H, DNA-DNA hybridization; Fn, Fusobacterium nucleatum; I, implant; Lb, Leptotrichia buccalis; NR, not reported; Pg, Porphyromonas gingivalis; Pi, Prevotella intermedia; Pm, Peptostreptococcus micros; Si, Streptococcus intermediate; Strep spp, Streptococcus subspecies; T, teeth; Td, Treponema denticola; Tf, Tannerella forsynthesis.

The microbiota associated with healthy peri-implant tissues are dominated by gram-positive facultative cocci and rods and by low proportions of gram-negative anaerobic rods.[15,16] Initial colonization of peri-implant sites with periodontitis-associated bacteria (eg, *Porphyromonas gingivalis, Treponema denticola, Tannerella forsythensis*) is detected as early as 2 weeks after placement.[17] The composition of bacteria around healthy teeth and around healthy implant sites is reported to remain similar for as long as 2 years.[17–19] However, the sum of bacterial counts of 40 periodontopathogenic species analyzed with DNA-DNA hybridization was higher around normal teeth than at implant sites both at baseline (immediately after implant placement) and 1 year later.[19] Also, the most predominant microbes around implants 1 year after placement were *Peptostreptococcus micros, Leptotrichia buccalis, Capnocytophaga sputigena*, and *Prevotella intermedia* ($>30 \times 10^5$ cells), whereas the most predominant microbes at tooth sites were *Streptococcus goordinii* and *Fusobacterium nucleatum* subspecies *polymorphum*, and *vincentii* ($>50 \times 10^5$ cells).[19] However, the presence of putative periodontal pathogens at peri-implant sites does not dictate loss or failure of an implant attachment, provided proper oral hygiene measures and periodontal supportive therapy are maintained.[18,20] Two follow-up studies of clinical, radiographic, and microbiological parameters of osseointegrated implants in partially edentulous patients treated for periodontal disease did not report marked differences in microbial flora between healthy implants and teeth at baseline and 10 years later.[21,22] In fact, putative bacterial species, including *P gingivalis, P intermedia, Aggregatibacter actinomycetemcomitans, Capnocytophaga* spp, and *Campylobacter rectus*, were present at clinically healthy implant sites at a 10-year examination. Therefore, it is suggested that periodontopathogens are present at implant sites as part of the normal resident microbiota and are not the sole factor affecting the long-term outcome of implant treatment.[22]

Microbial Composition Around Implants Associated with Peri-implantitis

Today, it is well accepted that peri-implant mucositis and peri-implantitis are induced by biofilm.[8,23] Although no single candidate bacterium is responsible for the infection of any implant system (**Table 2**), *Staphylococcus aureus* has been suggested to be important for dental implant failure because its specific affinity for titanium surfaces.[24] Recent reports have shown that *S aureus* is an early colonizer of implant surfaces. It is found at implant sites 3 months to 1 year after implant placement.[19,25] Early implant failures are reported to be associated with *S aureus* because of low serum antibody titers, which suggests an impaired host response to this microorganism.[26] A cluster of bacteria, including *S aureus*, has been found to be more prevalent at sites of peri-implantitis (30.2%) than at healthy implant sites (14.1%),[25] and the absence of *S aureus* is suggested to indicate implant health.[19] However, a recent study investigating the presence of opportunistic bacteria at peri-implantitis sites found *Pseudomonas aeruginosa* in 3 of the 31 patients examined and *S aureus* in only one.[27] Therefore, although *S aureus* and other opportunistic bacteria appear to play a role in select cases of peri-implantitis and implant failure, additional investigations are required because of the limited number of studies addressing this problem and the differences in the methods used.

In addition to opportunistic bacteria, specific periodontal pathogens have been identified at healthy implant sites, peri-implant mucositis sites, and peri-implantitis sites.[21,28] Several studies identified increased levels of red complex bacteria (*P gingivalis, T denticola, T forsythensis*) and *P gingivalis* at peri-implantitis sites.[25,27,29–31] Because of the similarity of the microbiota around normal teeth and adjacent implants, it has been suggested that bacterial flora at the adjacent tooth site can act as a

Table 2
Case-control and retrospective human studies on microbial composition in peri-implantitis

Authors	Implants (Patients)	Method	S	PDx	Clinical Measures	Results
Albertini et al,[27] 2014	48 PI 33 T (n = 33)	PCR Culture	Yes	Yes	BOP/SUP Radiograph	*Pg, Pi, Tf, Td* prevalence was similar at Peri-I and T sites. *Pa* (12%), *Ca* (3%), and *Sa* (3%) were detected Peri-I group.
Persson & Renvert,[25] 2013	166 PI 47 HI (n = 213)	DNA-H	Yes	Yes	PPD Radiograph	A cluster of bacteria including *Tf, Pg, Ts, Sa, Si,* and *Hi* were higher at Peri-I sites compared with HI (30.4% vs 14.1%). History of PDx, age, and *Tf* were found associated with Peri-I.
Heuer et al,[33] 2012	9 G 9 PM (n = 9)	DNA-H	NR	No	PD BOP Plaque	Microbial diversity of G sites was more complex than PM sites. *Fusobacterium, Prevotella, Porphyromonas, Streptococcus, Campylobacter,* and *Neisseria* were most prevalent at PM sites.
Dabdoub et al,[35] 2013	33 HT/HI 23 HT/DI 8 DT/HI 17 DT/DT (n = 81)	16S RNA Pyroseq.	NR	Yes	PD BOP/SUP GI Mobility Radiograph	Periodontal pathogens are found in 37% of the DI sites. *Staphylococcus* and *Treponema* are associated with DI compared with T sites. Most abundant species remain different between I and T sites. Geographic proximity is not sufficient to explain peri-implant microbial composition.
Koyanagi et al,[37] 2013	6 PI 6 PDx (n = 6)	16S RNA	No	Yes	PD BOP/SUP Radiograph	Microbial composition of Peri-I sites was more diverse than PDx. Periodontopathogens were detected in lower amounts in Peri-I sites.
Cortelli et al,[36] 2013	53 HI/53 HT 50 PM/50 G 50 PI/50 PDx (n = 306)	16S RNA	No	Yes	PD CAL BOP/SUP Radiograph	Peri-implant mucositis and Peri-I shared similar microbial composition. Composition of bacterial species was different between PI and PDx. Bacterial frequency was higher in teeth compared with implants *Pg* was associated with Peri-I.
Kumar et al,[34] 2012	10 PDx 10 PI 10 HI 10 HT (n = 40)	16S RNA Pyroseq	NR	Yes	PD CAL BOP Plaque	Peri-I and HI biofilms are less diverse than PDx and HT-related biofilms. PI had higher levels of *Actinomyces, Peptococcus, Mycoplasma, Eubacterium, Campylobacter, Butyrivibrio, S mutans,* and *Treponema* compared with HI and HT. Peri-I is a microbiologically heterogenous gram-negative infection.

Study	Sample	Method			Parameters	Findings
Renvert et al,[28] 2007	31 PI, 127 PM, 55 HI (n = 231)	DNA-H	NR	Yes	PPD, BOP, Radiograph	Edentulous and dentate subjects showed similar microbial profiles. Peri-I, PM, and HI sites had similar bacterial profile regardless of implant disease status.
Shibli et al,[30] 2008	22 PI, 22 HI (n = 44)	DNA-H	No	No	Radiograph, BOP/SUP	HI sites had similar supra/subgingival plaque composition. Peri-I sites had higher levels of red complex bacteria in supra/subgingival plaque. Peri-I sites had different bacterial composition between subra- and subgingival plaque.
Botero et al,[29] 2005	16 PI, 15 HI, 23 T (n = 19)	Culture	NR	NR	PD, BOP/SUP, Radiograph	Peri-I sites showed increased levels of gram-enteric rods and Pg. A correlation was found between subgingival colonization in PI and neighboring T sites for enteric rods and Pg.
Hultin et al,[31] 2002	45 PI, 53 HI, 133 T (n = 36)	DNA-H	Yes	No	PPD, GI, Plaque, Radiograph	Pg, Pi, Bf, Aa, and Td were detected in HI and PI sites and around teeth. Pg, Pi, Bf, Aa, and Td were detected $>10^6$ in PI sites. Peri-I is a site-specific infection rather than a specific host response.
Leonhardt et al,[16] 1999	NR (n = 88)	Culture	Yes	Yes	PD, BOP/SUP, Radiograph	Edentulous patients have not harbored periodontopathogens. Enterics were found commonly in Peri-I sites compared with HI sites. PI sites carried more periodontopathogens HI sites.
Sbordone et al,[38] 1995	19 FI (n = 13)	Culture	NR	NR	PD, PAL, BOP/SUP, Plaque, GI	Fusiform bacteria, spirochetes, and motile curved rods were isolated at failing implant sites.

Abbreviations: Aa, Aggregatibacter actinomycetemcomitans; BOP, bleeding on probing; Ca, Candida albicans; Cr, Campylobacter rectus; Cs, Capnocytophaga sputigena; C ssp, Capnocytophaga subspecies; DNA-C, DNA-DNA checkerboard; DNA-H, DNA-DNA hybridization; Fn, Fusobacterium nucleatum; G, gingivitis; Hi, Haemophilus intermedia; HI, healthy implants; HT, healthy teeth; I, Implants; Lb, Leptotrichia buccalis; NR, not reported; Pa, Pseudomonas aeruginosa; PDx, periodontal disease; Peri-I, peri-implantitis; Pg, Porphyromonas gingivalis; Pi, Prevotella intermedia; Pm, Peptostreptococcus micros; PM, peri-implant mucositis; PPD, periodontal probing depth; Pyroseq, Pyrosequencing; S, Smoking; Si, Streptococcus intermediate; Strep spp, Streptococcus subspecies; SUP, suppuration; Td, Treponema denticola; Tf, Tannerella forsynthesis; Ts, Treponema socranskii.

reservoir for the implant sulcus.[32] However, increasing evidence suggests that the immunology, histology, and microbiology of peri-implant diseases are different from those of periodontal diseases.[22,33–35] In a case-control study, peri-implant, mucositis lesions, characterized by bleeding and inflammation of the peri-implant mucosa, contained fewer diverse microbes (6 microbial genera) than gingivitis lesions (19 microbial genera). The most common genera found at peri-implant mucositis lesions were *Fusobacterium, Prevotella, Porphyromonas, Streptococcus, Campylobacter,* and *Neisseria.*[33] Similarly, the microbial composition of peri-implantitis lesions was less diverse than that of periodontitis lesions, and periodontal pathogens were detected at lower frequencies around peri-implantitis sites than around natural teeth.[34–37] Most of the abundant species in peri-implant lesions are reported to be different from those around natural teeth.[35] For example, peri-implantitis lesions contained higher levels of *Actinomyces, Peptococcus, Campylobacter, Butyrivibrio, Streptococcus mutans,* and nonmutans *Streptococcus* than healthy implant sites. Peri-implantitis sites also yielded higher levels of *Peptostreptococcus, Mycoplasma, Eubacterium, Campylobacter, S mutans,* and *Treponema* than did periodontitis sites.[34] Of potential importance with respect to biomarkers is the finding that enteric bacteria, spirochetes, and opportunistic bacteria have often been detected as the most abundant members of the microbiota at the sites of failed implants.[16,29,38]

The available information about whether the presence of a single bacterium or a cluster of bacteria can be used as a biomarker for distinguishing peri-implant disease from peri-implant health appears to be limited and requires further evaluation. Identifying good biomarkers of peri-implantitis and implant failure is difficult because investigators have used various methods of sampling and methods for analyzing bacteria (eg, bacterial culture, DNA hybridization, and 16S RNA), and have used small, geographically restricted patient populations. These problems have prevented conclusions regarding the specificity of the peri-implant microbiota. In addition, it is thought that structural and topographic differences between implant surfaces and natural tooth surfaces may influence a unique and unknown bacterial composition that has not yet been identified.[39] Thus, additional studies that recognize these concepts are needed so that we can fully characterize the microbiota related to peri-implant disease. As a result, these studies can lead to better prevention and management strategies for peri-implantitis.

PROTEINS AS BIOLOGICAL MARKERS FOR PERI-IMPLANTITIS

Peri-implantitis is a progressive condition that, if left untreated, involves 3 biological phases: inflammation, connective tissue destruction, and bone resorption. As such, researchers have sought concentrations of biological molecules associated with these 3 biological phases in oral fluids, with the goal of finding early predictors of susceptibility and detecting the molecules associated with the early, intermediate, and late endpoints of this disease. With the identification of specific molecular markers of peri-implantitis, clinicians should be able to monitor disease progression and devise preventive strategies and interventional therapies that can limit the progression of this disease. In addition, biomarkers should help define the interval for periodic recall and the response to therapies. This section provides an overview of protein biomarkers, associated with the host response, that are detected in the oral fluid of patients with peri-implantitis. **Table 3** provides details of studies that have investigated the biomarkers found in the crevicular fluid surrounding healthy and failing implants.

Inflammatory Biomarkers

The immune system responds predictably to infection and injury with inflammation in the affected area. Accordingly, microbial biofilm on peri-implant surfaces induces an inflammatory response in susceptible hosts; this response involves features shared with and distinct from features of periodontitis.[40,41] The classic inflammatory peptides and proteins that respond to bacterial inflammation are cytokines and chemokines produced by T lymphocytes and monocytes/macrophages. In addition, many nonspecific markers of inflammation make up the inflammatory milieu. These proteins appear in peri-implant crevicular fluid (PICF) or gingival crevicular fluid (GCF) samples taken from the area around the implant and could serve as markers of inflammation and early detection.[42] In addition, the volume of PICF is increased during peri-implantitis, and this information can be informative to the clinician.[43]

The proteins myeloperoxidase (MPO) and lactoferrin are found in the granules of neutrophils that are released after tissue injury and inflammation. MPO is a marker of inflammation that also serves as a biomarker of cardiovascular disease,[44] whereas lactoferrin is known to regulate the immune response and protect against bacterial infection.[45] The utility of these 2 proteins as biomarkers of peri-implantitis has been suggested. Liskmann and colleagues[46] collected clinical measures of periodontal health and PICF from 24 adults with 64 oral implants. They found that MPO levels were significantly higher around inflamed implants than around healthy implants and were associated with increased pocket depth, a higher gingival index, and bleeding on probing. Similarly, Hultin and colleagues[31] found that in 17 patients, the concentrations of lactoferrin were higher in PICF from peri-implantitis sites than in PICF from stable implant sites.

Prostaglandins are produced by cyclooxygenases during inflammation and contribute to the clinical features of inflammation.[47] They are found at higher concentrations in fluids emanating from sites of gingivitis and periodontitis,[5] and they were recently detected in PICF. Basegmez and colleagues[48] detected higher levels of prostaglandin E2 around implants as probing depths and time after implantation increased.

IL-1β, a proinflammatory cytokine, is known to be important in the pathogenesis of periodontal disease.[49] It contributes to the activation of osteoclasts, bone resorption, and down-regulation of type 1 collagen expression in bone.[50] IL-1β has been detected at higher levels in GCF and saliva associated with severe periodontitis, periodontal disease progression, and, recently, peri-implantitis.[1,51,52] A study involving 13 patients with 50 implants found that the concentrations of IL-1β were 3 to 9 times higher at peri-implantitis sites than at healthy implant sites.[53] Similarly, a study involving 16 patients with 34 endoseous titatnium implants, found that mean levels of IL-1β in PICF were significantly higher at the 6 peri-implantitis sites than at the 20 healthy implant sites.[43] In contrast, Hultin and colleagues[31] studied 17 patients with 45 implants and found that the concentrations of IL-1β at peri-implantitis sites were not different from those at stable implant sites.

As time progresses and the inflammatory phase matures, peri-implantitis involves the connective tissue destruction phase. This phase is associated with neutrophil- and macrophage-derived enzymes that degrade collagen and extracellular matrices. Thus, the predominant enzymes involved are MMPs. This family of enzymes has been detected in saliva and GCF from patients with periodontal disease[1,54] and recently in PICF from patients with severe peri-implantitis and during periods of ongoing bone loss activity. Arakawa and colleagues[55] used Western blot analysis in a study involving 64 patients. They found that MMP-8 was the main collagenase in PICF from severe peri-implantitis sites and during periods of ongoing bone loss activity. Concentrations

Table 3
Relevant studies involving protein biomarkers of peri-implantitis

Authors	Biomarker	Study Design	Implants (Patients)	Implant Function/ Year	Smoker	Clinical Measures	Outcome
Panagakos et al,[53] 1996	IL-1β	Case control study	17 HI 33 Peri-I (n = 13)	7–30 mo	NR	PI GI BOP PD	Increased levels of IL-1β and pro– IL-1β is detected in Peri-I sites compared with HI.
Hultin et al,[31] 2002	IL-1β	Cross-sectional study	45 implants (n = 17)	2–13 y	NR	Radiographic BL Inflammation Suppuration	Level of IL-1β was found similar in stable and diseased sites.
Murata et al,[43] 2002	Osteocalcin Dpd IL-1β	Cross-sectional case control study	20 HI 6 Peri-I 8 PM (n = 16)	9–112 mo	Nonsmokers	BL PD PI GI	Osteocalcin was significantly higher in PM sites compared with HI. IL-1β was significantly higher in Peri-I sites compared with PM and HI sites. Dpd was not detected in either PICF or GCF.
Liskmann et al,[46] 2004	MPO	Cross-sectional study	31 HI 34 Peri-I (n = 40)	NR	NR	PG GI BOP	MPO activity is increasing with increasing PD and GI. MPO activity is higher when BOP is present.
Arikan et al,[57] 2008	sRANKL, OPG	Cohort study	79 HI 3 Peri-I 4 PM (n = 39)	12–16 mo	Nonsmokers	Radiographic BL BOP PD Suppuration	OPG needs further investigation as a possible biomarker of implant health status.

Study	Markers	Study design	Sample	Duration	Smoking	Clinical parameters	Findings
Arikan et al,[56] 2011	ICTP, sRANKL, OPG, Albumin	Case control study	21 HI 18 Peri-I (n = 28)	2–17 y	Nonsmokers	Radiographic BL CAL PD BOP GI	PI group showed lower amounts and concentrations of OPG and higher amounts and concentrations of ICTP. Local levels of OPG and ICTP reflect alveolar bone resorption.
Arakawa et al,[55] 2012	MMP-1, MMP-8, MMP-13	Case control study	162 implants 4 HI 4 Peri-I (n = 64)	1–7.4 y	NR	Radiographic BL	Incidence of Peri-I was 3.7% of implants. MMP-8 only biomarker detected in PICF from Peri-I sites.
Basegmez et al,[48] 2012	PGE2, MMP-8	Longitudinal study	72 HI (n = 28)	18 mo	Nonsmokers	PI GI PD	MMP-8 levels in PICF showed a significant correlation between PD and GI. MMP-8 seems to be an early marker of connective tissue destruction.
Rakic et al,[58] 2013	sRANKL RANK OPG	Cross-sectional study	25 HI 23 Peri-I 22 CP (n = 70)	≥2 y	Nonsmokers	PD rCAL BOP PI	sRANK/RANK/OPG levels were higher in PI group compared with HI. sRANK/RANK/OPG levels correlated with clinical parameters, BOP, PD, rCAL. RANK levels were associated with PI compared with CP.
Rakic et al,[59] 2014	sRANKL RANK OPG Catepsin-K Sclerostin	Cross-sectional study	58 HI 52 Peri-I 54 PM (n = 164)	≥2 y	Nonsmokers	Radiographic BL rCAL PD BOP PI	Increased sRANKL, OPG and sclerostin levels were associated with Peri-I sites. Increased cathepsin-C levels were associated with PM.

Abbreviations: BL, bone loss; BOP, bleeding on probing; CAL, clinical attachment level; CP, chronic periodontitis; Dpd, Deoxypyridinoline; HI, healthy implant; NR, not reported; PD, probing depth; Peri-I, peri-implantitis; PI, plaque index; PM, peri-mucositis; rCAL, relative clinical attachment level.

of MMP-8 were higher in PICF from 72 implants at 6 and 18 months after implantation, a period coincident with the maturation of the inflammatory phase.[48] The activity of elastase (MMP-12) is also found to be higher at peri-implantitis sites than at healthy control implant sites.[31] In contrast, MMP-1 and MMP-13 have not been detected at peri-implantitis sites.[55]

The advanced stages of peri-implantitis are associated with bone remodeling, radiographic evidence of bone loss, and implant mobility. Osteoclasts, osteoblasts, and bone signaling molecules are active during this phase. A study by Murata and colleagues[43] (2002) was one of the first to detect osteocalcin, a biomarker of bone formation, in PICF from peri-implant mucositis sites. However, these investigators did not detect deoxypyridinoline, a marker of bone resorption, in PICF from peri-implantitis sites. Another marker and by-product of bone resorption is C-telopeptide pyridinoline cross-links of type I collagen (ICTP). Concentrations of ICTP are significantly higher in PICF from patients with peri-implantitis than in PICF from patients with healthy implants[56]; however, little consistent information is available about ICTP concentrations at specific peri-implantitis sites. Osteoprotegerin (OPG), a decoy receptor for the receptor activator of nuclear factor-kappa B ligand (RANKL), has been detected in PICF from implants sites,[57] and concentrations of OPG are reported to be significantly lower in patients with peri-implantitis than in patients with healthy implants.[56] However, findings regarding OPG are conflicting. In a study involving 70 patients, Rakic and colleagues[58] found that concentrations of OPG were significantly higher in PICF from 23 peri-implantitis sites than in PICF from 25 healthy peri-implant sites.

Like OPG, the role of soluble RANKL as a biomarker of the bone resorption phase of peri-implantitis is controversial. Arikan and colleagues[56] found that the concentrations of soluble RANKL were significantly lower in PICF with peri-implantitis sites than in PICF from healthy implant sites. In contrast, Rakic and colleagues[58] detected soluble RANKL at higher concentrations in PICF from peri-implantitis sites than in PICF from healthy implant sites. In a recent study involving 52 patients with peri-implantitis, 54 patients with mucositis, and 58 patients with healthy peri-implant tissue, Rakic and colleagues[59] validated their earlier findings, that is, they found that the concentrations of OPG, RANK, and soluble RANKL were significantly higher in patients with peri-implantitis than in patients with healthy peri-implant tissues. Rakic and colleagues also found that sclerostin concentrations were significantly higher in the PICF of patients with peri-implantitis than in PICF of patients with healthy peri-implant tissues.

Currently, few studies have validated biomarkers of peri-implantitis, and few interventional studies have examined microbes and biomarkers. Thus, at this time, the information about biomarkers of peri-implantitis appears to be preliminary, and additional studies are necessary for confirming the specificity of the biomarkers. Benefits will be gained from prospective studies that involve larger numbers of patients and use robust assay techniques. In addition, it is likely that specificity will be gained from using a panel of biomarkers that target each of the 3 phases of peri-implantitis: inflammation, connective tissue destruction, and bone resorption.

SUMMARY
Microbiology

- Bacterial accumulation at peri-implant sites begins soon after implant placement.
- Similar bacterial species are detected at implant sites and tooth sulcus sites, yet the complexity of the microbiota around teeth is greater than that around implants in both health and disease.

- Increased numbers of red complex bacteria, specifically *P gingivalis*, are detected at peri-implantitis sites.
- Peri-implant disease and periodontal disease are associated with different bacterial compositions, a finding indicating that the microbiology of peri-implant disease is different from that of periodontitis.
- A few studies report that enteric rods, spirochetes, and opportunistic bacteria, including *S aureus* are associated with peri-implantitis and implant failure.
- Future studies involving large study populations that use optimal bacterial sampling and analyses are necessary for identifying specific microbiota and biomarkers of peri-implantitis and failing implants.

Protein Biomarkers

- Inflammatory biomarkers (MPO, lactoferrin, IL-1β, prostaglandins) appear to be early indicators of peri-implantitis.
- MMP-8 seems to be useful for monitoring the connective tissue destruction phase of peri-implant disease, but this finding requires validation.
- The bone remodeling biomarkers OPG, RANK, and soluble RANKL are promising biomarkers that may be associated with bone loss around implants.
- Additional studies involving larger numbers of subjects are necessary for validating biomarkers of peri-implantitis.

REFERENCES

1. Miller CS, King CP Jr, Langub MC, et al. Salivary biomarkers of existing periodontal disease: a cross-sectional study. J Am Dent Assoc 2006;137(3):322–9.
2. Al-Sabbagh M, Alladah A, Lin Y, et al. Bone remodeling-associated salivary biomarker MIP-1alpha distinguishes periodontal disease from health. J Periodontal Res 2012;47(3):389–95.
3. Giannobile WV, McDevitt JT, Niedbala RS, et al. Translational and clinical applications of salivary diagnostics. Adv Dent Res 2011;23(4):375–80.
4. Fine DH, Markowitz K, Furgang D, et al. Macrophage inflammatory protein-1alpha: a salivary biomarker of bone loss in a longitudinal cohort study of children at risk for aggressive periodontal disease? J Periodontol 2009;80(1):106–13.
5. Syndergaard B, Al-Sabbagh M, Kryscio RJ, et al. Salivary biomarkers associated with gingivitis and response to therapy. J Periodontol 2014;85:e295–303.
6. Elemek E, Almas K. Peri-implantitis: etiology, diagnosis and treatment: an update. N Y State Dent J 2014;80(1):26–32.
7. Lang NP, Berglundh T, Working Group 4 of Seventh European Workshop on Periodontology. Periimplant diseases: where are we now?—Consensus of the Seventh European Workshop on Periodontology. J Clin Periodontol 2011; 38(Suppl 11):178–81.
8. Lindhe J, Meyle J, Group D of European Workshop on Periodontology. Peri-implant diseases: Consensus Report of the Sixth European Workshop on Periodontology. J Clin Periodontol 2008;35(8 Suppl):282–5.
9. Quirynen M, De Soete M, van Steenberghe D. Infectious risks for oral implants: a review of the literature. Clin Oral Implants Res 2002;13(1):1–19.
10. Heitz-Mayfield LJ. Peri-implant diseases: diagnosis and risk indicators. J Clin Periodontol 2008;35(8 Suppl):292–304.
11. Esposito M, Hirsch J, Lekholm U, et al. Differential diagnosis and treatment strategies for biologic complications and failing oral implants: a review of the literature. Int J Oral Maxillofac Implants 1999;14(4):473–90.

12. Esposito M, Hirsch JM, Lekholm U, et al. Biological factors contributing to failures of osseointegrated oral implants. (II). Etiopathogenesis. Eur J Oral Sci 1998;106(3):721–64.
13. Tonetti MS, Schmid J. Pathogenesis of implant failures. Periodontol 2000 1994;4:127–38.
14. Misch CE, Perel ML, Wang HL, et al. Implant success, survival, and failure: the International Congress of Oral Implantologists (ICOI) Pisa Consensus Conference. Implant Dent 2008;17(1):5–15.
15. Furst MM, Salvi GE, Lang NP, et al. Bacterial colonization immediately after installation on oral titanium implants. Clin Oral Implants Res 2007;18(4):501–8.
16. Leonhardt A, Renvert S, Dahlen G. Microbial findings at failing implants. Clin Oral Implants Res 1999;10(5):339–45.
17. Quirynen M, Vogels R, Peeters W, et al. Dynamics of initial subgingival colonization of 'pristine' peri-implant pockets. Clin Oral Implants Res 2006;17(1):25–37.
18. Sbordone L, Barone A, Ciaglia RN, et al. Longitudinal study of dental implants in a periodontally compromised population. J Periodontol 1999;70(11):1322–9.
19. Salvi GE, Furst MM, Lang NP, et al. One-year bacterial colonization patterns of Staphylococcus aureus and other bacteria at implants and adjacent teeth. Clin Oral Implants Res 2008;19(3):242–8.
20. van Winkelhoff AJ, Goene RJ, Benschop C, et al. Early colonization of dental implants by putative periodontal pathogens in partially edentulous patients. Clin Oral Implants Res 2000;11(6):511–20.
21. Hultin M, Gustafsson A, Klinge B. Longterm evaluation of osseointegrated dental implants in the treatment of partially edentulous patients. J Clin Periodontol 2000;27(2):128–33.
22. Leonhardt A, Grondahl K, Bergstrom C, et al. Long-term follow-up of osseointegrated titanium implants using clinical, radiographic and microbiological parameters. Clin Oral Implants Res 2002;13(2):127–32.
23. Pye AD, Lockhart DE, Dawson MP, et al. A review of dental implants and infection. J Hosp Infect 2009;72(2):104–10.
24. Harris LG, Richards RG. Staphylococci and implant surfaces: a review. Injury 2006;37(Suppl 2):S3–14.
25. Persson GR, Renvert S. Cluster of bacteria associated with peri-implantitis. Clin Implant Dent Relat Res 2013. [Epub ahead of print].
26. Kronstrom M, Svenson B, Hellman M, et al. Early implant failures in patients treated with Branemark System titanium dental implants: a retrospective study. Int J Oral Maxillofac Implants 2001;16(2):201–7.
27. Albertini M, Lopez-Cerero L, O'Sullivan MG, et al. Assessment of periodontal and opportunistic flora in patients with peri-implantitis. Clin Oral Implants Res 2014. [Epub ahead of print].
28. Renvert S, Roos-Jansaker AM, Lindahl C, et al. Infection at titanium implants with or without a clinical diagnosis of inflammation. Clin Oral Implants Res 2007;18(4):509–16.
29. Botero JE, Gonzalez AM, Mercado RA, et al. Subgingival microbiota in peri-implant mucosa lesions and adjacent teeth in partially edentulous patients. J Periodontol 2005;76(9):1490–5.
30. Shibli JA, Melo L, Ferrari DS, et al. Composition of supra- and subgingival biofilm of subjects with healthy and diseased implants. Clin Oral Implants Res 2008;19(10):975–82.
31. Hultin M, Gustafsson A, Hallstrom H, et al. Microbiological findings and host response inpatients with peri-implantitis. Clin Oral Implants Res 2002;13(4):349–58.

32. Mombelli A, Marxer M, Gaberthuel T, et al. The microbiota of osseointegrated implants in patients with a history of periodontal disease. J Clin Periodontol 1995;22(2):124–30.
33. Heuer W, Kettenring A, Stumpp SN, et al. Metagenomic analysis of the peri-implant and periodontal microflora in patients with clinical signs of gingivitis or mucositis. Clin Oral Investig 2012;16(3):843–50.
34. Kumar PS, Mason MR, Brooker MR, et al. Pyrosequencing reveals unique microbial signatures associated with healthy and failing dental implants. J Clin Periodontol 2012;39(5):425–33.
35. Dabdoub SM, Tsigarida AA, Kumar PS. Patient-specific analysis of periodontal and peri-implant microbiomes. J Dent Res 2013;92(12 Suppl):168S–75S.
36. Cortelli SC, Cortelli JR, Romeiro RL, et al. Frequency of periodontal pathogens in equivalent peri-implant and periodontal clinical statuses. Arch Oral Biol 2013; 58(1):67–74.
37. Koyanagi T, Sakamoto M, Takeuchi Y, et al. Comprehensive microbiological findings in peri-implantitis and periodontitis. J Clin Periodontol 2013;40(3):218–26.
38. Sbordone L, Barone A, Ramaglia L, et al. Antimicrobial susceptibility of periodontopathic bacteria associated with failing implants. J Periodontol 1995; 66(1):69–74.
39. Renvert S, Aghazadeh A, Hallstrom H, et al. Factors related to peri-implantitis - a retrospective study. Clin Oral Implants Res 2014;25(4):522–9.
40. Becker ST, Beck-Broichsitter BE, Graetz C, et al. Peri-implantitis versus periodontitis: functional differences indicated by transcriptome profiling. Clin Implant Dent Relat Res 2014;16(3):401–11.
41. Belibasakis GN. Microbiological and immuno-pathological aspects of peri-implant diseases. Arch Oral Biol 2014;59(1):66–72.
42. Javed F, Al-Hezaimi K, Salameh Z, et al. Proinflammatory cytokines in the crevicular fluid of patients with peri-implantitis. Cytokine 2011;53(1):8–12.
43. Murata M, Tatsumi J, Kato Y, et al. Osteocalcin, deoxypyridinoline and interleukin-1beta in peri-implant crevicular fluid of patients with peri-implantitis. Clin Oral Implants Res 2002;13(6):637–43.
44. Anatoliotakis N, Deftereos S, Bouras G, et al. Myeloperoxidase: expressing inflammation and oxidative stress in cardiovascular disease. Curr Top Med Chem 2013;13(2):115–38.
45. Ward PP, Paz E, Conneely OM. Multifunctional roles of lactoferrin: a critical overview. Cell Mol Life Sci 2005;62(22):2540–8.
46. Liskmann S, Zilmer M, Vihalemm T, et al. Correlation of peri-implant health and myeloperoxidase levels: a cross-sectional clinical study. Clin Oral Implants Res 2004;15(5):546–52.
47. Ricciotti E, FitzGerald GA. Prostaglandins and inflammation. Arterioscler Thromb Vasc Biol 2011;31(5):986–1000.
48. Basegmez C, Yalcin S, Yalcin F, et al. Evaluation of periimplant crevicular fluid prostaglandin E2 and matrix metalloproteinase-8 levels from health to periimplant disease status: a prospective study. Implant Dent 2012;21(4):306–10.
49. Graves DT, Cochran D. The contribution of interleukin-1 and tumor necrosis factor to periodontal tissue destruction. J Periodontol 2003;74(3):391–401.
50. Stashenko P, Dewhirst FE, Peros WJ, et al. Synergistic interactions between interleukin 1, tumor necrosis factor, and lymphotoxin in bone resorption. J Immunol 1987;138(5):1464–8.
51. Engebretson SP, Grbic JT, Singer R, et al. GCF IL-1beta profiles in periodontal disease. J Clin Periodontol 2002;29(1):48–53.

52. Mogi M, Otogoto J, Ota N, et al. Interleukin 1 beta, interleukin 6, beta 2-micro-globulin, and transforming growth factor-alpha in gingival crevicular fluid from human periodontal disease. Arch Oral Biol 1999;44(6):535–9.

53. Panagakos FS, Aboyoussef H, Dondero R, et al. Detection and measurement of inflammatory cytokines in implant crevicular fluid: a pilot study. Int J Oral Maxillofac Implants 1996;11(6):794–9.

54. Sorsa T, Mantyla P, Ronka H, et al. Scientific basis of a matrix metalloproteinase-8 specific chair-side test for monitoring periodontal and peri-implant health and disease. Ann N Y Acad Sci 1999;878:130–40.

55. Arakawa H, Uehara J, Hara ES, et al. Matrix metalloproteinase-8 is the major potential collagenase in active peri-implantitis. J Prosthodont Res 2012;56(4): 249–55.

56. Arikan F, Buduneli N, Lappin DF. C-telopeptide pyridinoline crosslinks of type I collagen, soluble RANKL, and osteoprotegerin levels in crevicular fluid of dental implants with peri-implantitis: a case-control study. Int J Oral Maxillofac Implants 2011;26(2):282–9.

57. Arikan F, Buduneli N, Kutukculer N. Osteoprotegerin levels in peri-implant crevicular fluid. Clin Oral Implants Res 2008;19(3):283–8.

58. Rakic M, Lekovic V, Nikolic-Jakoba N, et al. Bone loss biomarkers associated with peri-implantitis. A cross-sectional study. Clin Oral Implants Res 2013; 24(10):1110–6.

59. Rakic M, Struillou X, Petkovic-Curcin A, et al. Estimation of bone loss biomarkers as a diagnostic tool for peri-implantitis. J Periodontol 2014;1–12 [Epub ahead of print].

Prosthetic Failure in Implant Dentistry

Ramtin Sadid-Zadeh, DDS, MS[a], Ahmad Kutkut, DDS, MS[b,*], Hyeongil Kim, DDS, MS[a]

KEYWORDS

- Single implant restoration • Partial fixed dental prosthesis • Prosthetic complication
- Prosthetic failure

KEY POINTS

- Although osseointegrated dental implants have become a predictable and effective modality for the treatment of single or multiple missing teeth, their use is associated with clinical complications.
- Such complications can be biologic, technical, mechanical, or esthetic and may compromise implant outcomes to various degrees.
- Our review showed that six categories of technical or mechanical complications were associated with single implant restorations and partial fixed implant-supported prostheses: loosening of screws, fracture of screw, fracture of framework, fracture of abutment, chipping or fracture of veneering material, and decementation.

INTRODUCTION

Biomechanics of Implant-Supported Restorations in Partially Edentulous Patients

The diagnosis and treatment planning of single restorations and partial fixed prostheses supported by dental implants require comprehensive scientific knowledge and a clear plan for definitive restorations before treatment begins. One of the most important factors in minimizing the incidence of biomechanical complications of single-implant restorations (SIRs) and partial fixed implant-supported prostheses (PFISPs) is to decrease the resistance to adverse leverage forces during function.[1] To minimize adverse leverage forces on anterior SIRs and PFISPs, implants should be placed as vertical as possible to the forces applied during function, and the fabrication of incisal guidance should be shallow.[1] For posterior SIRs and PFISPs, implants should be centered mesiodistally and as perpendicular as possible to the occlusal surface so

Authors reported no conflict of interest.

[a] Department of Restorative Dentistry, School of Dental Medicine, The State University of New York at Buffalo, 3435 Main Street, 215 Squire Hall, Buffalo, NY 14214, USA; [b] Division of Restorative Dentistry, Department of Oral Health Practice, College of Dentistry, University of Kentucky, 800 Rose Street, Lexington, KY 40536-029, USA
* Corresponding author.
E-mail address: ahmad.kutkut@uky.edu

that leverage can be minimized during function.[1] Other factors that may affect biomechanical forces on SIRs and PFISPs are cuspal inclination, implant inclination, horizontal offset of the implant, and apical offset of the implant.[2] Weinberg and Kruger[2] reported that every 10-degree increase in cusp inclination leads to a 30% increase in the torque applied to the restoration during function (**Fig. 1**). Also, every 10-degree increase in implant inclination may lead to a 5% increase in the torque applied to the restoration during function (**Fig. 2**). Moreover, a 1-mm increase in the horizontal offset of an implant restoration introduces a 15% increase in torque during function, and a 1-mm increase in the vertical offset introduces a 5% increase (**Figs. 3** and **4**). Biomechanically, the functional load applied to an implant restoration is directed to the coronal portion of the crestal bone around the body of the implant.[3] Therefore, extra care should be taken when multiple factors are present, such as heavy occlusal forces, a laterally positioned implant, and steep cuspal inclination, because the stress is concentrated at the abutment-implant connection, the point at which complications may occur.[1–3] This concentration of functional load at the crestal bone and at the connection between the crown or abutment and the implant increases when the vertical interarch space increases.[4] Finite element analysis of implant-supported restorations has shown that the largest amount of stress is concentrated at the coronal part of the alveolar bone at the implant-bone interface. This stress level increases with the vertical interarch space.[4]

Complications Associated with Implant-Supported Restorations in Partially Edentulous Patients

Although osseointegrated dental implants have become a predictable and effective method for treatment of missing teeth, they are accompanied by clinical complications.[5,6] In the literature, clinical complications have been reported to be biologic, technical or mechanical, esthetic, or phonetic. These complications may compromise the outcome of dental implants to various degrees.[7]

Endosseous implants can be restored with screw-retained or cement-retained restorations.[8] The choice between cement-retained and screw-retained restorations seems to be based primarily on the clinician's preference.[9] Screw-retained restorations offer the advantage of retrievability; they are also simple to replace and maintain. For a PFISP, such restorations also offer more stability and security at the interface between the implant abutment and the prosthesis.[10–15] Screw-retained restorations, however, require precise implant placement and optimal location of the

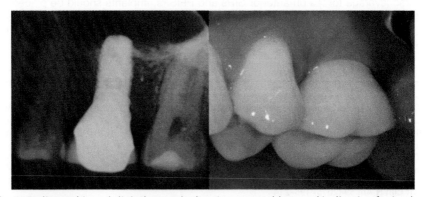

Fig. 1. Radiographic and clinical example showing acceptable cuspal inclination for implant-supported ceramometal crown restoration in first molar region.

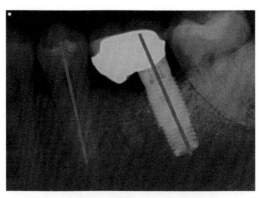

Fig. 2. Radiographic example showing unnecessary inclination in implant position, which may lead to an increase in the torque applied to the implant during function.

screw-access hole; otherwise, the restoration is unaesthetic.[16] However, cement-retained restorations offer good esthetic and occlusal contacts because of the absence of a screw-access hole.[10,17,18] Another advantage of cement-retained restorations may be the potential for passive fitting of a PISFP.[19] However, cement-retained restorations require adequate interarch space to allow fabrication of an abutment with a 3- to 4-mm axial wall.[19,20] This wall provides adequate surface area for the retention of an anterior, premolar, or molar crown. The difficulty associated with the removal of excess cement has been seen as a drawback of cement-retained restorations.[20]

For many years, metal ceramic restorations were the gold standard in dentistry.[8,21] However, patients' esthetic demands have driven dentists to use all-ceramic restorations.[22] In parallel with the application of zirconia (Zr) for tooth-borne restorations, Zr implant abutments have been fabricated for use instead of titanium abutments for cemented restorations or with direct veneering for screw-retained restorations.[23] Currently, most implant systems offer prefabricated titanium or Zr abutments. In addition, computer aided design (CAD)/computer aided manufacturing (CAM) technology has allowed the creation of custom-designed milled abutments that can fit individual needs. These custom-designed abutments can be fabricated of Zr, Zr with a titanium

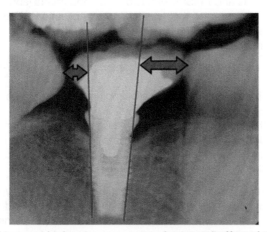

Fig. 3. Radiographic example showing unnecessary horizontal offset of the implant, which may lead to an increase in the torque applied to the implant during function.

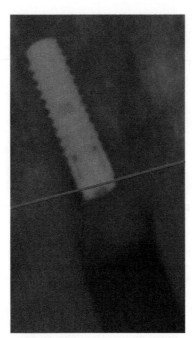

Fig. 4. Radiographic example showing unnecessary vertical offset of the implant, which may lead to an increase in the torque applied to the implant during function.

insert, or titanium. In addition, Ivoclar Vivadent (Amherst, NY) recently introduced custom-designed lithium disilicate abutments with titanium insert (**Figs. 5–8**).[24]

This article reviews the technical and mechanical complications associated with SIRs and PFISPs.

MEDLINE SEARCH

We initiated separate MEDLINE searches for English-language publications reporting clinical studies of SIRs and PFISPs with two-piece abutments (abutment and screw), their success, their failure, and their associated complications. The literature search covered the years 1990 to March 2014. Published articles were required to meet the following criteria for inclusion in this study:

- Publications had to present clinical data with a mean follow-up of more than 1 year.
- Publications had to identify the type of implant placed and the number of restorations performed, how long they had been in place, and how many were affected by the type of prosthetic or by technical complications.
- If a study reported repeated follow-up data, the most current report was used.
- PFISP was defined as two or more restorations connected to or supported by one or more implant fixtures, with or without cantilever.

If a published article met the inclusion criteria, we recorded the type of technical or mechanical complications that occurred. The raw data associated with a particular complication were combined, and a mean incidence of complications was calculated. So that we could calculate the mean incidence of each technical or prosthetic complication, we considered a certain complication to be not reported if the study did not

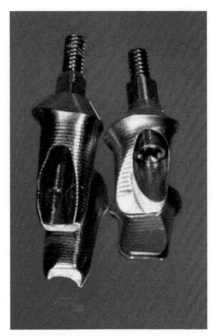

Fig. 5. Custom-designed titanium abutment with or without gold plating.

measure the complication. The incidence of a certain complication was reported to be zero if the published study mentioned that the complication was measured but did not provide the measurement in the results or discussion sections. For SIRs, if the study did not define the type of restoration, if metal restorations were mixed with the types of restorations, if no definite number of restorations was given, or if ceramic chipping or fracture was reported, the study was not considered when ceramic chipping or

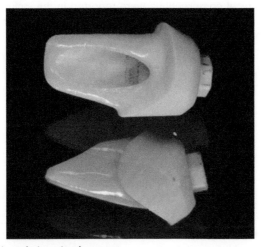

Fig. 6. Custom-designed zirconia abutment.

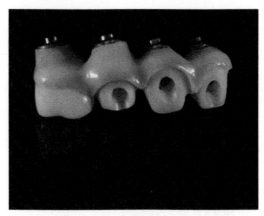

Fig. 7. Custom-designed zirconia abutment with titanium insert.

fracture complications were reported. For PFISPs, chipping or fracture of the veneering material was reported instead of a ceramic chipping or fracture complication.

The criterion for including a specific complication in this review was that three or more published studies had to report data related to the incidence of that particular complication. Certain complications were reported in a large number of studies, whereas others were presented in only three published articles. The incidence of each complication was compared for the purpose of establishing a trend for ranking the technical and prosthetic complications. Therefore, the percentages presented in this review suggest trends rather than absolute incidence values. The trends should be interpreted cautiously because of the large variation in the numbers of restorations evaluated and the absence of statistical analysis.

Single-Implant Restorations

A large number of published studies provide data about technical and mechanical complications with root-form SIR. We reviewed a total of 728 abstracts; of these, 48 introduced articles that fulfilled the inclusion criteria.[5,25–71] Our main categories of technical or mechanical complications were reported in the included studies: loosening of the abutment or screw, fracture of the veneering ceramic or the crown, decementation, fracture of the abutment or the coronal fixture, and abutment screw fracture.

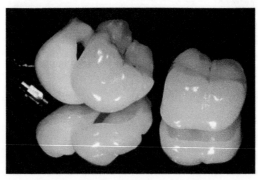

Fig. 8. Custom-designed lithium disilicate abutment with titanium insert.

Few published studies simultaneously evaluated all of the reported complications. The data regarding technical and mechanical complications are reported by category and were obtained by combining data from the various studies.

Loosening of the abutment screw or the abutment

Loosening of the abutment screw or the abutment is a frequently reported complication associated with SIRs; this complication occurred in 368 of the reported 6544 restorations (5.6%) within a mean of 4.8 years (**Table 1**). The incidence of this complication with SIRs was found to be as high as 59.6% within 15 years.[25] The design of the implant connection substantially affected the incidence of this complication: the incidence associated with external-connection (EC) implants was 18.3% at a mean of 5.3 years (217 of 1183 restorations; maximum, 59.9%),[25–41] whereas that associated with internal-connection (IC) implants was 2.7% at a mean of 4.5 years (142 of 5235 restorations; maximum, 31.6%).[42–69] It is noteworthy that many of the earlier studies did not apply standardized protocols for tightening the titanium screws with countertorque devices at predetermined torque levels. The incidence of this complication seemed to be reduced by the use of gold alloy screws if they were properly tightened.[25,39] Our calculations showed that this complication occurred with 147 of 4686 (3.1%) cement-retained restorations at a mean of 5.1 years,[25–28,31–46,48–61,64–69] and with 83 of 979 (8.5%) screw-retained restorations at a mean of 3.8 years.[26–30,34–38,46,58,59] Only three studies reported the use of screw-retained restorations with IC implants: screw loosening occurred in 17 of 665 total restorations (2.6%).[46,58,59]

Most of the articles included in this review reported studies of cement-retained restorations in conjunction with IC implants. The articles reported a total of 3921 restorations, of which only 48 (1.2%) were associated with loosening of the abutment screw or the abutment.[42–46,48–51,53–61,64,66–68] The highest incidence of screw loosening was associated with screw-retained restorations using EC implants (66 of 314 restorations; 21%)[25–28,31–36,38–42]; the second-highest incidence was associated with cement-retained restorations using EC implants (99 of 763 restorations; 13%).[26,28–30,34–38] A systematic review by Sailer and colleagues[72] reported that the incidence of screw loosening associated with SIRs was significantly higher for screw-retained restorations; however, a cross-sectional randomized controlled trial involving 18 patients found no significant difference between cement-retained and screw-retained restorations after a 10-year follow-up period.[26]

With regard to positioning of the implants, 24 published studies separated the incidence of the complication of loosening of abutment screws or abutments by anterior or posterior restorations. The mean incidence of this complication for anterior restorations (12.8%; 51 of 398 restorations)[25,26,39–42,46,52,53,57,60] was higher than that for posterior restorations (4.8%; 144 of 2972 restorations)[26,29,30,39,42,48,50,52–58,60–63,66,69,70]; however, screw loosening in the anterior region was associated primarily with the abutment design of the EC implant (39%; 49 of 127 restorations).[25,26,39,41] With IC implants, this complication was more common in the posterior region (4.3%) than in the anterior region (0.7%).[42,46,48,50,54–63,65,69]

To evaluate the influence of the material used to fabricate the abutment on the incidence of loosening of abutment screws or abutments, we categorized abutments as either Zr or metal alloy (MA) in the 47 studies that reported the material used.[25–36,38–40,42–51,59–62,64,66,68–70] The incidence of this complication was 4.4% with metal abutments and 2.1% with Zr abutments. When we categorized the same 47 studies by implant design (IC or EC), we found that the incidence of this complication was more strongly associated with the implant connection type than with the

Table 1
Studies reporting technical and mechanical complications for single-implant restorations, presented in chronologic order

Publication (48 Studies)	Number of Restorations	Type of Connection	Position of Restoration	Mean Time (y)	Screw or Cement Retained	Type of Restoration	Type of Abutment	Technical and Mechanical Complication
Jemt & Pettersson,[39] 1993	69	EC	44 A, 25 P	3	C	NR	MA	31
Ekfeldt et al,[38] 1994	93	EC	A, P	1.5	54 S, 39 C	70 MCC, 23 GA	MA	40
Becker & Becker,[30] 1995	24	EC	P	2	S	NR	MA	1
Henry et al,[5] 1996	106	EC	60 A, 47 P	5	NR	NR	NR	86
Muftu & Chapman,[61] 1998	404	IC	P	4	C	MCC	MA	7
Scheller et al,[31] 1998	65	EC	NR	5	C	ACC, MCC	MA	16
Polizzi et al,[41] 1999	30	EC	A	5.2	C	MCC	MA	2
Scholander,[32] 1999	258	EC	A, P	5	C	ACC, MCC, GA	MA	18
Mangano & Bartolucci,[60] 2001	80	IC	23 A, 57 P	3.5	C	ACC	MA	3
Mericske-Stern et al,[62] 2001	109	IC	P	4.2	102 S, 7 C	MCC	MA	20
Levine et al,[58] 2002	671	IC	P	1.8	600 S, 71 C	NR	MA	25
Krennmair et al,[59] 2002	146	IC	43 A, 103 P	3	93 C, 53 S	27 ACC, 119 MCC	MA	18
Haas et al,[37] 2002	71	EC	50 A, 21 P	5	S	NR	MA	19
Duncan et al,[46] 2003	34	IC	A	3	12 S, 22 C	MCC	MA	2
Simon,[70] 2003	126	EC, IC	P	3.8	8 S, 118 C	NR	MA	37
Döring et al,[68] 2004	250	IC	A, P	3.2	C	MCC, ACC	264 MA, 11 Zr	2
Glauser et al,[27] 2004	53	EC	39 A. 15 P	4	C	ACC	Zr	5
Gotfredsen,[43] 2004	20	IC	18 A, 2 P	5	C	MCC	MA	8
Brägger et al,[65] 2005	69	IC	NR	10	67 C, 2 S	MCC	NR	6
Drago & O'Connor,[47] 2006	82	IC	A, P	1.5	NR	NR	MA	1
Bischof et al,[55] 2006	157	IC	P	5	149 C, 8 S	MCC	MA	11
Norton,[69] 2006	181	IC	P	7.5	C	MCC	NR	44
Hall et al,[29] 2007	28	EC	A	1	S	MCC	MA	1

Study								
Cooper et al,[57] 2007	51	IC	A	3	C	MCC, ACC	MA	5
Mangano et al,[42] 2008	314	IC	116 A, 198 P	1	C	A/ACC, P/MCC	A/Zr, P/MA	2
Jemt,[25] 2008	47	EC	A	15	C	MCC	MA	29
Jemt,[28] 2009	41	EC	A, P	10	18 S, 23 C	MCC	MA	5
Nothdurft & Pospiech,[71] 2010	40	IC	P	1	C	ACC	Zr	4
Mangano et al,[45] 2010	302	IC	113 A, 189 P	4	C	A/ACC, P/MCC	MA	2
Krennmair et al,[67] 2010	112	IC	A, P	5.7	C	MCC, ACC	NR	16
Bonde et al,[40] 2010	49	EC	38 A, 11 P	10	C	ACC	MA	5
Kim et al,[63] 2010	94	IC	P	2	NR	CCC, MCC	NR	14
Hosseini et al,[66] 2011	75	IC	P	1	C	38 ACC, 37 MCC	38 Zr, 37 MA	2
Mangano et al,[49] 2011	531	IC	NR	3	C	MCC	MA	2
Vigolo et al,[26] 2012	36	EC	6A, 30 P	10	18 S, 18 C	MCC	MA	0
Schwarz et al,[53] 2012	232	IC	25 A, 117 P	5.8	C	179 MCC, 53 ACC	NR	57
Bergenblock et al,[33] 2012	65	EC	A, P	5	C	62 ACC, 3 MCC	MA	4
Montero et al,[34] 2012	93	EC	A, P	2.2	9 C, 84 S	MCC	MA	11
Vandeweghe et al,[35] 2012	15	EC	5 A, 10 P	1	S	ACC	Zr	5
Hosseini et al,[51] 2013	98	IC	A, P	3	C	64 ACC, 34 MCC	Zr, MA	3
Nothdurft et al,[50] 2014	40	EC	A, P	5	38 C, 2 S	21 MCC, 19 ACC	20 Zr, 20 MA	10
Lops et al,[54] 2013	81	IC	P	5	C	44 MCC, 37 ACC	44 MA, 37 Zr	9
Zembic et al,[36] 2013	40	IC	P	3	C	ACC	Zr	5
Lai et al,[56] 2013	229	IC	P	7.2	C	MCC	NR	29
Cha et al,[52] 2013	136	IC	22 A, 114 P	5	106 S, 30 C	CCC, MCC, ACC	Zr, MA	54
Mangano et al,[48] 2014	212	IC	P	10	C	MCC	MA	3
Spies et al,[44] 2014	47	IC	A, P	4.8	C	ACC	Zr	22
Mangano et al,[64] 2014	478	IC	A, P	10	C	MCC	MA	13

Abbreviations: A, anterior; ACC, all ceramic crown; C, cement-retained; CCC, complete cast crown; EC, external connection; GA, gold acrylic; IC, internal connection; MA, metal alloy; MCC, metal ceramic crown; NR, not reported; P, posterior; S, screw-retained; Zr, zirconia.

material used to fabricate the abutment (MA-EC, 15.1%; Zr-EC, 6.8%; MA-IC, 1.5%; and Zr-IC, 0.9%).[25–36,38–40,42–51,59–62,64,66,68–70]

To reduce the incidence of screw loosening, we recommend torqueing the abutment or the screw-retained crown twice to the specifications recommended by manufacturer with 5-minute intervals. In addition, using implant with IC, reducing the cuspal inclinations, and eliminating heavy occlusal contacts may reduce the incidence of the screw loosening.

Fracture of the veneering ceramic or the crown

Fracture of the veneering ceramic or the crown was the second most frequently reported complication associated with SIRs in 35 of the studies we reviewed. This complication occurred in 172 of 5052 (3.4%) ceramic and metal-ceramic restorations at a mean of 5 years.[5,25–29,31–36,38,40–45,48,50,51,53–59,61,64–66,68,69,71] Twenty-nine studies reported this complication separately in a ceramic or a metal-ceramic restoration. The incidence of this complication was higher for ceramic restorations (8.3%; 62 of 746 restorations)[27,33,35,36,40,42,44,45,50,51,53,54,66,71] than for metal-ceramic restorations (2.3%; 64 of 2759 restorations).[25,26,29,33,34,36,38,41,43,45,48,51,53–56,59,61,64–66,69]

We calculated the incidence of fracture of the veneering ceramic or the crown in the 19 studies that reported this complication separately for anterior and posterior SIRs. The incidence of the complication was 3.1% (82 of 2634 restorations) for posterior SIRs and 1.7% (7 of 421 restorations) for anterior SIRs.[25,26,28,35,42,45,48,50,51,53–58,61,66,69,71]

To evaluate the influence of implant connection on fractures of the veneering ceramic or the crown, we separated the reports of IC and EC implants. The incidence of this complication was higher in association with EC implants (5.4%; 52 of 955 restorations after 5.4 years) than with IC implants (2.9%; 120 of 4095 restorations after 4.7 years).[5,25–27,29,31–36,38–45,48,50,51,53–59,61,64–66,68,69,71]

The incidence of this complication was higher in association with cement-retained restorations (3.4%; 128 of 3810 restorations)[25–27,31–35,40–45,48,50,53,54,56–59,61,64,66,68,69,71] than with screw-retained restorations (0.6%; 5 of 798 restorations).[26,29,34,35,58,59] A systematic review by Sailer and colleagues[72] found that chipping of the veneering ceramic tended to occur more frequently with screw-retained SIRs; however, no fractures of the veneer were reported in a cross-sectional randomized controlled trial comparing cement-retained with screw-retained restorations at 10-year follow-up.[26]

To reduce the incidence of the fracture of the veneering ceramic or the crown, it is recommended to reduce the size of the occlusal table, create shallow cusp height, lighten the occlusal contacts, and provide uniform thickness and appropriate support for the veneering ceramic.

Other technical and mechanical complications

Decementation was reported by 21 studies.[26,27,31,32,36,41,43,44,53,56–59,61,62,64–67,69,70] Of 2394 restorations, 159 were dislodged during a mean of 5.2 years, for a 6.1% incidence of this complication. The incidence of decementation was negligible when glass ionomer or resin cements were used.[26,27,31,32,43,44,51,53,56–58,70] We recommend using resin-reinforced cement to reduce the chance of decementation.

Fracture of the abutment or the coronal fixture was reported to occur in 25 of 3695 restorations at a mean of 4.4 years (incidence, 0.5%).[5,27,30–33,36,42,45,48–52,54,56,58,60,61,63–67,71] The incidence of fracture of the abutment screw in 17 studies was reported to be 0.3% (7 of 2185 restorations).[5,30–33,35,43,48–52,62,65–68]

Partial Fixed Implant-Supported Prosthesis

Several studies provided data about technical and mechanical complications associated with PFISPs supported by one or more root-form implants. We reviewed 708 abstracts, 29 of which met the inclusion criteria.[44,46,49,73–98] Six categories of technical or mechanical complications were reported: (1) loosening of screws, (2) fracture of screws, (3) fracture of framework, (4) fracture of abutment, (5) chipping or fracture of veneering material, and (6) decementation.

Not many studies simultaneously evaluated all of the listed complications. The data regarding technical or mechanical complications are reported by category and were obtained by combining data from the 29 studies.

Technical and mechanical complications

Table 2 lists the studies that met the inclusion criteria. The 29 studies reported a total of 2998 PFISPs, 482 (16.1%) of which were associated with technical or mechanical complications over a mean of 5.4 years.[44,46,49,73–98] The most frequently reported complication was chipping or fracturing of veneering material, which was observed in 251 PFISPs (8%). The second most frequently reported complication was screw loosening, which occurred in 151 PFISPs (5%).

The design of the implant connection substantially affected the incidence of technical or mechanical complications. The incidence of such complications was higher for PFISPs restored with an EC implant (20.9%)[73,74,76,78,80,84,85,87,89–91,95,97,98] than for those restored with an IC implant (9.3%).[44,46,49,75,77,79,81–83,86,88,92–94,96]

Chipping or fracturing of veneering material was reported in association with 12.4% of the PFISPs over a mean of 5.7 years (251 of 2026 PFISPs).[44,73–79,81–90,92,94–97] The incidence of this complication was comparable for PFISPs restored with IC implants (11.3%)[44,75,77,79,81–83,86,88,94,96] and those restored with EC implants (13%).[73,74,76,78,84,85,87,89,90,95,97]

The second most frequently reported technical or mechanical complication associated with PFISPs was screw loosening (6.1%; 154 of 2511 restorations at a mean of 5.3 years).[46,73–78,81,84–90,92–98] When studies were separated by the design of the implant connection, screw loosening occurred more frequently in PFISPs restored with EC implants (120 of 1327 PFISPs) than in those restored with IC implants (34 of 1184 PFISPs). The incidence was more than three times as high in association with EC implants: approximately 9% for EC implants and 2.9% for IC implants over a mean of more than 5 years.[46,73–78,81,84–90,92–98]

Fourteen studies reported screw fracture, with an incidence of 3.2% over 5.4 years. The incidence of this complication in association with PFISPs was 3.6% (55 of 1517 PFISPs).[73,74,76,78,80,84,85,89,90,92,95–98]

To evaluate the influence of cement-retained or screw-retained restorations on the incidence of technical or mechanical complications associated with PFISPs, we found 11 published articles that reported the type of restoration (cement-retained or screw-retained) and the incidence of technical or mechanical complications.[44,49,77–79,81,83,86,90,95,98] When studies were separated by the type of retention, the total incidence of this complication was higher for screw-retained PFISPs (34.8%)[77,78,90,98] than for cement-retained PFISPs (6.3%)[44,49,79,81,83,86,95] at a mean of 5 years. The difference between retention types was particularly noticeable in the complication of screw loosening: cement-retained PFISPs resulted in only two loose prostheses, whereas screw-retained PFISPs resulted in 46 loose prostheses. A long-term study reported by Nissan and colleagues[99] compared the complication outcome associated with cement-retained and screw-retained PFISPs. The study found that the incidence of ceramic fracture and screw loosening was significantly higher for PFISPs restored with screw-retained implants than for those restored with cement-retained implants.[99]

Table 2

Studies reporting technical and mechanical complications for partial fixed implant-supported prostheses, presented in chronologic order

Publication (29 Studies)	Number of Restorations	Type of Connection	Mean Time (y)	Screw or Cement Retained	Type of Restoration	Technical and Mechanical Complication
Henry et al,[73] 1993	187	EC	3	NR	MA, different veneering	51
Gunne et al,[89] 1994	197	EC	3	NR	MA, different veneering	51
Wyatt & Zarb,[90] 1998	97	EC	5.4	S	MA, different veneering	50
Ortorp & Jemt,[74] 1999	68	EC	5	NR	MA, different veneering	12
Lekholm et al,[84] 1999	163	EC	10	NR	MA, different veneering	15
Andersson et al,[91] 1999	36	EC	2	S, C	NR	1
Wennerberg & Jemt,[97] 1999	133	EC	5	NR	MA, different veneering	43
Snauwaert et al,[80] 2000	308	EC	8	NR	NR	14
Jemt et al,[85] 2000	63	EC	3	NR	MCC	9
Lindh et al,[98] 2001	26	EC	2	S	MCC	5
Jemt et al,[76] 2003	63	EC	5	NR	MCC	22
Duncan et al,[46] 2003	25	IC	3	S, C	MCC	3
Wennström et al,[77] 2004	56	IC	5	S	MCC	6
Becker,[88] 2004	60	IC	10	S, C	MCC	3
Romeo et al,[92] 2004	179	IC	3.8	S, C	MCC	14

Eliasson et al,[78] 2006	146	EC	9.4	S	MA, different veneering	52
Romeo et al,[82] 2006	59	IC	8.5	S, C	MCC	3
Romeo et al,[93] 2006	115	IC	7	S, C	NR	13
Nedir et al,[94] 2006	93	IC	8	C	MCC	24
Kreissl et al,[95] 2007	66	EC	5	NR	MCC	21
Hälg et al,[79] 2008	32	IC	5.3	C	MCC	4
Romeo et al,[96] 2009	59	IC	8.2	S, C	MCC	24
Wahlström et al,[75] 2010	46	IC	5	S, C	MCC	20
Larsson & Vult von Steyern,[83] 2010	25	IC	5	C	ACC	11
Mangano et al,[49] 2011	462	IC	3.5	C	MCC	0
Pozzi et al,[81] 2012	37	IC	3.6	C	ACC	3
Vanlıoğlu et al,[86] 2013	52	IC	5	C	MCC	4
Kowar et al,[87] 2013	118	EC	5	NR	MA, different veneering	4
Spies et al,[44] 2014	27	IC	5	C	ACC	0

Abbreviations: ACC, all ceramic crown; C, cement-retained; EC, external connection; IC, internal connection; MA, metal alloy; MCC, metal ceramic crown; NR, not reported; S, screw-retained.

SUMMARY

The overall incidence of technical or mechanical complications in the articles reviewed is 10.8% for SIRs (714 of 6584 restorations over a mean of 4.7 years) and 16.1% for PFISPs (482 of 2998 restorations over a mean of 5.4 years). This cumulative complication rate should be considered with caution for several reasons: some studies did not report each category of technical or mechanical complications, the evaluation time differed for each study, the study methodology differed across studies, and the studies were performed during various eras of the development of implant dentistry.

Our review of the literature showed that the following six categories of technical or mechanical complications were associated with SIRs and PFISPs: (1) loosening of screws, (2) fracture of screw, (3) fracture of framework, (4) fracture of abutment, (5) chipping or fracture of veneering material, and (6) decementation.

The most common complication associated with SIRs was loosening of the screw (5.6%), whereas fracture of the veneering material (12.4%) was the most common complication of PFISPs. The reason for these differences may be that the various types veneering materials used in PFISPs, including acrylic and composite resins, was included in the calculation of the incidence of complications; in contrast, only ceramic veneering materials were included in this calculation for SIRs. Additional studies are needed, because ceramic abutments and all-ceramic implant supports are becoming increasingly popular for SIRs and PFISPs. When clinicians are determining whether to use SIRs or PFISPs for their patient, they should be aware of and should inform the patient of the possibility of complications. A routine follow-up examination should be considered for exploring and repairing the possible complications. One study has recommended that patients with implant-supported restorations should be followed up within 6 months of the restoration and at least annually thereafter.[100]

REFERENCES

1. Katona TR, Goodacre CJ, Brown DT, et al. Force-moment systems on single maxillary anterior implants: effects of incisal guidance, fixture orientation, and loss of bone support. Int J Oral Maxillofac Implants 1993;8:512–22.
2. Weinberg LA, Kruger B. A comparison of implant/prosthesis loading with four clinical variables. Int J Prosthodont 1995;8:421–33.
3. Rieger MR, Mayberry M, Brose MO. Finite element analysis of six endosseous implants. J Prosthet Dent 1990;63:671–6.
4. Naveau A, Renault P, Pierrisnard L. Effects of vertical interarch space and abutment height on stress distributions: a 3D finite element analysis. Eur J Prosthodont Restor Dent 2009;17:90–4.
5. Henry PJ, Laney WR, Jemt T, et al. Osseointegrated implants for single-tooth replacement: a prospective 5-year multicenter study. Int J Oral Maxillofac Implants 1996;11:450–5.
6. Taylor RC, McGlumphy EA, Tatakis DN, et al. Radiographic and clinical evaluation of single-tooth Biolok implants: a 5- year study. Int J Oral Maxillofac Implants 2004;19:849–54.
7. Goodacre CJ, Bernal G, Rungcharassaeng K, et al. Clinical complications with implants and implant prostheses. J Prosthet Dent 2003;90:121–32.
8. Hebel KS, Gajjar RC. Cement-retained versus screw-retained implant restorations: achieving optimal occlusion and esthetics in implant dentistry. J Prosthet Dent 1997;77:28–35.
9. Taylor TD, Agar JR, Vogiatzi T. Implant prosthodontics: current perspectives and future directions. Int J Oral Maxillofac Implants 2000;15:66–75.

10. Michalakis KX, Hirayama H, Garefis PD. Cement-retained versus screw-retained implant restorations: a critical review. Int J Oral Maxillofac Implants 2003;18: 719–28.
11. Zarb GA, Smith A. The longitudinal clinical effectiveness of osseointegrated dental implants: the Toronto study Part III: problems and complications encountered. J Prosthet Dent 1990;64:185–94.
12. Rangert B, Jemt T, Jörneus L. Forces and moments on Branemark implants. Int J Oral Maxillofac Implants 1989;4:241–7.
13. Zarb GA, Schimdt A. The longitudinal clinical effectiveness of osseointegrated dental implants: the Toronto study. Part II: Prosthetic results. J Prosthet Dent 1990;64:53–61.
14. Jemt T. Failures and complications in 391 consecutively inserted fixed prostheses supported by Brånemark implants in edentulous jaws: a study of treatment from the time of prosthesis placement to the first annual checkup. Int J Oral Maxillofac Implants 1991;6:270–6.
15. Chiche GJ, Pinault A. Considerations for fabrication of implant-supported posterior restorations. Int J Prosthodont 1991;4:37–44.
16. Walton JN, MacEntee MI. Problems with prostheses on implants: a retrospective study. J Prosthet Dent 1994;71:283–8.
17. Misch CE. Contemporary implant dentistry. St Louis (MO): Mosby-Year Book; 1993. p. 651–85.
18. Andersson B, Odman P, Lindvall AM, et al. Cemented single crowns on osseointegrated implants after 5 years: results from a prospective study on CeraOne. Int J Prosthodont 1998;11:212–8.
19. Chee W, Felton DA, Johnson PF, et al. Cemented versus screw-retained implant prostheses: which is better? Int J Oral Maxillofac Implants 1999;14:137–41.
20. Sadig WM, Al Harbi MW. Effects of surface conditioning on the retentiveness of titanium crowns over short implant abutments. Implant Dent 2007;16:387–96.
21. Segal BS. Retrospective assessment of 546 all-ceramic anterior and posterior crowns in a general practice. J Prosthet Dent 2001;85:544–50.
22. Paul SJ, Pietrobon N. Aesthetic evolution of anterior maxillary crowns: a literature review. Pract Periodontics Aesthet Dent 1998;10:87–94.
23. Ekfeldt A, Fürst B, Carlsson GE. Zirconia abutments for single-tooth implant restorations: a retrospective and clinical follow-up study. Clin Oral Implants Res 2011;22:1308–14.
24. Hatai Y. Extreme masking: achieving predictable outcomes in challenging situations with lithium disilicate bonded restorations. Int J Esthet Dent 2014;9: 206–22.
25. Jemt T. Single implants in the anterior maxilla after 15 years of follow-up: comparison with central implants in the edentulous maxilla. Int J Prosthodont 2008; 21:400–8.
26. Vigolo P, Mutinelli S, Givani A, et al. Cemented versus screw-retained implant-supported single-tooth crowns: a 10-year randomised controlled trial. Eur J Oral Implantol 2012;5:355–64.
27. Glauser R, Sailer I, Wohlwend A, et al. Experimental zirconia abutments for implant-supported single-tooth restorations in esthetically demanding regions: 4-year results of a prospective clinical study. Int J Prosthodont 2004;17: 285–90.
28. Jemt T. Cemented CeraOne and porcelain fused to TiAdapt abutment single-implant crown restorations: a 10-year comparative follow-up study. Clin Implant Dent Relat Res 2009;11:303–10.

29. Hall JA, Payne AG, Purton DG, et al. Immediately restored, single-tapered implants in the anterior maxilla: prosthodontic and aesthetic outcomes after 1 year. Clin Implant Dent Relat Res 2007;9:34–45.
30. Becker W, Becker BE. Replacement of maxillary and mandibular molars with single endosseous implant restorations: a retrospective study. J Prosthet Dent 1995;74:51–5.
31. Scheller H, Urgell JP, Kultje C, et al. A 5-year multicenter study on implant-supported single crown restorations. Int J Oral Maxillofac Implants 1998;13:212–8.
32. Scholander S. A retrospective evaluation of 259 single-tooth replacements by the use of Brånemark implants. Int J Prosthodont 1999;12:483–91.
33. Bergenblock S, Andersson B, Fürst B, et al. Long-term follow-up of CeraOne single-implant restorations: an 18-year follow-up study based on a prospective patient cohort. Clin Implant Dent Relat Res 2012;14:471–9.
34. Montero J, Manzano G, Beltrán D, et al. Clinical evaluation of the incidence of prosthetic complications in implant crowns constructed with UCLA castable abutments. A cohort follow-up study. J Dent 2012;40:1081–9.
35. Vandeweghe S, Cosyn J, Thevissen E, et al. A 1-year prospective study on Co-Axis implants immediately loaded with a full ceramic crown. Clin Implant Dent Relat Res 2012;14:e126–38.
36. Zembic A, Bösch A, Jung RE, et al. Five-year results of a randomized controlled clinical trial comparing zirconia and titanium abutments supporting single-implant crowns in canine and posterior regions. Clin Oral Implants Res 2013;24:384–90.
37. Haas R, Polak C, Fürhauser R, et al. long-term follow-up of 76 Bränemark single-tooth implants. Clin Oral Implants Res 2002;13:38–43.
38. Ekfeldt A, Carlsson GE, Börjesson G. Clinical evaluation of single-tooth restorations supported by osseointegrated implants: a retrospective study. Int J Oral Maxillofac Implants 1994;9:179–83.
39. Jemt T, Pettersson PA. 3-year follow-up study on single implant treatment. J Dent 1993;21:203–8.
40. Bonde MJ, Stokholm R, Isidor F, et al. Outcome of implant-supported single-tooth replacements performed by dental students. A 10-year clinical and radiographic retrospective study. Eur J Oral Implantol 2010;3:37–46.
41. Polizzi G, Fabbro S, Furri M, et al. Clinical application of narrow Brånemark System implants for single-tooth restorations. Int J Oral Maxillofac Implants 1999;14:496–503.
42. Mangano C, Mangano F, Piatelli A, et al. Single-tooth Morse taper connection implants after 1 year of functional loading: a multicentre study on 302 patients. Eur J Oral Implantol 2008;1:305–15.
43. Gotfredsen KA. 5-year prospective study of single-tooth replacements supported by the Astra Tech implant: a pilot study. Clin Implant Dent Relat Res 2004;6:1–8.
44. Spies BC, Stampf S, Kohal RJ. Evaluation of zirconia-based all-ceramic single crowns and fixed dental prosthesis on zirconia implants: 5-year results of a Prospective Cohort Study. Clin Implant Dent Relat Res 2014. [Epub ahead of print].
45. Mangano C, Mangano F, Piattelli, et al. Prospective clinical evaluation of 307 single-tooth Morse taper-connection implants: a multicenter study. Int J Oral Maxillofac Implants 2010;25:394–400.
46. Duncan JP, Nazarova E, Vogiatzi T, et al. Prosthodontic complications in a prospective clinical trial of single-stage implants at 36 months. Int J Oral Maxillofac Implants 2003;18:561–5.

47. Drago CJ, O'Connor CG. A clinical report on the 18-month cumulative survival rates of implants and implant prostheses with an internal connection implant system. Compend Contin Educ Dent 2006;27:266–71.
48. Mangano FG, Shibli JA, Sammons RL, et al. Short (8-mm) locking-taper implants supporting single crowns in posterior region: a prospective clinical study with 1-to 10-years of follow-up. Clin Oral Implants Res 2014;25:933–40.
49. Mangano C, Mangano F, Shibli JA, et al. Prospective evaluation of 2,549 Morse taper connection implants: 1- to 6-year data. J Periodontol 2011;82:52–61.
50. Nothdurft FP, Nonhoff J, Pospiech PR. Pre-fabricated zirconium dioxide implant abutments for single-tooth replacement in the posterior region: success and failure after 3 years of function. Acta Odontol Scand 2014;72:392–400.
51. Hosseini M, Worsaae N, Schiødt M, et al. A 3-year prospective study of implant-supported, single-tooth restorations of all-ceramic and metal-ceramic materials in patients with tooth agenesis. Clin Oral Implants Res 2013;24:1078–87.
52. Cha HS, Kim YS, Jeon JH, et al. Cumulative survival rate and complication rates of single-tooth implant; focused on the coronal fracture of fixture in the internal connection implant. J Oral Rehabil 2013;40:595–602.
53. Schwarz S, Schröder C, Hassel A, et al. Survival and chipping of zirconia-based and metal-ceramic implant-supported single crowns. Clin Implant Dent Relat Res 2012;14:e119–25.
54. Lops D, Bressan E, Chiapasco M, et al. Zirconia and titanium implant abutments for single-tooth implant prostheses after 5 years of function in posterior regions. Int J Oral Maxillofac Implants 2013;28:281–7.
55. Bischof M, Nedir R, Abi Najm S, et al. A five-year life-table analysis on wide neck ITI implants with prosthetic evaluation and radiographic analysis: results from a private practice. Clin Oral Implants Res 2006;17:512–20.
56. Lai HC, Si MS, Zhuang LF, et al. Long-term outcomes of short dental implants supporting single crowns in posterior region: a clinical retrospective study of 5-10 years. Clin Oral Implants Res 2013;24:230–7.
57. Cooper LF, Ellner S, Moriarty J, et al. Three-year evaluation of single-tooth implants restored 3 weeks after 1-stage surgery. Int J Oral Maxillofac Implants 2007;22:791–800.
58. Levine RA, Clem D, Beagle J, et al. Multicenter retrospective analysis of the solid-screw ITI implant for posterior single-tooth replacements. Int J Oral Maxillofac Implants 2002;17:550–6.
59. Krennmair G, Schmidinger S, Waldenberger O. Single-tooth replacement with the Frialit-2 system: a retrospective clinical analysis of 146 implants. Int J Oral Maxillofac Implants 2002;17:78–85.
60. Mangano C, Bartolucci EG. Single tooth replacement by Morse taper connection implants: a retrospective study of 80 implants. Int J Oral Maxillofac Implants 2001;16:675–80.
61. Muftu A, Chapman RJ. Replacing posterior teeth with freestanding implants: four-year prosthodontic results of a prospective study. J Am Dent Assoc 1998;129:1097–102.
62. Mericske-Stern R, Grütter L, Rösch R, et al. Clinical evaluation and prosthetic complications of single tooth replacements by non-submerged implants. Clin Oral Implants Res 2001;12:309–18.
63. Kim YK, Kim SG, Yun PY, et al. Prognosis of single molar implants: a retrospective study. Int J Periodontics Restorative Dent 2010;30:401–7.

64. Mangano F, Macchi A, Caprioglio A, et al. Survival and complication rates of fixed restorations supported by locking-taper implants: a prospective study with 1 to 10 years of follow-up. J Prosthodont 2014;23(6):434–44.

65. Brägger U, Karoussis I, Persson R, et al. Technical and biological complications/failures with single crowns and fixed partial dentures on implants: a 10-year prospective cohort study. Clin Oral Implants Res 2005;16:326–34.

66. Hosseini M, Worsaae N, Schiodt M, et al. A 1-year randomised controlled trial comparing zirconia versus metal-ceramic implant supported single-tooth restorations. Eur J Oral Implantol 2011;4:347–61.

67. Krennmair G, Seemann R, Schmidinger S, et al. Clinical outcome of root-shaped dental implants of various diameters: 5-year results. Int J Oral Maxillofac Implants 2010;25:357–66.

68. Döring K, Eisenmann E, Stiller M. Functional and esthetic considerations for single-tooth Ankylos implant-crowns: 8 years of clinical performance. J Oral Implantol 2004;30:198–209.

69. Norton MR. Multiple single-tooth implant restorations in the posterior jaws: maintenance of marginal bone levels with reference to the implant-abutment microgap. Int J Oral Maxillofac Implants 2006;21:777–84.

70. Simon RL. Single implant-supported molar and premolar crowns: a ten-year retrospective clinical report. J Prosthet Dent 2003;90:517–21.

71. Nothdurft F, Pospiech P. Prefabricated zirconium dioxide implant abutments for single-tooth replacement in the posterior region: evaluation of peri-implant tissues and superstructures after 12 months of function. Clin Oral Implants Res 2010;21:857–65.

72. Sailer I, Mühlemann S, Zwahlen M, et al. Cemented and screw-retained implant reconstructions: a systematic review of the survival and complication rates. Clin Oral Implants Res 2012;23:163–201.

73. Henry PJ, Tolman DE, Bolender C. The applicability of osseointegrated implants in the treatment of partially edentulous patients: three-year results of a prospective multicenter study. Quintessence Int 1993;24:123–9.

74. Ortorp A, Jemt T. Clinical experiences of implant-supported prostheses with laser-welded titanium frameworks in the partially edentulous jaw: a 5-year follow-up study. Clin Implant Dent Relat Res 1999;1(2):84–91.

75. Wahlström M, Sagulin GB, Jansson LE. Clinical follow-up of unilateral, fixed dental prosthesis on maxillary implants. Clin Oral Implants Res 2010;21:1294–300.

76. Jemt T, Henry P, Lindén B, et al. Implant-supported laser-welded titanium and conventional cast frameworks in the partially edentulous law: a 5-year prospective multicenter study. Int J Prosthodont 2003;16:415–21.

77. Wennström JL, Ekestubbe A, Gröndahl K, et al. Oral rehabilitation with implant-supported fixed partial dentures in periodontitis-susceptible subjects. A 5-year prospective study. J Clin Periodontol 2004;31:713–24.

78. Eliasson A, Eriksson T, Johansson A, et al. Fixed partial prostheses supported by 2 or 3 implants: a retrospective study up to 18 years. Int J Oral Maxillofac Implants 2006;21:567–74.

79. Hälg GA, Schmid J, Hämmerle CH. Bone level changes at implants supporting crowns or fixed partial dentures with or without cantilevers. Clin Oral Implants Res 2008;19:983–90.

80. Snauwaert K, Duyck J, van Steenberghe D, et al. Time dependent failure rate and marginal bone loss of implant supported prostheses: a 15-year follow-up study. Clin Oral Investig 2000;4:13–20.

81. Pozzi A, Sannino G, Barlattani A. Minimally invasive treatment of the atrophic posterior maxilla: a proof-of-concept prospective study with a follow-up of between 36 and 54 months. J Prosthet Dent 2012;108:286–97.
82. Romeo E, Ghisolfi M, Rozza R, et al. Short (8-mm) dental implants in the rehabilitation of partial and complete edentulism: a 3- to 14-year longitudinal study. Int J Prosthodont 2006;19:586–92.
83. Larsson C, Vult von Steyern P. Five-year follow-up of implant-supported Y-TZP and ZTA fixed dental prostheses. A randomized, prospective clinical trial comparing two different material systems. Int J Prosthodont 2010;23:555–61.
84. Lekholm U, Gunne J, Henry P, et al. Survival of the Brånemark implant in partially edentulous jaws: a 10-year prospective multicenter study. Int J Oral Maxillofac Implants 1999;14:639–45.
85. Jemt T, Henry P, Lindén B, et al. A comparison of laser-welded titanium and conventional cast frameworks supported by implants in the partially edentulous jaw: a 3-year prospective multicenter study. Int J Prosthodont 2000;13:282–8.
86. Vanlıoğlu B, Özkan Y, Kulak-Özkan Y. Retrospective analysis of prosthetic complications of implant-supported fixed partial dentures after an observation period of 5 to 10 years. Int J Oral Maxillofac Implants 2013;28:1300–4.
87. Kowar J, Eriksson A, Jemt T. Fixed implant-supported prostheses in elderly patients: a 5-year retrospective comparison between partially and completely edentulous patients aged 80 years or older at implant surgery. Clin Implant Dent Relat Res 2013;15:37–46.
88. Becker CM. Cantilever fixed prostheses utilizing dental implants: a 10-year retrospective analysis. Quintessence Int 2004;35:437–41.
89. Gunne J, Jemt T, Lindén B. Implant treatment in partially edentulous patients: a report on prostheses after 3 years. Int J Prosthodont 1994;7:143–8.
90. Wyatt CC, Zarb GA. Treatment outcomes of patients with implant-supported fixed partial prostheses. Int J Oral Maxillofac Implants 1998;13:204–11.
91. Andersson B, Schärer P, Simion M. Ceramic implant abutments used for short-span fixed partial dentures: a prospective 2-year multicenter study. Int J Prosthodont 1999;12:318–24.
92. Romeo E, Lops D, Margutti E, et al. Long-term survival and success of oral implants in the treatment of full and partial arches: a 7-year prospective study with the ITI dental implant system. Int J Oral Maxillofac Implants 2004;19:247–59.
93. Romeo E, Lops D, Amorfini L, et al. Clinical and radiographic evaluation of small-diameter (3.3-mm) implants followed for 1-7 years: a longitudinal study. Clin Oral Implants Res 2006;17:139–48.
94. Nedir R, Bischof M, Szmukler-Moncler S, et al. Prosthetic complications with dental implants: from an up-to-8-year experience in private practice. Int J Oral Maxillofac Implants 2006;21:919–28.
95. Kreissl ME, Gerds T, Muche R, et al. Technical complications of implant-supported fixed partial dentures in partially edentulous cases after an average observation period of 5 years. Clin Oral Implants Res 2007;18:720–6.
96. Romeo E, Tomasi C, Finini I, et al. Implant-supported fixed cantilever prosthesis in partially edentulous jaws: a cohort prospective study. Clin Oral Implants Res 2009;20:1278–85.
97. Wennerberg A, Jemt T. Complications in partially edentulous implant patients: a 5-year retrospective follow-up study of 133 patients supplied with unilateral maxillary prostheses. Clin Implant Dent Relat Res 1999;1:49–56.
98. Lindh T, Bäck T, Nyström E, et al. Implant versus tooth-implant supported prostheses in the posterior maxilla: a 2-year report. Clin Oral Implants Res 2001;12:441–9.

99. Nissan J, Narobai D, Gross O, et al. Long-term outcome of cemented versus screw-retained implant-supported partial restorations. Int J Oral Maxillofac Implants 2011;26:1102–7.
100. Academy of Osseointegration. 2010 guidelines of the Academy of Osseointegration for the provision of dental implants and associated patient care. Int J Oral Maxillofac Implants 2010;25:620–7.

Complications Associated with Implant-Retained Removable Prostheses

Farhad Vahidi, DMD, MSD[a],*, Gitanjali Pinto-Sinai, DDS[b]

KEYWORDS

- Implant mechanical complications • Implant-supported overdenture
- Implant-supported removable prostheses
- Implant-supported removable partial dentures

KEY POINTS

- Implant-supported removable prostheses improve patients' satisfaction with treatment and quality of life.
- These prostheses are associated with biological and mechanical complications.
- The mechanical complications associated with implant-supported overdentures and implant-supported removable partial dentures include loss of retention of attachment systems, the need to replace retention elements and to reline or repair the resin portion of the denture and implant fracture.
- Implant-supported removable prostheses are very successful but require periodic maintenance.

INTRODUCTION

The changing demographics of the population in the United States and other Western countries have created a shift in the rates and patterns of edentulism.[1] Although the overall trend is toward a decrease in complete edentulism, the group in greatest need of complete or partial oral rehabilitation is the rapidly growing aging population. A study conducted by Douglass and colleagues[1] in 2002 concluded that, "The 10% decline in edentulism experienced each decade for the past 30 years will be more than offset by the 79% increase in the adult population older than 55 years.[1]"

Conventional complete and partial dentures have historically been the treatment options of choice for patients desiring removable prostheses. These options have been suitable for patients with limited financial resources who prefer noninvasive treatment. However, these treatment options are not without complications. In general, the

[a] Department of Prosthodontics, New York University, College of Dentistry, 380 2nd Avenue, Room 302, New York, NY 10010, USA; [b] Division of Restorative Dentistry, Department of Oral Health Practice, University of Kentucky, College of Dentistry, 800 Rose Street, Lexington, KY 40536, USA
* Corresponding author.
E-mail address: Fv1@nyu.edu

Dent Clin N Am 59 (2015) 215–226
http://dx.doi.org/10.1016/j.cden.2014.08.001
0011-8532/15/$ – see front matter © 2015 Elsevier Inc. All rights reserved.

dental.theclinics.com

success of conventional complete dentures depends on starting with appropriate oral anatomy, such as minimally resorbed ridges, arch forms resistant to displacement, and palate forms conducive to denture stability. Of course, obtaining the ideal oral anatomy is rarely possible, especially if a patient has remained edentulous for several years before wearing dentures. The resulting complete dentures may lack stability and retention, affecting mastication and speech, and the overall effect has been a negative on the patient's quality of life. Patients may withdraw socially if they have a fear of being unable to eat or of losing their dentures when speaking. The edentulous mandible tends to be of more concern to denture wearers than the edentulous maxilla.

Conventional partial dentures, especially those with mandibular distal extension bases, present their own set of complications, primarily rotation around the distal abutment, which creates discomfort because of an unstable denture base. This problem can call for periodic relining of the denture for the purpose of maintaining occlusal contacts and avoiding traumatic occlusal forces that cause ridge resorption or damage to abutment teeth because of the difference in resilience between teeth and mucosa.

With advances in osseointegrated implants and the success of fixed dental prostheses has come a change in treatment options for patients who desire removable prostheses but who have completely or partially edentulous ridges. Treatment options include complete or partial dentures retained by single or multiple endosseous implants, which may or may not be splinted, and a variety of attachments, such as ball attachments, Locator abutments, bar attachments, and even magnets.

A panel of subject experts at a 2002 symposium[2] in Montreal, Ontario, Canada, concluded that "The evidence currently available suggests that the restoration of the edentulous mandible with a conventional denture is no longer the most appropriate first choice prosthodontic treatment. There is now overwhelming evidence that a two-implant overdenture should become the first choice of treatment for the edentulous mandible." A subsequent statement was released after the 2009 meeting of The British Society for the Study of Prosthetic Dentistry in York, United Kingdom.[3] This panel concluded that "A substantial body of evidence is now available demonstrating that patient's satisfaction and quality of life with ISOD (implant-supported overdentures) is significantly greater than for conventional dentures." Although the ISOD has not yet been deemed the gold standard of care, it is certainly seen as the first choice for removable prostheses.

Even with the progress of implant dentistry, complications are associated with implant-retained removable prostheses. Such complications may arise from the integration of the implants themselves, or from the design of the prosthesis. Failures or complications may result from a variety of factors, such as the number of implants placed and their location. For instance, the number of implants required for a successful prosthesis may vary depending on occlusal forces and the quality and quantity of bone present. The types of attachments selected by the operator may result in various degrees of stability. The content of this article is intended to focus on the failures and complications associated with implant-retained prostheses and to provide some insight into the prevention of complications and solutions to the problems when failures do occur.

NUMBER AND LOCATION OF IMPLANTS
Overdentures

The issues associated with stability and retention of conventional complete dentures, especially those in the mandible, have resulted in new treatment options. In the 1960s, clinicians began using natural tooth roots that had undergone root canal treatment as abutments for dentures; this procedure became a means of increasing the retention of dentures. With few available studies to guide the methodology for choosing the abutments, the standard protocol was to use anterior teeth, typically at least 2 teeth, especially in the mandible. This protocol was based on the fact that mandibular anterior teeth were usually the last to be lost and the easiest to treat endodontically. However, during the 1970s and 1980s the trend for denture abutments began to move away from natural abutments and toward implant abutments. This change coincided with the increase in published studies related to implant placement.

During treatment planning for an overdenture (OD), it is important to question not only whether there are an ideal number of implants that will maximize the retention of an ISOD but also how their location (maxilla or mandible) affects the outcome.

Mandible

The compact bone structure of the mandible and its dense cortical plates make the largest facial bone a good recipient for implants. Several published studies have shown that patient satisfaction is higher with mandibular implant-retained ODs than with conventional dentures in the areas of stability, retention, chewing function, and even esthetics. In determining the design of a mandibular implant OD, the clinician must consider how many implants are necessary to create improved function without subjecting the patient to excessive surgical procedures.

In 1987, Van Steenberghe and colleagues[4] were among the first authors to support the placement of only 2 mandibular implants for an OD. They reported a 98% success rate with a 52-month follow-up. A 2012 review of the McGill and York consensus statement[3] also concluded, on the basis of the results of several randomized controlled studies, that the placement of 2 mandibular implants for an OD is a minimum standard for patient satisfaction with regard to improved function. Does this mean that the placement of additional mandibular implants is considered unnecessary? According to the findings of a literature review by Sadowsky,[5] which cited a study by Jacobs and colleagues[6], the annual posterior mandible resorption rate was 2 to 3 times higher for patients with OD than for those with conventional complete dentures. Although anterior mandibular bone resorption decreased from 0.4 mm annually to approximately 0.1 mm annually (Atwood and Coy[7] and Tallgren[8]) with the placement of anterior interforaminal implants, this was not the case in the posterior mandible without implants. Sadowsky[5] concluded that, for younger patients or those edentulous for less than 10 years, an OD with 2 implants may actually be contraindicated. Instead, using more implants in the posterior mandible to create a fixed prosthesis not only preserved bone but helped to regenerate bone.[9]

The opposing arch also appears to affect the design of mandibular ODs. Placing a mandibular OD against a conventional complete maxillary denture can generate sufficient occlusal force to the premaxilla area to cause bone resorption and soft tissue inflammation. This problem, as reported by Haraldson and colleagues,[10] can lead to a higher incidence of midline fracture of the maxillary prostheses. To reduce this combination syndrome[11] effect, Thiel and colleagues[12] recommend using an occlusal design, removing anterior contacts in centric relation, and minimizing excursive contacts.

A study by Merickse-Stern[13] concluded that retention, stability, and occlusal equilibration of dentures improve only slightly with an increasing number of implants. Another in vivo study by Fontijn-Tekamp[14] compared the placement of 2 or 4 transmandibular implants and found that the masticatory forces were not significantly different between implant-supported and soft tissue implant dentures. Sadowsky[5] concluded that, although the use of 2 implants does improve function, some scenarios call for the placement of more implants in the mandible, such as a maxilla with natural teeth, which would increase the masticatory forces on the mandible; implants that are less than 8 mm in length or less than 3 mm in width; soft tissue that would be sensitive to occlusal loading; high muscle attachments or sharp mylohyoid projections; large V-shaped ridges; and patients' demand for high retention.

Although 2-implant and-4 implant designs seem to be the most discussed for mandibular ISODs, in 2010 Gonda and colleagues[15] performed a study comparing the use of a single implant in the mandibular midline area to the use of 2 implants. Differences in the rates of fracture of the denture acrylic base were not statistically significant; thus, the authors concluded that, for patients who are older, with larger financial constraints, and the inability to undergo more involved surgical procedures, a single mandibular implant may be adequate for OD retention.

In 2002 the McGill consensus statement[16] concluded that "OD treatment of the mandible having more than two implants does not lead to a more satisfied individual in terms of denture and social function." However, Fitzpatrick[17] states, in his "Standard of care for the edentulous mandibles" that "No single treatment modality or technique for tooth replacement can fit all patient requirements." Therefore, it is good data collection, discussion with the patient of desires and goals, and treatment of the mandible as a component of the entire oral makeup instead of on its own that will allow the clinician to construct an OD design with an appropriate number of implants for a specific patient.

The number of implant fixtures required for a mandibular OD will vary based on the amount of remaining bone that supports the basal seat of the denture, width and the length of the implants to be used. The patient's general health condition is also a contributing factor.

Maxilla

Although numerous studies report significant improvement in denture function with the placement of implants in the mandible, the same cannot be said for the maxilla. De Albuquerque Junior and colleagues[18] reported that implant prostheses in the maxilla will probably have the most impact when a patient is struggling with conventional maxillary dentures. Maxillary trabecular bone is not naturally conducive to primary implant stability, and bone resorption patterns can create unfavorable occlusal forces.[19] Many studies[20–22] have reported that lower maxillary implant survival rates are correlated with decreased quality and quantity of bone, implant angulation that follows the resorption pattern of bone, and increased abutment length caused by thickened maxillary mucosa. Therefore, an ISOD may not be the best choice if appropriate bony support is available for a conventional denture. The clinician should evaluate an existing denture for stability, retention, and overall function and relate those findings to the patient's complaints.[23] Because maxillary ODs do not have palate extension, they are preferred by patients who cannot tolerate palatal coverage (**Fig. 1**).

If the existing denture is ill-fitting or the esthetics are unacceptable to the patient, a new denture must be fabricated. At the wax try-in, the patient must be satisfied with the arrangement of the teeth so that a duplicated denture can be used as a surgical guide for implant placement. The arrangement of the teeth will also determine the space available for retainers and attachments.

When working with the maxilla, the clinician must contend with cavities specific to that bone, such as sinuses and the nasal cavity. It is the anatomy of the jaw that drives the location and placement options for implants, which in turn drive the design of the prosthetic. Therefore, before designing a maxillary prosthesis or placing implants, the

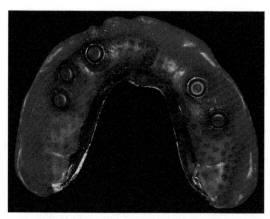

Fig. 1. Maxillary OD, palate-less, with free-standing attachments.

clinician must focus treatment planning on data collection using appropriate radiographic tools, such as computed tomographic scans, for measuring the volume of available bone for implants.

The resorption pattern is important for implant placement. Anterior-posterior resorption of more than 10 mm or substantial maxillary vertical resorption that renders the implant components visible during speech can dictate anterior implant positioning. If too much maxillary anterior bone is present, the clinician may opt to avoid placing implants in the premaxilla to avoid detrimental impacts on OD frameworks that are space-sensitive.[23] In such a case, the posterior ridges may be favored over the anterior ridges for implant placement.

The resorption pattern of the maxillary posterior ridges is medial and superior. Relative to the mandibular arch, the resulting jaw/tooth relationship may be jeopardized, placing undue force on prostheses or implants.

Once the diagnostic data have been collected and evaluated, implant placement can be determined and the prosthetic can be designed, with constant focus on the esthetic goals of the clinician and the patient. Although Branemark and colleagues[24] consider 4 ideally placed implants to be sufficient for prostheses, Eckert and Carr[25] advocate at least 6 maxillary implants for prosthetic success. The primary reason for this difference in recommendation is that failure of 1 of 4 implants will result in the loss of an important component that was integral to the design of the prosthetic, whereas the loss of 1 of 6 implants may still give the clinician room to modify the design.

Per Boucher,[26] the hard palate is the primary *supporting* area of a maxillary denture. Thus, the authors recommend that a palate-less denture be supported by at least 6 implants.[27]

Damghani and colleagues[27] found that the prosthetic design is affected not only by the number of implants placed but also by the distance between them. An in vitro study showed that the decrease in the difference of force to the palatal area was larger with 4 implants placed a maximum of 8 mm apart than with 2 implants. The overall difference in force on the palate was highest with 4 implants placed a maximum of 24 mm apart, but this difference was not statistically significantly different from that achieved with 4 implants spaced 8 mm apart.

If total support by implants is not attainable, the clinician should consider retentive elements that allow prosthetic movement. This choice will serve to remove high stress around the terminal implants that could cause, at the least, fracture of the OD acrylic base and, at most, fracture of retentive elements or loss of the implant (**Fig. 2**).

Eckert and Carr[25] recommend that multiple implants should be left unsplinted if an implant has failed before prosthodontic fabrication.

MECHANICAL COMPLICATIONS OF IMPLANT SUPPORTED OVERDENTURES

A review of the published literature showed that implant-supported mandibular ODs are successful both biologically and mechanically. Andreiotelli and colleagues[28] reported that implant-supported ODs in the mandible provide predictable results. A lower rate of implant survival and a higher rate of mechanical complications seen for implant-supported maxillary ODs.

The following mechanical complications of ISODs have been reported: loss of retention of attachment systems, replacement or activation of retentive elements, loosening of screws, the need for relining or repairing the resin portion of the denture base, pop-out of denture teeth, and implant fracture (**Figs. 3–5**).[29] Various attachment systems have been used with ISODs, such as ball attachments, bar systems, and Locator attachments (Zest Anchors, Inc, Escondido, CA, USA). The most common mechanical complication associated with OD is maladjustment of the attachment system, regardless of the type of attachment used.

An important question is whether the attachment systems should be splinted or left unsplinted. Stoumpis and Kohal[30] reported no difference in implant survival rates between splinted and unsplinted systems. They also concluded that an unsplinted design requires more prosthetic maintenance. Naert and colleagues[31] found that the most common problem with mandibular ODs is replacement of the O-ring on ball attachments. The Locator attachment, which was introduced in 2001, is usually unsplinted. The attachment is a self-aligning, resilient dual retention system. It is available in various heights to fit several implant systems or brands.[32] Cakarer and colleagues[33] reported that the number of mechanical complications associated with the Locator attachment is lower than that for ball or bar attachments. Kleis and colleagues[34] compared 3 types of attachments on ODs supported by 2 implants and reported that all systems required maintenance of retentive elements within 1 year of follow-up.

The complications associated with the bar attachment system (splinted) are its bulk, the possibility of mucosal hyperplasia around the bar, oral hygiene problems, and the need for adjustment of the clip. In a systematic review of maxillary ISODs with a mean

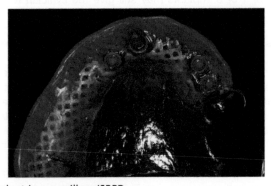

Fig. 2. Loss of implant in a maxillary ISRPD.

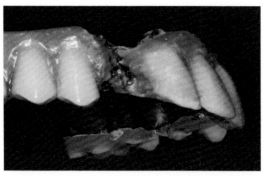

Fig. 3. Resin fracture and pop-out of a tooth in an implant-supported OD.

observation of at least 1 year after placement, Slot and colleagues[35] found that the use of 6 implants splinted with a bar was the most successful system. Bar attachments also require more laboratory technique than other system.

Mechanical failure of bar attachments for ODs is caused by insufficient metal thickness, inferior solder joints, excessive cantilever length, and incorrect location of the implant.[36] Cakarer and colleagues[33] found that implant fractures most commonly occur with the ball attachment; they found no implant fractures with the Locator attachment (**Fig. 6**).

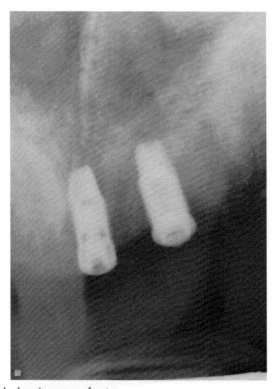

Fig. 4. Radiograph showing screw fracture.

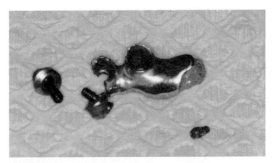

Fig. 5. Bar and screw fracture in an OD.

There is no doubt that ISODs require mechanical maintenance. To reduce the frequency of these mechanical problems, practitioners must identify problems and find a simple solution to them.

The following are some recommended solutions for reducing the incidence of or solving the mechanical problems associated with ISODs:

1. The ODs must have proper extension and basal support. The fit of the denture base must be checked periodically. If necessary, the denture base should be relined or rebased as indicated.
2. The retentive elements of the attachment system must be checked and replaced as necessary.
3. To avoid fracture of the denture base, ISODs should contain a metal framework. The design and thickness of the metal skeleton must allow sufficient thickness of the acrylic resin.[37]
4. Instruction in oral hygiene and maintenance of soft tissue around the attachment systems are essential, especially with bar systems.
5. The distal extension of a bar attachment in resorbed mandibular ridges must not be too long. The use of the proper length will prevent bar fracture. Merickse-Stern[38] recommended that the cantilever part of the bar must not extend beyond the first premolars (**Fig. 7**).
6. Fabricating bar systems with CAD-CAM technology may lead to fewer mechanical failures.
7. The placement of multiple implants for supporting an OD, specifically in the maxilla, will simplify the repair of the prosthesis if an implant fails or fractures.

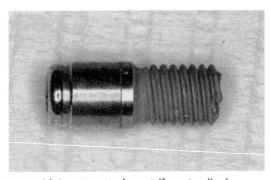

Fig. 6. Implant fracture with Locator attachment (free-standing).

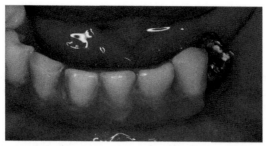

Fig. 7. Fracture of the distal cantilever of the metal skeleton of prosthesis.

IMPLANT-SUPPORTED REMOVABLE PARTIAL DENTURE

Prosthetic management of partial edentulism is still challenging. Traditionally, the condition of the abutment teeth surrounding the prosthesis and the length of the edentulous span dictate the design of removable partial dentures (RPDs).

Differences in the viscoelastic responses of the abutment teeth and mucosal tissue to occlusal loading result in the transmission of torque forces to the abutment teeth. Such forces can increase the mobility of abutment teeth and decrease the retention and stability of the RPD. Torque force on the mucosa can create a shearing force on the underlying alveolar ridges, leading to increased bone resorption and requiring periodic relining of the posthesis to improve stability.[39]

The use of osseointegrated implants as direct retainers in implant-supported removable partial dentures (ISRPDs) has been indicated.[32] The use of implants in the distal extension areas within class I and II Kennedy RPDs has been recommended.[39,40] Such implant will increase the stability of the RPD, preserve bone, and increase retention.

In an in vitro study, Sato and colleagues[41] found that placing implant at the distal edentulous ridge can prevent displacement of the denture's distal extension bases. They found that the load on the bilateral first molar areas of ISRPDs is significantly less than that with conventional RPDs. Implant-retained or implant-supported RPDs improve retention and stability, minimize rotational movement, and significantly increase patient satisfaction.[42] Campos and colleagues[43] concluded that the use of implants with ball attachment retainers over a free-end RPD allowed patients to select harder foods to chew and resulted in smaller particle sizes at the time of swallowing than did conventional free-end RPDs.

Cunha and colleagues[44] reported that placing the implant closer to the abutment tooth placed less load on the supporting structures of that tooth. In addition, placing at least one implant in the edentulous area resulted in a lower stress load to the supporting tissues than that associated with distal extension RPDs. The use of free-standing resilient attachments is preferred within ISRPDs.[32,40,41]

COMPLICATIONS ASSOCIATED WITH IMPLANT-SUPPORTED REMOVABLE PARTIAL DENTURES

Mechanical complications associated with ISRPDs are similar to those associated with ISODs. In a systematic review of ISRPDs with distal extension, de Freitas and colleagues[45] found an implant survival rate of 95% to 100%. They reported that the complications associated with ISRPDs include the need for repairing or relining the prosthesis, the replacement of attachments, loosening of screws, and the need for repair of the acrylic denture base. Regardless of these mechanical complications, these prostheses are low in cost and beneficial to the patient. The use of ISRPDs increases patient satisfaction.

SUMMARY

Implant-supported removable prostheses improve patients' satisfaction with treatment and quality of life. Improvements of implant surface and in attachment elements have made this treatment method very successful. Even so, these prostheses are associated with biological and mechanical complications. The mechanical complications associated with ISODs and ISRPDs include loss of retention of attachment systems, the need to replace retention elements and to reline or repair the resin portion of the denture, and implant fracture. Implant-supported removable prostheses are very successful but require periodic maintenance.

REFERENCES

1. Douglass CW, Shih A, Ostry L. Will there be a need for complete dentures in the United States in 2020? J Prosthet Dent 2002;87(1):5–8.
2. Thomason JM, Feine J, Exley C, et al. Mandibular two implant-supported overdentures as the first choice standard of care for edentulous patients – the York Consensus Statement. Br Dent J 2009;207:185–6.
3. Thomason JM, Kelly SA, Bendkowski A, et al. Two implant retained overdentures–a review of the literature supporting the McGill and York consensus statements. J Dent 2012;40(1):22–34. http://dx.doi.org/10.1016/j.jdent.2011.08.017.
4. Van Steenberghe D, Quirynen M, Calberson L, et al. A prospective evaluation of the fate of 697 consecutive intra-oral fixtures ad modum Branemark in the rehabilitation of edentulism. J Head Neck Pathol 1987;6:53–8.
5. Sadowsky SJ. Mandibular implant-retained overdentures: a literature review. J Prosthet Dent 2001;86(5):468–73.
6. Jacobs R, Schotte A, van Steenberghe D, et al. Posterior jaw bone resorption in osseointegrated implant-supported overdentures. Clin Oral Implants Res 2001; 12:19–25.
7. Atwood DA, Coy WA. Clinical, cephalometric, and densitrometic study of reduction of residual ridges. J Prosthet Dent 1971;26:280–95.
8. Tallgren A. The continuing reduction of residual alveolar ridges in complete denture wearers: a mixed-longitudinal study covering 25 years. J Prosthet Dent 1972;27:120–32.
9. Davis WH, Lam PS, Marshall MW, et al. Using restorations borne totally by anterior implants to preserve the edentulous mandible. J Am Dent Assoc 1999;130: 1183–9.
10. Haraldson T, Jemt T, Stalblad PA, et al. Oral function in subjects with overdentures supported by osseointegrated implants. Scand J Dent Res 1988;96:235–42.
11. Kelly E. Changes caused by a mandibular removable partial denture opposing a maxillary complete denture. J Prosthet Dent 1972;27:140–50.
12. Thiel CP, Evans DB, Burnett RR. Combination syndrome associated with a mandibular implant-supported overdenture: a clinical report. J Prosthet Dent 1996;75:107–13.
13. Merickse-Stern R. Clinical evaluation of overdenture restorations supported by osseointegrated titanium implants: a retrospective study. Int J Oral Maxillofac Implants 1990;5(4):375–83.
14. Fontijn-Tekamp FA, Slagter AP, van't Hof MA, et al. Bite forces with mandibular implant-retained overdentures. J Dent Res 1998;77:1832–9.

15. Gonda T, Maeda Y, Walton JN, et al. Fracture incidence in mandibular over-dentures retained by one or two implants. J Prosthet Dent 2010;103(3):178–81.
16. Thomason JM. The McGill consensus statement on overdentures. Mandibular 2-implant overdentures as first choice standard of care for edentulous patients. Eur J Prosthodont Restor Dent 2002;10:95–6.
17. Fitzpatrick B. Standard of care for the edentulous mandible: a systematic review. J Prosthet Dent 2006;95:71–8.
18. De Albuquerque Junior RF, Lund JP, Tang L, et al. Within-subject comparison of maxillary long-bar implant-retained prostheses with and without palatal coverage: patient-based outcomes. Clin Oral Implants Res 2000;11:555–65.
19. Klemetti E. Is there a certain number of implants needed to retain an overdenture? J Oral Rehabil 2008;35(Suppl 1):80–4.
20. Chan MF, Närhi TO, de Baat C, et al. Treatment of the atrophic edentulous maxilla with implant-supported overdentures: a review of the literature. Int J Prosthodont 1998;11(1):7–15.
21. Razavi R, Zena RB, Khan Z, et al. Anatomic site evaluation of edentulous maxillae for dental implant placement. J Prosthodont 1995;4(2):90–4.
22. Rangert B. Biomechanics of the Brånemark system. Aust Prosthodont J 1995; 9(Suppl):39–48.
23. Drago C, Carpentieri J. Treatment of maxillary jaws with dental implants: guidelines for treatment. J Prosthodont 2011;20(5):336–47.
24. Brånemark PI, Svensson B, Van Steenberghe D. Ten-year survival rates of fixed prostheses on four or six implants ad modum Brånemark in full edentulism. Clin Oral Implants Res 1995;6:227–31.
25. Eckert SE, Carr AB. Implant-retained maxillary overdentures. Dent Clin North Am 2004;48(3):585–601.
26. Boucher C. A critical analysis of the mid-century impression techniques for full dentures. J Prosthet Dent 1951;1:472–92.
27. Damghani S, Masri R, Driscoll CF, et al. The effect of number and distribution of unsplinted maxillary implants on the load transfer in implant-retained maxillary overdentures: an in vitro study. J Prosthet Dent 2012;107(6):358–65.
28. Andreiotelli M, Att W, Strub JR. Prosthodontic complications with implant over-dentures: a systematic review. Int J Prosthodont 2010;23(3):195–203.
29. Goodacre CJ, Bernal G, Rungchara Ssaeng K, et al. Clinical complications with implants and implant prostheses. J Prosthet Dent 2003;90(2):121–32.
30. Stoumpis C, Kohal J. To splint or not to splint oral implants in the implant-supported overdenture therapy? A systematic review. J Oral Rehabil 2011;38:857–69.
31. Naert I, Alssadi G, Quirynen M. Prosthetic aspects and patients' satisfaction with two implant –retained mandibular overdentures: a ten year randomized clinical study. Int J Prosthodont 2004;17:401–10.
32. Chikunov I, Doan P, Vahidi F. Implant retained partial overdenture with resilient at-tachments. J Prosthet Dent 2008;17:141–8.
33. Cakarer S, Taylan K, Yaltirik M, et al. Complications associated with the ball, bar and Locator attachments for implant-supported overdentures. Med Oral Patol Oral Cir Bucal 2011;16(7):953–9.
34. Kleis WK, Kammaerer PW, Hartmann S, et al. A comparison of three different attachment systems for mandibular two implant overdentures: one year report. Clin Implant Dent Relat Res 2010;12(3):209–18.
35. Slot W, Raghoebar GM, Vissink A, et al. A systematic review of implant supported maxillary overdentures after a mean observation period of at least one year. J Clin Periodontol 2010;37:98–110.

36. Waddell JN, Payne AG, Swain MV. Physical and metallurgical considerations of failures of soldered bars in bar attachment systems for implant overdentures: a review of the literature. J Prosthet Dent 2006;96(4):283–8.

37. Choi M, Acharya V, Barg R, et al. Resinous denture base fracture resistance: effects of thickness and teeth. Int J Prosthodont 2012;25(1):53–8.

38. Merickse-Stern R. Prosthodontics management of maxillary and mandibular overdentures. In: Feine JS, Carlson GE, editors. Implant overdentures as the standard of case for edentulous patients. Chicago: Quintessence; 2003. p. 83–96.

39. Shahmiri R, Aarts JM, Bennani V, et al. Strain distribution in a Kennedy class I implant assisted removable partial denture under various loading conditions. Int J Dent 2013;22(7):550–5.

40. Kusmanovic DV, Payne AG, Purton DG. Distal implants to modify the Kennedy classification of a removable partial denture: a clinical report. J Prosthet Dent 2004;92(1):8–11.

41. Sato M, Suzuki X, Kurihara D, et al. Effects of implant support on mandibular distal extension removable partial dentures: relationship between denture supporting area and stress distribution. J Prosthodont Res 2013;57(2):109–12.

42. Goncalves TM, Campos CH, Rodrigues Garcia RC. Implant retention and support for distal extension partial removable denture prostheses: satisfaction outcomes. J Prosthet Dent 2014;112(2):334–9.

43. Campos CH, Goncalves TM, Rodrigues Garcia RC. Implant retainers for free-end removable partial dentures affect mastication and nutrient intake. Clin Oral Implants Res 2013;25:957–61.

44. Cunha LD, Pellizzer EP, Verri FR, et al. Evaluation of the influences of location of osseointegrated implants associated with mandibular removable partial dentures. Implant Dent 2008;17(3):278–87.

45. de Freitas RF, de Carvalho DK, da Fonte Porto Carreiro A, et al. Mandibular implant-supported removable partial denture with distal extension: a systematic review. J Oral Rehabil 2012;39(10):791–8.

Esthetic Failure in Implant Dentistry

Rodrigo Fuentealba, DDS[a],*, Jorge Jofré, DDS, PhD[b]

KEYWORDS

- Esthetic zone • Dental implants • Esthetic failure • Patient satisfaction
- Prosthetically driven implant placement • PES/WES

KEY POINTS

- In today's dentistry, it is not enough to simply assess the clinical parameters of a dental implant restoration in the rehabilitation of missing teeth.
- Although the dental literature contains information about esthetic failure in general dentistry, no clear consensus is available regarding esthetic failure of dental implants.
- Both objective and subjective parameters are important in determining the esthetic success or failure of an implant-supported crown.
- On the basis of objective indices, esthetic failures in implant dentistry can be categorized as pink-tissue failures and white-tissue failures.
- Pink-tissue failures are more common; they include facial recession, gingival asymmetry, papillary deficiency, and graying of the gingival tissue.

Osseointegrated endosseous dental implants have been deemed an innocuous and predictable form of rehabilitation that can be used to replace dentition in patients who are completely or partially edentulous and those who are missing only a single tooth. The average survival rate of multiple-implant designs is higher than 90%.[1–3] The success rate of such implants has also been evaluated, although various criteria have been used and these have changed over time.[4] The criteria for implant success in 1979 permitted 1 mm or less of mobility with some radiographic radiolucency and bone loss, whereas it currently includes absence of mobility, absence of radiographic radiolucency, and minimal bone loss.[5,6]

Even though the parameters of success have evolved, the early concern in implant dentistry was primarily osseointegration, and even today, osseointegration remains the predominant parameter of success in implant dentistry. However, because of

The authors have nothing to disclose.
[a] Restorative Division, University of Kentucky College of Dentistry, 800 Rose Street, D642, Lexington, KY 40356-0297, USA; [b] Center for Advanced Prosthodontics and Implant Dentistry, University of Concepcion, Victoria 232 Barrio Universitario Concepción, Concepcion 4030000, Chile
* Corresponding author.
E-mail address: rodrigo.fuentealba@uky.edu

patient and clinician demands and the increased certainty of osseointegration, new parameters are now being used to assess implant success. Some examples of these parameters are peri-implant soft-tissue level, prosthesis level, and patient's subjective assessments; these parameters should be considered by dentists in evaluating the success or failure of implant dentistry. The focus is shifting from implant survival to the creation of lifelike implant restorations with natural-looking peri-implant soft tissues.[4] Patients today have a high demand for esthetics and want not only improved function but also normal appearance.[7]

Esthetics plays an important role in any implant placement but is crucial for implants placed in the anterior maxilla. An anterior single implant-supported crown restoration must meet a particularly high standard of esthetic quality because the adjacent natural teeth provide an immediate comparison to the crown.[8] Overall, implant dentistry in the esthetic zone is challenging because the implant restoration and surrounding tissues will be visible when the patient smiles fully and because it will be placed in an area of esthetic importance for the patient.[9] According to the Straightforward, Advanced, and Complex International Team for Implantology (ITI) classification, any implant in the esthetic zone must be classified as either advanced or complex, a classification deriving from the technique sensitivity required for replacing missing teeth in the anterior maxilla.[10]

Patients' and clinicians' high demands and expectations for esthetics have expanded the criteria for the success of implants from osseointegration alone to a harmonious and natural blending of the restoration with the surrounding tissues and dentition.[11] Higginbottom and colleagues[9] defined an esthetic implant restoration as one that resembles a natural tooth in all aspects. Acknowledging that patients and clinicians consider the esthetics of an implant very important, it should be determined when an implant is considered a failure from an esthetic point of view.

Although the dental literature contains information about esthetic failure in general dentistry, to the authors' knowledge, no clear consensus is available regarding esthetic failure of dental implants. Late in the 1990s, el Askary and colleagues[12] defined an implant failure as failure of the implant to fulfill its purpose (functional, esthetic, or phonetic). However, the only types of failures associated by the authors were absence of osseointegration, prosthetic fracture, gingival bleeding, and infection. Furthermore, until recently an implant was considered a failure when it was lost, fractured, or mobile, or a source of irreversible pain or infection.[13] In summary, the word failure as applied to dental implants is frequently used in the dental literature to indicate the loss of osseointegration; it has seldom been used to describe a lack of esthetic success. In fact, the word complication is often used when a problem occurs with any of the replaceable components of the implant system.[12,14]

Most dictionaries define failure as "lack of success." If this definition is extrapolated to esthetics and dental implants, esthetic failure in implant dentistry would refer to a lack of success in achieving esthetics with dental implant restorations. Consequently, success in implant dentistry needs to be redefined.

The dental literature demonstrates the lack of a consensus about the parameters used to determine esthetic success or esthetic failure in implant dentistry. As mentioned, some authors apparently do not consider these parameters important, because they consider only osseointegration when evaluating the success of their treatments.[13] Other authors report esthetic failures but fail to provide adequate information about how these failures were evaluated.[15] Henry and colleagues[16] reported an esthetic failure rate of 10% in a 5-year multicenter study; nevertheless, the authors did not report the parameters used to determine the cause of these esthetic failures. Similarly, Goodacre and colleagues[17] did not describe poor esthetic outcomes as failures but rather as esthetic complications. As examples of such complications, they reported improper restoration contour, poor shade, and exposure of implant components because of gingival recession.

Esthetics refers to the response of the mind and the emotions to beauty. As Lew Wallace wrote, "Beauty is altogether in the eye of the beholder." Two important factors influence this concept in dentistry: the patient and the clinician. Esthetics is a subjective perception that varies from individual to individual and is also influenced by sociocultural values.[18] Chang and colleagues[8] demonstrated that the appreciation of esthetic outcomes is higher among patients than among prosthodontists. They indicated that the factors considered by clinicians to be important for an acceptable esthetic result of restorative therapy may not be imperative for patient satisfaction. Dueled and colleagues,[19] on the other hand, found a positive linear correlation between professional and patient evaluations of esthetic outcomes, but this correlation was not statistically significant. In most studies, patients were more satisfied with the overall outcome than was the professional examiner.[20–22]

OBJECTIVE ESTHETIC INDICES

The dental literature has described several systems for evaluating esthetic outcomes of implant restorations in the esthetic zone.

In 1997, Jemt[23] proposed an index to assess the size of the interproximal gingival papillae adjacent to single implant restorations. This index has been used in several studies evaluating esthetics in dental implant dentistry because it was one of the first to consider the papilla in relation to implant restorations.[19,24,25] Jemt's Papilla Index (JPI) categorizes the presence of interdental papilla on a scale ranging from 0 to 4, assigning a rating of 0 for no papillae and a rating of 4 for hyperplastic papillae. However, the JPI does not consider the entire contour of the soft tissue around the implant.[23]

Fürhauser and colleagues[26] developed the pink esthetic score (PES) for evaluating the soft tissue around single-tooth implant crowns. They objectively assessed the esthetic outcome of the soft tissues contouring a dental implant restoration, addressing crucial problems that are easily overlooked in a general assessment. The PES criteria are based on 7 variables: mesial papilla, distal papilla, soft-tissue level, soft-tissue contour, alveolar process deficiency, soft-tissue color, and texture. Each variable is given a score of 2, 1, or 0 with 2 as the best score and 0 as the worst score, for a maximal possible score of 14. All variables except papilla are assessed by comparison with a reference tooth. The PES index not only includes more variables than the JPI but also evaluates the height, level, color, and texture of the peri-implant soft tissues. Others have used this index successfully[27–32] and have indicated that the appearance of the peri-implant soft tissue and the dental restoration is the "difference maker" between a successful and an unsuccessful outcome.[27]

Evans and Chen[24] developed the subjective esthetic score (SES) as a complement to the JPI. Their objective was to rate the esthetic outcome of immediate implant placement on the basis of the vertical change in the position of the mucosal margin and the fullness of tissue after the restoration. The SES has proved to be a good complement to the JPI because it assesses the soft tissue surrounding the implant restoration as a whole. Furthermore, this index is useful in evaluations of esthetics because it assesses gingival recession after implant placement.

Meijer and colleagues[33] developed the Implant Crown Aesthetic index as an objective index for rating the esthetic outcomes of implant-supported single crowns and adjacent soft tissues. They rated 9 variables, 5 related to the crown (mesiodistal dimension, position of the incisal edge, labial convexity, color/translucency, and surface) and 4 relating to the surrounding soft tissue (position of the labial margin of the peri-implant mucosa, position of the mucosa in the approximal embrasures, contour of the labial surface of the mucosa/color, and surface of the labial mucosa). This index considers the adjacent and contralateral teeth as a reference and scores the esthetics of the restoration on a scale ranging from 0 to 5: 0, excellent; 1 to 2, satisfactory; 3 to 4, moderate; and 5 poor. This index was an improvement because it incorporated variables relating to both the surrounding soft tissues and the hard-tissue restorations in the determination of esthetic outcomes. Other authors have used this index successfully.[34]

Dueled and colleagues[19] developed an objective scoring system for evaluating the esthetic outcomes of oral rehabilitation for patients with tooth agenesis. Their score incorporates mucosal discoloration, crown morphology, crown color match, and symmetry/harmony. It also evaluates the level of the papilla by using a modified JPI. Each variable is assessed with a score ranging from 1 to 4, with 1 as the optimal score and 4 as the poorest.

Belser and colleagues[35] developed an objective comprehensive esthetic index that incorporates the PES with a white esthetic score (PES/WES). The authors' objective was to develop an index that evaluates the relevant peri-implant soft tissues and specifically evaluates the parameters inherent to the restoration. The index is easy to use and reproducible, and it can be used in research and in clinical practice. The authors modified Fürhauser's PES by decreasing the number of variables from 7 to 5: mesial papilla, distal papilla, curvature of the facial mucosa, level of the facial mucosa, and root convexity/soft tissue color and texture at the facial aspect of the implant site. All variables except the papilla are assessed by comparison with a reference tooth. Each variable is rated on a 2-1-0 scale, with 2 as the best score and 0 as the poorest; this rating results in a maximal possible score of 10. The authors set the threshold of clinical acceptability at 6. The WES focuses on the visible part of the implant restoration and is based on 5 variables: general tooth form, outline/volume of the clinical crown, color (hue/value), surface texture, and translucency/characterization. Each variable is rated on the same 2-1-0 scale, for a maximal possible score of 10. Again, the authors set the threshold of clinical acceptance at 6. When the PES and the WES are combined, the maximal score is 20, which indicates that the peri-implant soft tissues and the clinical single-tooth implant crown are a close match for the contralateral natural tooth. The authors arbitrarily set the clinically acceptability at 60%.

The PES/WES index was the first attempt at determining esthetic failure. It can be inferred that any score lower than 6 on either scale or lower than 12 on the combined index can be assessed as an esthetic failure. Although a score higher than 6 or 12 implies an esthetic success, acceptability should be based on a score of 6 for each scale separately and not on a combined score of 12. A dental implant restoration should be considered a failure (or deemed unacceptable) if the score on either index is lower than 6. Of all available indices, the PES/WES index has been the most widely used and accepted by the research community for evaluating the esthetic outcomes of various implant placement and restorative techniques.[29-31,34,36-44]

Cosyn and colleagues[29-31] used Fürhauser's PES with 7 parameters. Each parameter is assessed with a 2-1-0 scale. The authors set the threshold for clinical acceptance at a score of 8 of the possible total of 14 points; they considered a score of 12 or higher to be (almost) perfect and a score lower than 8 to be a failure. They also used the WES, maintaining Belser's requirement of a score of 6 or higher for clinical acceptability and establishing a new threshold score of 9 or higher for results considered (almost) perfect. Cosyn determined that a WES lower than 6 represented an esthetic failure and evaluated each case for metal exposure. To the authors' knowledge, Cosyn and colleagues are the only authors to have clearly reported an objective value for an esthetic failure.

PATIENTS' SUBJECTIVE EVALUATIONS OF SATISFACTION WITH ESTHETICS

In today's dentistry, it is not enough to simply assess the clinical parameters of a dental implant restoration in the rehabilitation of missing teeth. Patient-reported outcome measures (PROMs) have become a relevant method of establishing the impact of implant dentistry on the patient's quality of life.[45] In 2006, Marshall and colleagues[46] reported the necessity of shifting into a patient-based health care model in which patient-reported assessments provide useful feedback that can assist clinicians in improving the quality of care. In 1989, Smith and Zarb[47] stated that, if an oral implant rehabilitation is to be considered a success, both the clinician and the patient should find the esthetics of the restoration acceptable. Although patient satisfaction is very important, it is difficult to assess because of its subjective and multifactorial nature. Patient satisfaction is related to many aspects of PROMs in implant dentistry, including increase in quality of life, mastication capabilities, economics, and esthetic satisfaction.[48] Although many of these aspects have been studied in relation to implant dentistry, evidence about the esthetic aspect of patient satisfaction is not only sparse but also widely diverse; no index and no agreed-on methods for measuring patient-reported esthetic success have been published in the dental literature.[49,50]

The current need for considering the patient's viewpoint in measures of treatment outcome has led many authors to incorporate patient-reported satisfaction within their outcome evaluations.[8,15,21,22,30,31,51,52] Patient satisfaction is influenced by many variables: confidence when smiling, comfort when chewing or biting, speaking well, and value for the price.[22] Most authors have found that patients are very satisfied with their esthetic outcomes, with 80% or more of the patients surveyed reporting satisfaction.[8,22,51,53] Most authors have also found poor correlations between professional esthetic evaluations and patient-reported esthetic outcomes.[8,19,22,30,52] Cosyn and colleagues[30] found no statistically significant correlation between objective PES and WES ratings and the patient's esthetic satisfaction as determined by a visual analog scale. Mazurat and Mazurat[54] indicated that the best way to improve patient satisfaction is to have a patient who is well informed and therefore has realistic expectations.

Much effort has gone into obtaining objective ratings of the esthetic outcome of an implant-supported single-tooth restoration, and the PES/WES index has proved to be a most useful tool in this regard. However, as clinicians, we must now find a way to combine the objectivity of the PES/WES index and the subjectivity of patient-reported esthetic satisfaction with the outcome. Only with such a combination can an index be created that will allow the inclusion of patient satisfaction in the evaluation of the success or failure of a restoration. In the meantime, esthetic failures in implant dentistry can be categorized on the basis of objective criteria. It is essential to recognize the causes of factors affecting these results and the possible treatment and prevention of these failures so that predictable peri-implant esthetic outcomes and patient satisfaction can be obtained.

The 2004 Consensus Statement of the ITI regarding esthetics indicated that objectively the esthetic zone is any dentoalveolar segment that is visible when the patient is fully smiling.[55] This muscular action around the lips is associated with brightening of the eyes and is one of the most important aspects of nonverbal communication. The smile line, which defines the esthetic zone, focuses on the position of the upper lip and falls into 1 of 3 categories[56]: a high smile (29% of the population), which reveals the total cervical incisal length of the maxillary anterior teeth and contiguous gingiva; an average smile (56% of the population), which reveals only 75%–100% of the maxillary anterior teeth and the interproximal gingiva; and a low smile (15% of the population), which reveals less than 75% of the anterior teeth. For prosthodontists, a high smile is challenging because it exposes the gingiva, and any soft-tissue deficiency will be highlighted. Even a low smile can be a challenge with a demanding patient. Therefore, the clinician should carefully inform the patient about the risks and possible outcomes of any planned procedure.

OBJECTIVE FAILURES IN IMPLANT DENTISTRY

On the basis of objective indices, esthetic failures in implant dentistry can be categorized as pink-tissue failures and white-tissue failures. The most frequently reported pink-tissue failures are facial recession, gingival asymmetry, papillary deficiency, and graying of the gingival tissue.

Pink-Tissue Failures: Factors, Prevention, and Treatment

Pink-tissue complications within the esthetic zone can be caused by various errors committed before, during, or after the placement of implant. Several factors can lead to these failures, but the incidence of these factors can be substantially reduced by proper implant spacing, cautious timing of site preparation, and careful implant placement.[57]

Implant position

The 3-dimensional positioning of a dental implant is a key factor in achieving an adequate esthetic result. The position of the implant dictates the emergence profile of the tooth to be replaced; for this reason, implants should be positioned properly in all 3 spatial directions. Furthermore, achieving a long-lasting esthetic outcome requires using the final restoration as the guide for implant placement and considering the form and position of the planned prosthesis for final restoration.[58–60] Over the past decade, advances in implant dentistry have helped create a greater appreciation for the esthetic demands of the clinician and the patient.[61] Because of these demands, implant dentistry has experienced a profound shift: from function, with a surgically driven approach, to esthetics, with a prosthetically and biologically driven approach.[62] In nature, what looks good usually works well. Applying this same premise to implant dentistry will allow a treatment outcome that balances esthetics with function.

The ideal positioning of an implant in all 3 dimensions, regardless of the implant system used, has been well described in the dental literature. Published reports have also described zones of comfort and danger in the placement of an implant in the esthetic zone.[63] Mesiodistally, the danger zones are located next to adjacent teeth. The facial danger zone is located anywhere facially to the imaginary line highlighted from the point of emergence of the adjacent teeth. The palatal danger zone begins 2 mm from the point of emergence and is associated with an increased risk of ridge-lap restoration.[63] Several guidelines have been suggested for optimizing esthetic results in implant placement. First, the position of the implant depends on the planned restoration that the implant will support. Second, the implant platform should be located 3 mm apical to the zeniths of the predetermined facial-gingival margins of the planned restorations. Third, the center of the implant should be placed at least 3 mm palatal to the anticipated facial margins. The objective is to avoid poor facial bone thickness and gingival recession. Special consideration should be given to the thin gingival biotype; in such cases, it may be necessary to place the body and shoulder of the implant slightly more palatially to mask any show-through of titanium.[63] Fourth, an interimplant spacing of 3 mm is required between adjacent implant platforms. A decrease in this spacing can cause resorption of the interproximal alveolar crest and a reduction in papillary height. Fifth, the implants should emerge through the palatal incisal edge of the ensuing crown positions.[62]

The risk of esthetic failure is higher when implants are placed "free hand," without surgical guides.[59,64] Reverse planning, starting from the final tooth position, allows determination of the exact location of the implant and assures an esthetic outcome. Careful planning and the use of a wax-up, a mock-up, and surgical guides will provide the surgeon with references for locating the implant properly in the 3 directions of the space: apico-occlusal, mesio-distal, and labio-palatal. In this manner, an esthetic result can be achieved. However, fabricating a guide from a wax-up is associated with certain limitations. If the planned position does not match the available bone, the clinician has few options for making small changes. The recent development of virtual restorative planning is promising, because it combines the ideal prosthetic position with the availability of bone. Computer technologies, applied with knowledge, make esthetic complications unlikely and provide optimal function and appearance.[65,66]

The failures that result from improper implant placement are many and can lead to all of the above-mentioned pink-tissue failures. Nevertheless, these failures can be avoided by thorough treatment planning, careful site development, the use of surgical guides, and a proper understanding of restorative aspects when the implant is placed.[60]

Multiple edentulous space replacement
When 2 anterior adjacent teeth are missing, the dental literature agrees that 2 implants should be placed if enough space is available (**Fig. 1**). However, when they are replacing multiple teeth, adjacent implants could compromise the interimplant crestal bone, resulting in resorption and soft-tissue loss. Maintaining or creating a proximal papilla between 2 implants is one of the most challenging aspects of such a procedure. Interimplant spacing of 3 mm is required between adjacent implant platforms so that interimplant bone and soft tissues can be preserved.[62,67,68] A distance of 5 mm or less from the base of the proximal contact to the crest of the bone is recommended for assuring the presence of a proximal papilla.[69] If a papillary deficiency is present when hard-tissue and soft-tissue augmentation procedures have failed, the restorative solution is to enlarge the proximal contact and locate it more apically, thereby allowing reduction of the cervical embrasure.[70]

When 3 or more anterior teeth are missing, the underlying alveolar bone crest is normally flat, and the mucosal profile between adjacent implants tends to level.[71] The consensus of the dental literature is that the fabrication of a fixed partial denture (FPD) with ovate pontics sculpting the intervening tissue may provide a better esthetic appearance than the placement of individual crowns. The placement of 2 implants and one pontic will create an illusion of papilla between an implant and an adjacent pontic (**Fig. 2**).[9,60]

When lateral and central incisors are missing, the best treatment option may be to place 2 implants in the lateral incisor position and 2 ovate pontics in the central position.[72,73] An excellent esthetic and functional result can be achieved by following the same principles as those followed when teeth are missing from canine to canine: the placement of 4 implants in the position of both canines and central incisors and the fabrication of 2 FPDs from the canine to the central incisor.

Timing of implant placement
The timing of postextraction implant placement is not an impediment to obtaining optimal esthetic results; however, various placement times generate different clinical

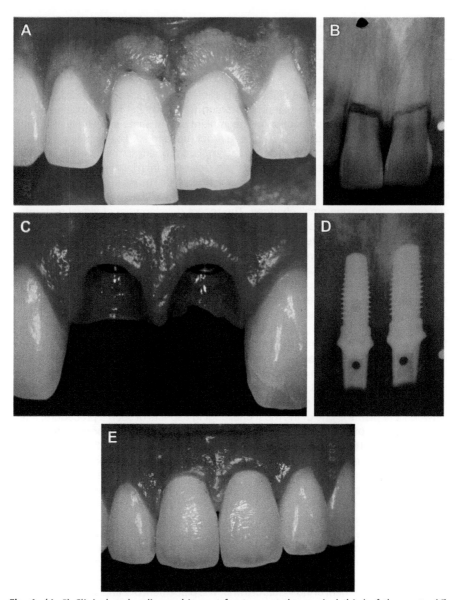

Fig. 1. (*A, B*) Clinical and radiographic root fractures at the cervical third of the roots. (*C*) Immediate implant placement. (*D*) Radiographic evaluation. (*E*) Final restoration with proper soft-tissue contours.

challenges that should be considered for optimizing the esthetic outcome.[74] Case reports have demonstrated that predictable esthetic outcomes can be attained with socket augmentation and immediate provisionalization of the implant.[75]

Immediate implant placement and provisionalization can result in predictable outcomes, including the maintenance of soft-tissue esthetics[76,77]; however, this procedure requires a high level of clinical competence.[24] Because it has been associated with great variability in outcomes,[78] the following clinical conditions must be met

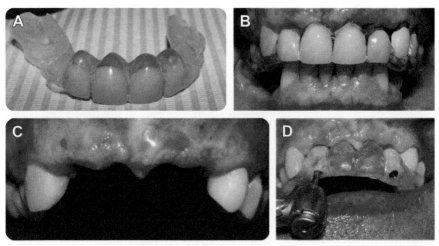

Fig. 2. (*A*) Interim removable partial denture with ovate pontics. (*B*) Interim removable partial denture with ovate pontic for sculpting the tissue and developing the illusion of a papilla between an implant and an adjacent pontic and between pontics. (*C*) Soft-tissue result after ovate pontic remodeling. (*D*) Implant placement in the area of the lateral incisors for a future FPD design using a surgical guide.

to ensure a good outcome: a facial bone wall at least 1 mm thick, a thick gingival biotype, and enough available bone to provide primary stability. If these conditions are not met, early or delayed implant placement should be considered.[74] Belser and colleagues[35] demonstrated that early implant placement for anterior maxillary single-tooth replacement is also a predictable treatment modality from an esthetic point of view. Furthermore, the outcomes of early and delayed placement of single implants in the anterior maxilla are comparable in terms of clinical response, soft-tissue appearance, and patient satisfaction.[30,79]

Although promising results are feasible for immediate, early, and delayed single implants in the esthetic zone, the question of which of these treatment methods would result in better treatment outcomes has not yet been definitively answered because of the lack of well-designed controlled clinical studies.[50]

The immediate placement of an implant in a fresh extraction socket in the anterior maxilla with no incisions or flap elevation is a surgical option that can ensure ideal healing of peri-implant tissues and can preserve the presurgical aspects of gingiva and bone (see **Fig. 1**; **Fig. 3**).[77,80] In delayed implantation, a flapless protocol may provide a better short-term esthetic result, although there appears to be no long-term advantage.[81]

Soft-tissue management

Soft tissue is of fundamental importance for esthetics, and the esthetics of a well-placed implant can be poor if the soft tissue is improperly managed. Soft tissue should be considered at the earliest stages of implant planning, before tooth extraction if possible.[60] Soft-tissue contours are influenced by the presence and the position of the bony anatomy. As with natural teeth, with implants the concept of biological width dictates that peri-implant soft tissues should consistently be approximately 3 mm thick around the implant and even thicker in interproximal areas. This thickness should be considered when an implant is placed, because the bone position will determine the soft-tissue position.[63]

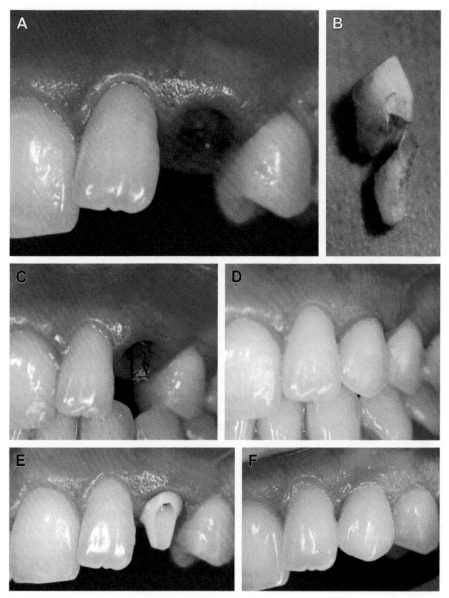

Fig. 3. (*A*, *B*) Atraumatic extraction. (*C*, *D*) Interim abutment and temporary crown forming the emergence profile. (*E*, *F*) All-ceramic abutment; final restoration with proper gingival contours.

The gingival biotype must also be considered when the goal is optimal esthetics. A thick biotype is considered favorable, especially with regard to gingival recession, the most common esthetic complication associated with dental implants.[82] A thin biotype with reduced tissue thickness and scalloped gingival architecture is the least favorable for consideration of esthetics. This biotype may require modifications of the gingival biotype, such as connective tissue grafting.[83] Care should be taken during these procedures to minimize the lack of blood supply, for instance, with flapless surgery.[84]

Establishing a soft-tissue contour with intact papillae is the most difficult factor in achieving an optimal esthetic result. The interproximal crestal bone level seems to be the primary factor in the presence of peri-implant papilla.[70] Studies have demonstrated that maintaining a distance of no more than 6 mm from the contact point to the alveolar crest neighboring the implant is necessary to obtain an intact papilla.[63] On the other hand, when an implant is replacing a single tooth, the peri-implant papilla is dependent not on the proximal bone next to the implant but instead on the bone level of the adjacent tooth.[85] Techniques for addressing a missing papilla because of the lack of vertical bone are very difficult to perform. One such technique is the orthodontic extrusion of natural teeth.[70] Other techniques have been proposed, but none of them are reasonably predictable.[86] The height and thickness of facial bone are important for long-term harmonious gingival margins. Therefore, the quality and quantity of facial bone should be considered before an implant is placed. An implant placed in an area containing a facial bone defect will lead to gingival recession. Various surgical techniques are available for overcoming facial bony defects, including onlay grafting, guided bone regeneration, a combination of block bone grafts and barrier membranes, and distraction osteogenesis (**Fig. 4**).[63]

A common pink-tissue failure is gingival asymmetry. Some options for correcting this failure are orthodontic movement and/or crown lengthening of the teeth in the esthetic zone. Orthodontic movement should be slow, and natural teeth in the esthetic zone can move vertically. This movement causes the soft and hard tissues to move in unison with the tooth being modified orthodontically. This technique can be complemented by periodontal plastic procedures such as crown lengthening. These options re-create the tissue architecture by modifying the position of the teeth and blending the soft tissues with the implant restoration within the esthetic zone.[87]

Careful and, as much as possible, a low-traumatic soft-tissue handling is essential for obtaining natural-looking results.[63] Mismanagement of the soft tissue often results in esthetically unacceptable restorations, and such situations are difficult to correct. An important step in decreasing scarring in the soft-tissue topography around the implant is making the incisions exclusively on the attached gingiva.[88] Transposing the palatal keratinized tissues labially also enhances the emergence contour (**Fig. 5**).[89]

The basic principles of reflecting the flap, handling the tissues, and closing the wound should be considered so that esthetic failures can be prevented. Many options for reconstructing the interdental papilla have been proposed, but none of them provide reasonable predictability.[86]

Hard-tissue management

In the past, the amount of available bone often dictated the placement of implants. Today, bone augmentation procedures are used to align the bone and to permit the precise placement of the dental implant, according to previous prosthetic planning (see **Fig. 2C**).

Advances in manufacturing bone substitutes and increases in knowledge about guided tissue regeneration procedures have made bone-grafting techniques more predictable and, therefore, have made implant placement prosthetically driven. On the other hand, advanced reconstructive surgery increases the risk of complications and compromised esthetics. Therefore, efforts have been made to avoid complex therapy by performing minimally invasive treatment of bone defects.[31]

Implant design (diameter)

Improper implant selection can also lead to esthetic failure. Initially, it was recommended that the size of the implant to replace a missing tooth should be similar to the

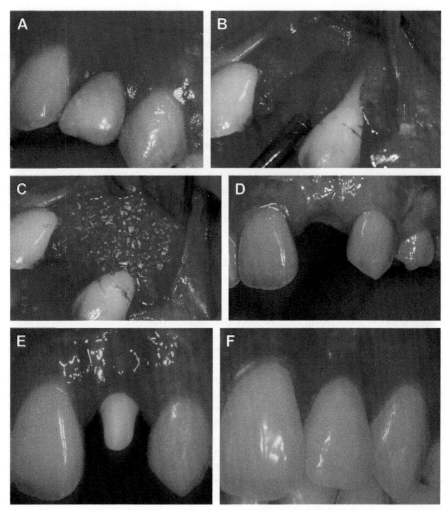

Fig. 4. (*A*) Preoperative view. (*B*) Facial bony defect. (*C*) Guided bone regeneration. (*D*) After reconstruction result. (*E*) All ceramic abutment. (*F*) Final restoration with proper soft-tissue contours.

diameter of the missing tooth at the bony crest. These wide-necked implants lead to less available bone on the facial aspect of the implant and to the esthetic failures described above. When multiple implants are placed, these wide-necked implants decrease the amount of bone between the implants and lead to bone resorption. However, in the past decade, emphasis has been placed on avoiding oversized implants in an effort to optimize esthetic results in the anterior maxilla.[63] Maintaining a generous amount of facial bone by using implants less than 4 mm in diameter appears to be beneficial for esthetics.[90]

Prosthetic considerations

Because the final restoration is the ultimate objective of implant procedures, implant position should always be considered from the perspective of achieving the optimal

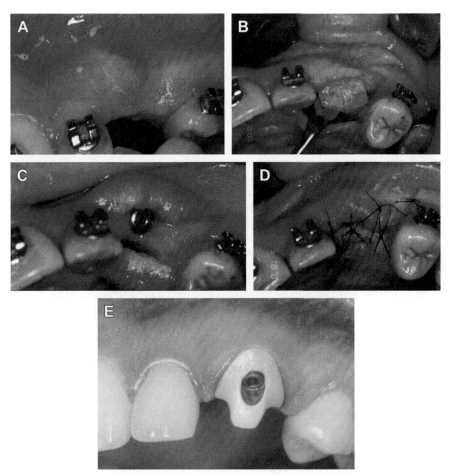

Fig. 5. (A) Implant in poor position, angled labially and exiting the ridge too coronally; thin gingival biotype. (B, C) Transposing the palatine keratinized tissues labially. (D) Closing the flap. (E) Final result of soft-tissue management.

restoration. After implant placement, many factors may affect the restorative phase, beginning with the healing abutment and the provisional restoration, which create the first gingival contour, followed by the abutment connection, the abutment diameter, and the shape and color of the final restoration. The abutment connection is important: an abutment connection in which the abutment is narrower than the implant offers distinct advantages, most notably less bone loss.[90]

The provisional stage of the treatment is another important factor that influences esthetics. It has been suggested that provisional restoration should be immediately inserted after implant fixation to guide the healing of gingival tissues with a proper emergence profile. This procedure also provides the patient with psychological comfort because the immediate esthetic reestablishment will be beneficial.[58,90,91] When implant placement is delayed, an emergence profile should be created by gradually increasing the cervical diameter of the provisional restoration until the expected soft gingival contour has been achieved. After the correct emergence profile has been created or maintained with the provisional implant restoration, the position of the soft tissue must be transferred to the master cast for fabrication of the abutment and the restoration. This procedure can be performed with a customized impression coping that duplicates the emergence profile achieved with the provisional restoration. The shape of the definitive abutments and the definitive restoration will be identical to that of the provisional restoration, thereby maintaining the exact soft-tissue architecture, optimizing esthetics, and minimizing gingival discrepancies.[92]

The restorative material of choice for the abutment and final crown could influence the color of the peri-implant soft tissues. Bressan and colleagues[93] determined that the color peri-implant tissues are different from that of the soft tissue around natural teeth regardless of the type of restorative material used. Jung and colleagues[94] associate this difference in color with the thickness of the soft tissues: when the tissues were more than 3 mm thick, no changes could be detected, but when they were 2 mm thick or less, the all-ceramic material exerted the least color change on the soft tissues. Therefore, when a thin biotype is present, a zirconia custom abutment with an all-ceramic crown should be the material of choice. Nevertheless, some patients still show color changes in the gingival tissues. In such cases, as a second option for masking these color changes when a thin biotype is present, some authors recommend staining the neck of the implant abutment with pink porcelain. This staining will minimize the change in the soft-tissue color.[95] A third option for a thin biotype is to undercontour the labial subgingival aspect of the abutment and, if necessary, the crown itself. This procedure allows space for the gingival tissue and maintains the soft-tissue contour. This concept is important for preserving the long-term stability of the soft tissue.[96,97]

The advantages and disadvantages of cement-retained and screw-retained restorations have been thoroughly discussed in the dental literature. Esthetically, when the access to the screw channel is through the esthetic area, the screw option should be ruled out. The option of angled or custom abutment will correct the malpositioning of the implant, achieving a better esthetic result.[98,99] One important factor regarding cemented restorations and esthetics is the difficulty of removing excess cement. Over the long term, the remaining cement may cause peri-implant inflammation and resorption of the peri-implant bone, leading to recession of the soft tissues and exerting a negative impact on esthetics.[99]

When the reconstruction of ridge defects fails or the patient does not want to explore a surgical approach, nonsurgical management is possible. Ridge and soft-tissue deficiencies can be managed prosthetically with the use of gingiva-colored porcelain placed onto the cervical collars of customized abutments and the cervical aspect of the final restoration.[100]

White-Tissue Failures

White-tissue failures are related to the general form of the tooth, the outline and volume of the clinical crown, color (hue and value), surface texture, and translucency and characterization. Butler and Kinzer[101] indicated that the restorative failures are easier to correct than malpositioning problems. Solutions to these failures must be addressed individually on a case-by-case basis. Nevertheless, most of these failures depend on technique and are fortunately always reversible. For avoiding white-tissue failures, a team approach is highly recommended. This team should include a dental technician, preferably one who has advanced knowledge and clinical experience.[63]

Several restorative materials can be used to restore an anterior implant. However, clinical reports[102] and randomized clinical trials[103] regarding final implant restorations have confirmed that the material chosen for fabricating an implant crown does not in itself ensure an optimal esthetic outcome.

Independent of their type, many failures can be avoided by proper workup and treatment planning. Each of these aspects of treatment should be considered so that esthetic failures can be avoided and the desired natural-looking outcome can be achieved. Replacing missing teeth in the anterior maxilla is a challenge and involves all of the aspects thoroughly discussed in this article, but this procedure also holds an artistic aspect that should not be underestimated. This aspect is reflected in the words of Ralph Waldo Emerson: "Love of beauty is taste. The creation of beauty is art."

REFERENCES

1. Branemark PI, Svensson B, van Steenberghe D. Ten-year survival rates of fixed prostheses on four or six implants ad modum Branemark in full edentulism. Clin Oral Implants Res 1995;6(4):227–31.
2. Dental endosseous implants: an update. ADA Council on Scientific Affairs. J Am Dent Assoc 1996;127(8):1238–9.
3. ADA Coucil on Scientific Affairs. Dental endosseous implants: an update. J Am Dent Assoc 2004;135(1):92–7.
4. Papaspyridakos P, Chen CJ, Singh M, et al. Success criteria in implant dentistry: a systematic review. J Dent Res 2012;91(3):242–8.
5. Dental implants. Benefit and risk. Natl Inst Health Consens Dev Conf Summ 1978;1(3):13–9.
6. Albrektsson T, Zarb G, Worthington P, et al. The long-term efficacy of currently used dental implants: a review and proposed criteria of success. Int J Oral Maxillofac Implants 1986;1(1):11–25.
7. Higginbottom FL. Implants as an option in the esthetic zone. J Oral Maxillofac Surg 2005;63(9 Suppl 2):33–44.
8. Chang M, Odman PA, Wennström JL, et al. Esthetic outcome of implant-supported single-tooth replacements assessed by the patient and by prosthodontists. Int J Prosthodont 1999;12(4):335–41.
9. Higginbottom F, Belser U, Jones JD, et al. Prosthetic management of implants in the esthetic zone. Int J Oral Maxillofac Implants 2004;19(Suppl):62–72.
10. Dawson A, Chen S, Buser D, et al. The SAC classification in implant dentistry. Berlin: Quintessence; 2009.
11. Holst S, Blatz MB, Hegenbarth E, et al. Prosthodontic considerations for predictable single-implant esthetics in the anterior maxilla. J Oral Maxillofac Surg 2005; 63(9 Suppl 2):89–96.
12. el Askary AS, Meffert RM, Griffin T. Why do dental implants fail? Part I. Implant Dent 1999;8(2):173–85.
13. Paquette DW, Brodala N, Williams RC. Risk factors for endosseous dental implant failure. Dent Clin North Am 2006;50(3):361–74, vi.
14. Porter JA, von Fraunhofer JA. Success or failure of dental implants? A literature review with treatment considerations. Gen Dent 2005;53(6):423–32 [quiz: 433, 446].
15. Ericsson I, Nilson H, Lindh T, et al. Immediate functional loading of Branemark single tooth implants. An 18 months' clinical pilot follow-up study. Clin Oral Implants Res 2000;11(1):26–33.
16. Henry PJ, Laney WR, Jemt T, et al. Osseointegrated implants for single-tooth replacement: a prospective 5-year multicenter study. Int J Oral Maxillofac Implants 1996;11(4):450–5.
17. Goodacre CJ, Kan JY, Rungcharassaeng K. Clinical complications of osseointegrated implants. J Prosthet Dent 1999;81(5):537–52.

18. Alkhatib MN, Holt R, Bedi R. Prevalence of self-assessed tooth discolouration in the United Kingdom. J Dent 2004;32(7):561-6.
19. Dueled E, Gotfredsen K, Trab Damsgaard, et al. Professional and patient-based evaluation of oral rehabilitation in patients with tooth agenesis. Clin Oral Implants Res 2009;20(7):729-36.
20. Kourkouta S, Dedi KD, Paquette DW, et al. Interproximal tissue dimensions in relation to adjacent implants in the anterior maxilla: clinical observations and patient aesthetic evaluation. Clin Oral Implants Res 2009;20(12):1375-85.
21. Meijndert L, Meijer HJ, Stellingsma K, et al. Evaluation of aesthetics of implant-supported single-tooth replacements using different bone augmentation procedures: a prospective randomized clinical study. Clin Oral Implants Res 2007; 18(6):715-9.
22. Suphanantachat S, Thovanich K, Nisapakultorn K. The influence of peri-implant mucosal level on the satisfaction with anterior maxillary implants. Clin Oral Implants Res 2012;23(9):1075-81.
23. Jemt T. Regeneration of gingival papillae after single-implant treatment. Int J Periodontics Restorative Dent 1997;17(4):326-33.
24. Evans CD, Chen ST. Esthetic outcomes of immediate implant placements. Clin Oral Implants Res 2008;19(1):73-80.
25. Misje K, Bjørnland T, Saxegaard E, et al. Treatment outcome of dental implants in the esthetic zone: a 12- to 15-year retrospective study. Int J Prosthodont 2013; 26(4):365-9.
26. Fürhauser R, Florescu D, Benesch T, et al. Evaluation of soft tissue around single-tooth implant crowns: the pink esthetic score. Clin Oral Implants Res 2005;16(6):639-44.
27. Gehrke P, Lobert M, Dhom G. Reproducibility of the pink esthetic score–rating soft tissue esthetics around single-implant restorations with regard to dental observer specialization. J Esthet Restor Dent 2008;20(6):375-84 [discussion: 385].
28. Lai HC, Zhang ZY, Wang F, et al. Evaluation of soft-tissue alteration around implant-supported single-tooth restoration in the anterior maxilla: the pink esthetic score. Clin Oral Implants Res 2008;19(6):560-4.
29. Cosyn J, Eghbali A, De Bruyn H, et al. Immediate single-tooth implants in the anterior maxilla: 3-year results of a case series on hard and soft tissue response and aesthetics. J Clin Periodontol 2011;38(8):746-53.
30. Cosyn J, Eghbali A, De Bruyn H, et al. Single implant treatment in healing versus healed sites of the anterior maxilla: an aesthetic evaluation. Clin Implant Dent Relat Res 2012;14(4):517-26.
31. Cosyn J, Eghbali A, Hanselaer L, et al. Four modalities of single implant treatment in the anterior maxilla: a clinical, radiographic, and aesthetic evaluation. Clin Implant Dent Relat Res 2013;15(4):517-30.
32. Luo Z, Zeng R, Luo Z, et al. Single implants in the esthetic zone: analysis of recent peri-implant soft tissue alterations and patient satisfaction. A photographic study. Int J Oral Maxillofac Implants 2011;26(3):578-86.
33. Meijer HJ, Stellingsma K, Meijndert L, et al. A new index for rating aesthetics of implant-supported single crowns and adjacent soft tissues–the Implant Crown Aesthetic Index. Clin Oral Implants Res 2005;16(6):645-9.
34. den Hartog L, Raghoebar GM, Slater JJ, et al. Single-tooth implants with different neck designs: a randomized clinical trial evaluating the aesthetic outcome. Clin Implant Dent Relat Res 2013;15(3):311-21.
35. Belser UC, Grütter L, Vailati F, et al. Outcome evaluation of early placed maxillary anterior single-tooth implants using objective esthetic criteria: a cross-sectional,

retrospective study in 45 patients with a 2- to 4-year follow-up using pink and white esthetic scores. J Periodontol 2009;80(1):140–51.

36. Taylor EJ, Yuan JC, Lee DJ, et al. Are predoctoral students able to provide single tooth implant restorations in the maxillary esthetic zone? J Dent Educ 2014;78(5):779–88.

37. Mangano C, Levrini L, Mangano A, et al. Esthetic evaluation of implants placed after orthodontic treatment in patients with congenitally missing lateral incisors. J Esthet Restor Dent 2014;26(1):61–71.

38. Cho HL, Lee JK, Um HS, et al. Esthetic evaluation of maxillary single-tooth implants in the esthetic zone. J Periodontal Implant Sci 2010;40(4):188–93.

39. Mangano FG, Mangano C, Ricci M, et al. Esthetic evaluation of single-tooth Morse taper connection implants placed in fresh extraction sockets or healed sites. J Oral Implantol 2013;39(2):172–81.

40. Gu YX, Shi JY, Zhuang LF, et al. Esthetic outcome and alterations of soft tissue around single implant crowns: a 2-year prospective study. Clin Oral Implants Res 2014. [Epub ahead of print].

41. Cristalli MP, Marini R, La Monaca G, et al. Immediate loading of post-extractive single-tooth implants: a 1-year prospective study. Clin Oral Implants Res 2014. [Epub ahead of print].

42. Buser D, Chappuis V, Bornstein MM, et al. Long-term stability of contour augmentation with early implant placement following single tooth extraction in the esthetic zone: a prospective, cross-sectional study in 41 patients with a 5- to 9-year follow-up. J Periodontol 2013;84(11):1517–27.

43. Bonde MJ, Stokholm R, Schou S, et al. Patient satisfaction and aesthetic outcome of implant-supported single-tooth replacements performed by dental students: a retrospective evaluation 8 to 12 years after treatment. Eur J Oral Implantol 2013; 6(4):387–95.

44. Mangano F, Mangano C, Ricci M, et al. Single-tooth Morse taper connection implants placed in fresh extraction sockets of the anterior maxilla: an aesthetic evaluation. Clin Oral Implants Res 2012;23(11):1302–7.

45. McGrath C, Lam O, Lang N. An evidence-based review of patient-reported outcome measures in dental implant research among dentate subjects. J Clin Periodontol 2012;39(Suppl 12):193–201.

46. Marshall S, Haywood K, Fitzpatrick R. Impact of patient-reported outcome measures on routine practice: a structured review. J Eval Clin Pract 2006;12(5): 559–68.

47. Smith DE, Zarb GA. Criteria for success of osseointegrated endosseous implants. J Prosthet Dent 1989;62(5):567–72.

48. Guckes AD, Scurria MS, Shugars DA. A conceptual framework for understanding outcomes of oral implant therapy. J Prosthet Dent 1996;75(6):633–9.

49. Fava J, Lin M, Zahran M, et al. Single implant-supported crowns in the aesthetic zone: patient satisfaction with aesthetic appearance compared with appraisals by laypeople and dentists. Clin Oral Implants Res 2014. [Epub ahead of print].

50. den Hartog L, Slater JJ, Vissink A, et al. Treatment outcome of immediate, early and conventional single-tooth implants in the aesthetic zone: a systematic review to survival, bone level, soft-tissue, aesthetics and patient satisfaction. J Clin Periodontol 2008;35(12):1073–86.

51. Kan JY, Rungcharassaeng K, Lozada J. Immediate placement and provisionalization of maxillary anterior single implants: 1-year prospective study. Int J Oral Maxillofac Implants 2003;18(1):31–9.

52. Gotfredsen K. A 5-year prospective study of single-tooth replacements supported by the Astra Tech implant: a pilot study. Clin Implant Dent Relat Res 2004;6(1):1–8.

53. De Rouck T, Collys K, Cosyn J. Immediate single-tooth implants in the anterior maxilla: a 1-year case cohort study on hard and soft tissue response. J Clin Periodontol 2008;35(7):649–57.

54. Mazurat NM, Mazurat RD. Discuss before fabricating: communicating the realities of partial denture therapy. Part II: clinical outcomes. J Can Dent Assoc 2003;69(2):96–100.

55. Belser U, Buser D, Higginbottom F. Consensus statements and recommended clinical procedures regarding esthetics in implant dentistry. Int J Oral Maxillofac Implants 2004;19(Suppl):73–4.

56. Dong JK, Jin TH, Cho HW, et al. The esthetics of the smile: a review of some recent studies. Int J Prosthodont 1999;12(1):9–19.

57. Wheeler SL. Implant complications in the esthetic zone. J Oral Maxillofac Surg 2007;65(7 Suppl 1):93–102.

58. Martin WC, Pollini A, Morton D. The influence of restorative procedures on esthetic outcomes in implant dentistry: a systematic review. Int J Oral Maxillofac Implants 2014;29(Suppl):142–54.

59. Almog DM, Torrado E, Meitner SW. Fabrication of imaging and surgical guides for dental implants. J Prosthet Dent 2001;85(5):504–8.

60. Chee W, Jivraj S. Failures in implant dentistry. Br Dent J 2007;202(3):123–9.

61. Al-Sabbagh M. Implants in the esthetic zone. Dent Clin North Am 2006;50(3): 391–407, vi.

62. Priest GF. The esthetic challenge of adjacent implants. J Oral Maxillofac Surg 2007;65(7 Suppl 1):2–12.

63. Buser D, Martin W, Belser UC. Optimizing esthetics for implant restorations in the anterior maxilla: anatomic and surgical considerations. Int J Oral Maxillofac Implants 2004;19(Suppl):43–61.

64. Noharet R, Pettersson A, Bourgeois D. Accuracy of implant placement in the posterior maxilla as related to 2 types of surgical guides: a pilot study in the human cadaver. J Prosthet Dent 2014;112(3):526–32.

65. de Almeida EO, Pellizzer EP, Goiatto MC, et al. Computer-guided surgery in implantology: review of basic concepts. J Craniofac Surg 2010;21(6):1917–21.

66. Katsoulis J, Pazera P, Mericske-Stern R. Prosthetically driven, computer-guided implant planning for the edentulous maxilla: a model study. Clin Implant Dent Relat Res 2009;11(3):238–45.

67. Grunder U, Gracis S, Capelli M. Influence of the 3-D bone-to-implant relationship on esthetics. Int J Periodontics Restorative Dent 2005;25(2):113–9.

68. Tarnow DP, Cho SC, Wallace SS. The effect of inter-implant distance on the height of inter-implant bone crest. J Periodontol 2000;71(4):546–9.

69. Siqueira S Jr, Pimentel SP, Alves RV, et al. Evaluation of the effects of buccal-palatal bone width on the incidence and height of the interproximal papilla between adjacent implants in esthetic areas. J Periodontol 2013;84(2):170–5.

70. Chow YC, Wang HL. Factors and techniques influencing peri-implant papillae. Implant Dent 2010;19(3):208–19.

71. Belser UC, Buser D, Hess D, et al. Aesthetic implant restorations in partially edentulous patients–a critical appraisal. Periodontol 2000;1998(17):132–50.

72. Krennmair G, Seemann R, Weinländer M, et al. Implant-prosthodontic rehabilitation of anterior partial edentulism: a clinical review. Int J Oral Maxillofac Implants 2011;26(5):1043–50.

73. Jivraj S, Chee W. Treatment planning of implants in the aesthetic zone. Br Dent J 2006;201(2):77–89.
74. Morton D, Chen ST, Martin WC, et al. Consensus statements and recommended clinical procedures regarding optimizing esthetic outcomes in implant dentistry. Int J Oral Maxillofac Implants 2014;29(Suppl):216–20.
75. Fu PS, Wu YM, Wang JC, et al. Optimizing anterior esthetics of a single-tooth implant through socket augmentation and immediate provisionalization: a case report with 7-year follow-up. Kaohsiung J Med Sci 2012;28(10):559–63.
76. De Rouck T, Collys K, Cosyn J. Single-tooth replacement in the anterior maxilla by means of immediate implantation and provisionalization: a review. Int J Oral Maxillofac Implants 2008;23(5):897–904.
77. Jofre J. A chairside technique to preserve the anatomy of the pre-existing crown in immediate implant provisionalization: a case report. International Journal of Odontostomatology 2010;4:291–4.
78. Chen ST, Buser D. Esthetic outcomes following immediate and early implant placement in the anterior maxilla–a systematic review. Int J Oral Maxillofac Implants 2014;29(Suppl):186–215.
79. Schropp L, Isidor F. Clinical outcome and patient satisfaction following full-flap elevation for early and delayed placement of single-tooth implants: a 5-year randomized study. Int J Oral Maxillofac Implants 2008;23(4):733–43.
80. Sammartino G, Marenzi G, di Lauro AE, et al. Aesthetics in oral implantology: biological, clinical, surgical, and prosthetic aspects. Implant Dent 2007;16(1):54–65.
81. Bashutski JD, Wang HL, Rudek I, et al. Effect of flapless surgery on single-tooth implants in the esthetic zone: a randomized clinical trial. J Periodontol 2013; 84(12):1747–54.
82. Kois JC. Predictable single-tooth peri-implant esthetics: five diagnostic keys. Compend Contin Educ Dent 2004;25(11):895–6, 898, 900 passim; [quiz: 906–7].
83. Fu JH, Lee A, Wang HL. Influence of tissue biotype on implant esthetics. Int J Oral Maxillofac Implants 2011;26(3):499–508.
84. Cabello G, Rioboo M, Fabrega JG. Immediate placement and restoration of implants in the aesthetic zone with a trimodal approach: soft tissue alterations and its relation to gingival biotype. Clin Oral Implants Res 2013;24(10):1094–100.
85. Kan JY, Rungcharassaeng K, Umezu K, et al. Dimensions of peri-implant mucosa: an evaluation of maxillary anterior single implants in humans. J Periodontol 2003;74(4):557–62.
86. Prato GP, Rotundo R, Cortellini P, et al. Interdental papilla management: a review and classification of the therapeutic approaches. Int J Periodontics Restorative Dent 2004;24(3):246–55.
87. Kan JY, Rungcharassaeng K, Fillman M, et al. Tissue architecture modification for anterior implant esthetics: an interdisciplinary approach. Eur J Esthet Dent 2009;4(2):104–17.
88. Sculean A, Gruber R, Bosshardt DD. Soft tissue wound healing around teeth and dental implants. J Clin Periodontol 2014;41(Suppl 15):S6–22.
89. Mohamed J, Alam N, Singh G, et al. Roll flap technique for anterior implant esthetics, case report. Indian J Med Sci 2012;2(1):393–5.
90. Rodriguez AM, Rosenstiel SF. Esthetic considerations related to bone and soft tissue maintenance and development around dental implants: report of the Committee on Research in Fixed Prosthodontics of the American Academy of Fixed Prosthodontics. J Prosthet Dent 2012;108(4):259–67.
91. Freitas Junior AC, Goiato MC, Pellizzer EP, et al. Aesthetic approach in single immediate implant-supported restoration. J Craniofac Surg 2010;21(3):792–6.

92. Ntounis A, Petropoulou A. A technique for managing and accurate registration of periimplant soft tissues. J Prosthet Dent 2010;104(4):276–9.

93. Bressan E, Paniz G, Lops D, et al. Influence of abutment material on the gingival color of implant-supported all-ceramic restorations: a prospective multicenter study. Clin Oral Implants Res 2011;22(6):631–7.

94. Jung RE, Holderegger C, Sailer I, et al. The effect of all-ceramic and porcelain-fused-to-metal restorations on marginal peri-implant soft tissue color: a randomized controlled clinical trial. Int J Periodontics Restorative Dent 2008;28(4): 357–65.

95. Ishikawa-Nagai S, Da Silva JD, Weber HP, et al. Optical phenomenon of peri-implant soft tissue. Part II. Preferred implant neck color to improve soft tissue esthetics. Clin Oral Implants Res 2007;18(5):575–80.

96. Chu SJ, Tarnow DP. Managing esthetic challenges with anterior implants. Part 1: midfacial recession defects from etiology to resolution. Compend Contin Educ Dent 2013;34(Spec No 7):26–31.

97. Mankoo T. Single-tooth implant restorations in the esthetic zone–contemporary concepts for optimization and maintenance of soft tissue esthetics in the replacement of failing teeth in compromised sites. Eur J Esthet Dent 2007; 2(3):274–95.

98. Hebel KS, Gajjar RC. Cement-retained versus screw-retained implant restorations: achieving optimal occlusion and esthetics in implant dentistry. J Prosthet Dent 1997;77(1):28–35.

99. Shadid R, Sadaqa N. A comparison between screw- and cement-retained implant prostheses. A literature review. J Oral Implantol 2012;38(3):298–307.

100. Kamalakidis S, Paniz G, Kang KH, et al. Nonsurgical management of soft tissue deficiencies for anterior single implant-supported restorations: a clinical report. J Prosthet Dent 2007;97(1):1–5.

101. Butler B, Kinzer GA. Managing esthetic implant complications. Compend Contin Educ Dent 2012;33(7):514–8, 520–2.

102. Tan PL, Dunne JT Jr. An esthetic comparison of a metal ceramic crown and cast metal abutment with an all-ceramic crown and zirconia abutment: a clinical report. J Prosthet Dent 2004;91(3):215–8.

103. Gallucci GO, Grütter L, Nedir R, et al. Esthetic outcomes with porcelain-fused-to-ceramic and all-ceramic single-implant crowns: a randomized clinical trial. Clin Oral Implants Res 2011;22(1):62–9.

Index

Note: Page numbers of article titles are in **boldface** type.

A

Alveolar nerve, inferior, injury to, 131–132, 133

B

Bacterial infection, implants and, 11
Biologic markers, of failing implants, **179–194**
    roles of, 179–180
Bisphosphonates, as risk factor for implant failure, 32
Bleeding, as complication of implant placement, 58–60
        in mandible, 59–60
        in maxilla, 59
Bone quality, implants and, 6–7, 8

C

Caldwell-Luc sinus augmentation, lateral wall, 101–114
        sinus membrane perforation during, 101, 113
            treatment of, 113–114
        technical complications of, 101–113
Cone beam computer tomography, applications of, 41–42
    artifacts on, and assessment of implant placement, 52–54
    comparison with other imaging modalities, 51–52
    cross-sectional, for postoperative assessment, 49, 50, 51, 52, 53
    indications for, 42–51
    limitations of, 42, 44–45, 46
    radiation dose and, 45
    to detect implant failure, 46–49, 50, 51, 52, 53
    to evaluate implants after placement, 50–51
    to measure bone mineral density, 42–44
    to select potential implant site, 42
    use of, in early detection of implant failure, **41–56**

D

Diabetes, as risk factor for implant failure, 30–31
    as risk factor for peridontitis, 30
    periodontal conditions in, 162

Dent Clin N Am 59 (2015) 247–253
http://dx.doi.org/10.1016/S0011-8532(14)00126-8
0011-8532/15/$ – see front matter © 2015 Elsevier Inc. All rights reserved.

dental.theclinics.com

Moving?

Make sure your subscription moves with you!

To notify us of your new address, find your **Clinics Account Number** (located on your mailing label above your name), and contact customer service at:

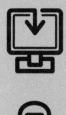

Email: journalscustomerservice-usa@elsevier.com

800-654-2452 (subscribers in the U.S. & Canada)
314-447-8871 (subscribers outside of the U.S. & Canada)

Fax number: 314-447-8029

Elsevier Health Sciences Division
Subscription Customer Service
3251 Riverport Lane
Maryland Heights, MO 63043

*To ensure uninterrupted delivery of your subscription, please notify us at least 4 weeks in advance of move.

Printed and bound by CPI Group (UK) Ltd, Croydon, CR0 4YY

07/10/2024

01040498-0011